RESOLVING THE ANTIBIOTIC PARADOX

Progress in Understanding Drug Resistance and Development of New Antibiotics

ADVANCES IN EXPERIMENTAL MEDICINE AND BIOLOGY

Recent Volumes in this Series

Volume 447
LIPOXYGENASES AND THEIR METABOLITES: Biological Functions
Edited by Santosh Nigam and Cecil R. Pace-Asciak

Volume 448
COPPER TRANSPORT AND ITS DISORDERS: Molecular and Cellular Aspects
Edited by Arturo Leone and Julian F. B. Mercer

Volume 449
VASOPRESSIN AND OXYTOCIN: Molecular, Cellular, and Clinical Advances
Edited by Hans H. Zingg, Charles W. Bourque, and Daniel G. Bichet

Volume 450
ADVANCES IN MODELING AND CONTROL OF VENTILATION
Edited by Richard L. Hughson, David A. Cunningham, and James Duffin

Volume 451
GENE THERAPY OF CANCER
Edited by Peter Walden, Uwe Trefzer, Wolfram Sterry, and Farzin Farzaneh

Volume 452
MECHANISMS OF LYMPHOCYTE ACTIVATION AND IMMUNE REGULATION VII:
Molecular Determinants of Microbial Immunity
Edited by Sudhir Gupta, Alan Sher, and Rafi Ahmed

Volume 453
MECHANISMS OF WORK PRODUCTION AND WORK ABSORPTION IN MUSCLE
Edited by Haruo Sugi and Gerald H. Pollack

Volume 454
OXYGEN TRANSPORT TO TISSUE XX
Edited by Antal G. Hudetz and Duane F. Bruley

Volume 455
RHEUMADERM: Current Issues in Rheumatology and Dermatology
Edited by Carmel Mallia and Jouni Uitto

Volume 456
RESOLVING THE ANTIBIOTIC PARADOX: Progress in Understanding Drug
Resistance and Development of New Antibiotics
Edited by Barry P. Rosen and Shahriar Mobashery

RESOLVING THE ANTIBIOTIC PARADOX
Progress in Understanding Drug Resistance and Development of New Antibiotics

Edited by

Barry P. Rosen and
Shahriar Mobashery

Wayne State University
Detroit, Michigan

KLUWER ACADEMIC / PLENUM PUBLISHERS
New York, Boston, Dordrecht, London, Moscow

Library of Congress Cataloging in Publication Data

Resolving the antibiotic paradox: progress in understanding drug resistance and development of new
    antibiotics / edited by Barry P. Rosen and Shahriar Mobashery.
        p.   cm.—(Advances in experimental medicine and biology; v. 456)
    "Proceedings of the Symposium on Resolving the Antibiotic Paradox: Progress in Drug Design and
Resistance, held May 29, 1997, at Wayne State University, Detroit, Michigan"—T.p. verso.
    Includes bibliographical references and index.
    ISBN 0-306-46039-4
    1. Drug resistance in microorganisms—Congresses. I. Rosen, Barry P. II. Mobashery, Shahriar. III.
Symposium on Resolving the Antibiotic Paradox: Progress in Drug Design and Resistance (1997: Wayne
State University) IV. Series.
    [DNLM: 1. Drug Resistance, Microbial—physiology congresses. 2. Antibiotics—pharmacology con-
gresses. 3. Drug Design congresses. W1 AD559 v.456 1998]
    QR177.R47   1998
    616'.01—dc21
    DNLM/DLC   98-46308
    for Library of Congress   CIP

Proceedings of the Symposium on Resolving the Antibiotic Paradox: Progress in Drug Design and
Resistance, held May 29, 1997, at Wayne State University, Detroit, Michigan

ISBN 0-306-46039-4

© 1998 Kluwer Academic / Plenum Publishers, New York
233 Spring Street, New York, N.Y. 10013

10 9 8 7 6 5 4 3 2 1

A C.I.P. record for this book is available from the Library of Congress.

Printed in the United States of America

PREFACE

Antibiotic resistance, once a term appreciated only by microbiologists, has become a common topic in the popular press. Stuart Levy, one of the contributors to this collection, bears some of the responsibility for increasing public awareness with the publication of his book "The Antibiotic Paradox" in 1992.[*] Misuse of antibiotics resulting in increased bacterial resistance had previously been recognized in the infectious disease community. However, Dr. Levy's eloquent public warning about the shrinking efficacy of our antibiotic armamentarium served to alert the lay person to the potential consequences of this demise in useful therapy.

Because of the proliferation of diverse antibiotic classes with increasing potency and broader activity spectra, it had been assumed that any ordinary bacterial infection could be eradicated with the proper selection of drug. However, it has become evident that we are surrounded by resistant bacteria, many of which were introduced unwittingly into our environment through the unnecessary use of antibiotics. When it became evident that a number of people were returning for multiple visits to their family physicians for persistent ear infections or non-responsive bronchitis, questions were raised about the antibiotic treatments that were being prescribed. Bacteria resistant to common antibiotic regimens were being isolated more frequently, often as organisms classified as "multi-resistant" with decreased susceptibilities to two or more structural classes of agents. Nosocomial spread of these resistances was aided by the transmission of plasmid-mediated resistance factors between species. In addition, colonizing bacteria in healthy patients were found to be carrying the same resistance factors in their normal flora. As people are exposed to increasing amounts of antibiotics, either through medical use, or through the overuse of these agents for other purposes, the potential for further mutations becomes greater, resulting in bacteria with even higher resistance. In this book Mazel and Davies present an overview describing the selection of antibiotic resistance, and Lerner presents the resistance picture as seen by a practicing infectious disease specialist. These chapters serve to put the current situation in perspective.

Development of new antibacterial agents has continued for over fifty years, with the early agents based on compounds that were isolated as fermentation products. With the exception of the quinolones, all the classes of antibacterial agents in widespread use today

---

[*] Levy, S. B., 1992, *The Antibiotic Paradox. How Miracle Drugs Are Destroying the Miracle;* Plenum Press, New York.

originated from natural products. Many of these agents such as the β-lactam antibiotics were later tailored to be active against subpopulations of resistant bacteria, based upon specific resistance mechanisms that were deemed to be of medical concern at the time. During the late 1970s and early 1980s an explosion of antibacterial agents targeting the same resistant populations reached the marketplace. As a result, some in the pharmaceutical industry perceived that there was now a glut of available antibiotics, and a number of antibacterial programs were curtailed or diminished, with resources diverted into anti-viral or anti-fungal programs. Those companies that remained actively looking for new drugs were not always searching for novel classes of compounds, so that the impact of many drug discovery programs was low. No obvious break-throughs were identified during this time.

During this perceived hiatus in antibiotic research, many other activities were occurring simultaneously. In the 1980s resistant bacteria were emerging as critical target pathogens, such as vancomycin-resistant enterococci, penicillin-resistant streptococci, methicillin-resistant staphylococci,and Gram-negative bacteria carrying extended-spectrum β-lactamases. Basic research groups in both the academic world and the pharmaceutical industry examined each of these groups of bacteria for novel approaches to therapeutic intervention. In this book both traditional and novel approaches to antimicrobial drug discovery are described to highlight some of the more successful strategies over the past few years.

More conventional drug discovery programs have involved structural modifications of compounds from the traditional classes of natural products. Often a specific type of resistance mechanism has been targeted in an attempt to regain the use of broad-spectrum agents. This kind of approach is discussed in the chapters herein describing novel tetracyclines with activity against tetracycline efflux pumps; the aminoglycoside antibiotics; and the β-lactams that have been designed to circumvent specific β-lactamase inactivation mechanisms. Chimeric drugs such as the quinolonyl lactones have been proposed to capture the activity of both quinolones and cephalosporins. In some cases, well-characterized pathways have been utilized to identify novel targets, as in the case of peptidoglycan biosynthesis.

Some of the more exciting aspects of the current book are the chapters dealing with novel chemical structures shown to have antibacterial activity. Of the agents discussed, the oxazolidinones have progressed the furthest, with linezolid currently in advanced clinical studies. This class of compound with a Gram-positive spectrum of activity represents an advance in structural novelty for antibacterial agents. The diphenolic methanes that have been described as antimicrobial agents working through inhibition of a two component transduction system represent another novel type of agent. Both the oxazolidinones and the bis-phenols are thought to affect bacterial processes that are not associated with the mechanism of action of other antibacterial agents. Therefore, it has been postulated that cross-resistance with other classes of antibiotics should be rare.

Antibacterial activity due to a novel mechanism is the goal of many in the drug discovery community. Resistance issues are perceived to be less, as there would be no drugs in use to pre-select a resistant population. Novel mechanisms that have not been effectively exploited as drug targets include transport mechanisms such as the multi-drug transport and metalloid transport systems described in this book. The newer tetracyclines that inhibit or evade efflux pumps may be included in this group.

Bacterial genomics offers the opportunity for drug discovery scientists to identify novel essential genes that can serve as drug targets. With the proliferation of genomic information that is becoming available, it is only a matter of time and patience before a number of novel targets can be identified. However, risks are always associated with the development of novel drugs. Cross-reactivity between prokaryotic and eukaryotic enzymes leading to toxicity is an issue that has already been successfully addressed by the current set of antibacterial agents. But, unless risks are taken, novelty will remain elusive.

In this book the issue of bacterial resistance has been addressed in ways that show both conventional, and precarious, drug discovery approaches. Although one can be assured that any new antibacterial agent will eventually select for a resistant bacterial population, we can hope that this process can be slowed by some of the agents described. Novelty has returned to the antimicrobial discovery process. We continue to hope that at least some of these novel agents will become commercial successes in order to provide us with a new generation of antimicrobial agents.

Karen Bush
R. W. Johnson Pharmaceutical Research Institute
June, 1998

CONTENTS

1. Antibiotic Resistance: The Big Picture   1
   Didier Mazel and Julian Davies

2. Clinical Impact of Antibiotic Resistance   7
   Stephen A. Lerner

3. Reversing Tetracycline Resistance: A Renaissance for the Tetracycline Family of
   Antibiotics   17
   Stuart B. Levy and Mark Nelson

4. Aminoglycoside Antibiotics: Structures, Functions, and Resistance   27
   Gerard D. Wright, Albert M. Berghuis, and Shahriar Mobashery

5. How β-Lactamases Have Driven Pharmaceutical Drug Discovery: From
   Mechanistic Knowledge to Clinical Circumvention   71
   Karen Bush and Shahriar Mobashery

6. Antifolate Resistance Mechanisms from Bacteria to Cancer Cells with Emphasis
   on Parasites   99
   Marc Ouellette, Éric Leblanc, Christoph Kündig, and Barbara Papadopoulou

7. Resistance to Antitubercular Drugs   115
   Luiz A. Basso and John S. Blanchard

8. Structure and Function of Multidrug Transporters   145
   Hendrik W. van Veen and Wil N. Konings

9. Metalloid Resistance Mechanisms   159
   Rita Mukhopadhyay, Jiaxin Li, Hiranmoy Bhattacharjee, and Barry P. Rosen

10. The Impact of Bacterial Genomics on Antibacterial Discovery   183
    David J. C. Knowles and Frank King

11. Peptidoglycan Biosynthesis: Unexploited Antibacterial Targets within a Familiar
    Pathway   197
    Kenny K. Wong and David L. Pompliano

12. Design, Synthesis, and Evaluation of Novel Oxazolidinone Antibacterial Agents
    Active against Multidrug-Resistant Bacteria   219
    Michael R. Barbachyn, Steven J. Brickner, Robert C. Gadwood,
    Stuart A. Garmon, Kevin C. Grega, Douglas K. Hutchinson,
    Kiyotaka Munesada, Robert J. Reischer, Mikio Taniguchi,
    Lisa M. Thomasco, Dana S. Toops, Hiromi Yamada, Charles W. Ford, and
    Gary E. Zurenko

13. Concept, Design, and Preclinical Evaluation of Quinolonyl Lactam
    Antibacterials   239
    Paul M. Hershberger and Thomas P. Demuth, Jr

14. Bacterial Two-Component Signalling as a Therapeutic Target in Drug Design:
    Inhibition of NRII by the Diphenolic Methanes (Bisphenols)   269
    John M. Domagala, Diane Alessi, Maxwell Cummings, Stephen Gracheck,
    Liren Huang, Michael Huband, Gregg Johnson, Eric Olson,
    Martin Shapiro, Rajeshwar Singh, Yuntao Song, Ruth Van Bogelen,
    Dean Vo, and Sara Wold

Index   287

ANTIBIOTIC RESISTANCE

The Big Picture

Didier Mazel [1] and Julian Davies [2]

[1]Institut Pasteur
75024 Paris France
[2]Department of Microbiology and Immunology
University of British Columbia
Vancouver, BC. V6R 1V3 Canada

The introduction of antibiotics for the treatment of bacterial diseases in the late 1940s was heralded as one of the great innovations of the modern world (on a par with radio and the internal combustion engine) and led many to believe that infectious diseases would be conquered once and for all. No longer would tuberculosis, dysentery, cholera, pneumonia, enteric diseases inflict their toll on humankind and its social systems -- or so it was thought. The use of antibiotics transformed medical practice to both advantage and disadvantage; previously untreatable diseases were now potentially controllable, but paradoxically, because antibiotics were easy to use and so successful, they may have become a substitute for good clinical practice in some instances. Certainly the use of antibiotics as preventatives (prophy-laxis) in human and animal medicine has had a negative effect on antibiotic therapy overall, the increasing number of treatment failures in hospitals and the community providing abun-dant evidence of this (Ciba, 1997).

It is unlikely that the problem of antibiotic resistance as it exists today could have been anticipated in the early days of antibiotic usage, although there were a few visionaries who recognised the threat and the factors that would promote its appearance.

It is to be hoped that penicillin will not be abused as were the sulfonamides ... too small doses lead to the production of resistant strains of bacteria. ... There is probably no chemo-therapeutic drug to which in suitable circumstances the bacteria cannot react by in some way acquiring 'fastness' (resistance). Sir Alexander Fleming 1946

We cannot be sure that the searchers for new drugs and antibiotics will always win the race. However hard and successfully we may work in the search for new drugs we shall therefore continue to labour under discouragement so long as we are faced with the bugbear of drug resistance. The problem is one of microbial biochemistry, physiology and genetics, and can only be solved by work in these fields. Until we understand the problem we shall have no hope of

Resolving the Antibiotic Paradox, edited by Rosen and Mobashery.
Kluwer Academic / Plenum Publishers, New York, 1998.

overcoming it, and until we overcome it we shall have no real sense of security in our chemotherapy. The subject ... is not only of the greatest scientific interest and importance; it has also
a background of practical medical urgency. Sir Charles Harington 1957

In more recent years, with widespread resistance to many valuable drugs being reported in learned publications and the popular press, many other physicians and scientists
have spoken out against the overuse, imprudent use, and outright abuse of antibiotics
(Levy, 1992). There is frequent mention of the end of the antibiotic era or the regression to
a pre-antibiotic state in infectious diseases treatment.

In spite of significant increases in knowledge of antibiotic resistance mechanisms
and their origins over the past few decades, our understanding is rudimentary, especially
with respect to the ecological aspects. Antibiotic resistance is currrently studied by analysis of the end-product -- the organism causing the therapeutic problem. In order to have
more control over the development of antibiotic resistance it is essential that an understanding of the earliest stages of the process be obtained. What happens (microbiologi-
cally) when a novel antibiotic is introduced for therapeutic use on a large scale? Where
and how does resistance first arise and how soon can the consequences be identified? Why
is resistance so stable and how do bacteria tolerate their increased genetic load or growth-
retarding mutations, in the competition for survival in highly competitive environments?
Until these questions can be answered, the approach to antibiotic therapy will remain one
of educated guesses with no real hope of controlling infectious disease on a large or even
small scale, despite the best-intentioned efforts.

Extensive studies of the antibiotic resistance genes, their expression and the mobile
genetic elements that carry them, have led to the genetic and biochemical characterisation
of resistance mechanisms in a broad spectrum of bacterial hosts (Davies, 1994). About ten
distinct biochemical mechanisms of antibiotic resistance have been identified. The widespread distribution of resistance determinants throughout the microbial population can be
readily explained by the pick-up of resistance genes by mobile genetic elements and resulting heterologous gene exchange. The existence of a resistance gene pool that is available to microbes in response to pressures of selection is generally accepted, but the origin
of the resistance genes is still unresolved. A number of suggestions have been made that
include (1) housekeeping genes (alternate substrates, mutation to new substrate recog-ni-
tion, etc.), (2) 'natural' resistance genes in soil communities and (3) antibiotic-producing
microbes (self-production). Any or all of these potential sources could be involved, but
evidence from comparative studies of the resistance enzymes and their genes supports the
notion that antibiotic-producing organisms represent the most likely generalised source
(Benveniste and Davies, 1973).

Resistance to the glycopeptide antibiotics (vancomycin, teichoplanin) in the enterococci has increased remarkably in recent years and the resistant strains constitute a significant nosocomial problem. Vancomycin blocks the synthesis of bacterial cell walls by
binding to a D-Ala-D-Ala moiety in the growing peptidoglycan structure; resistance arises
by the substitution of D-Ala-D-Lac, which is unable to bind the antibiotic effectively, with
the result that cell wall synthesis continues in the presence of inhibitor.

The *vanA* gene cluster found in the enterococci contains one of the more complex antibiotic resistance mechanisms so far identified (Leclercq and Courvalin, 1997, Walsh, et al.,
1996). It has been demonstrated that the different genes encode functions for (a) altering the
vancomycin binding site, (b) removing the endogenous binding sites and (c) regulating the
expression of the resistance genes through a two-component system (Figure 1). This gene
cluster and the related *vanB* cluster are carried by transposable elements.

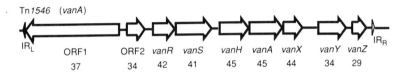

Figure 1. The vancomycin resistance gene cluster of TN*1546*. This gene cluster is responsible for glycopeptide resistance in *Enterococcus faecalis*. The functions of the various genes are: *vanR* and *vanS*, regulator and sensor of two component regulatory systems; *vanH*, dehydrogenase to convert pyruvate to lactate; *vanA*, ligase that inserts lactate into cell wall peptide through ester bond formation; *vanX* and *vanY*, hydrolases to remove the normal vancomycin-binding fragment. Open arrows indicate the open reading frames (ORF1, transposase; ORF2, resolvase). The percentage of guanosine plus cytosine is indicated below each ORF. IR are the inverted repeats. (For more complete information, see Leclercq et al., 1997.)

The evolutionary origin of the *vanA* cluster is of great interest, since it is probable that it was inherited intact rather than being assembled in response to selection. Studies from the laboratory of G. Wright (Marshall, et al., 1997; G. Wright, personal communication), have provided strong evidence that the *vanA*, *H* and *X* genes, whose products are central to the biochemical mechanism of vancomycin resistance, were probably acquired from glycopeptide-producing streptomycetes. The latter organisms possess a group of genes that include a close analogue of the *vanA* gene which, when cloned and expressed in a heterologous host, shows D-Ala-D-Lac synthetic activity. These studies of vancomycin resistance lend credence to the notion that antibiotic-producing bacteria are the foremost source of the antibiotic resistance determinants of bacterial pathogens; this is supported by the finding that antibiotic resistance mechanisms with common biochemical characteristics can be found in both producing organisms and clinical isolates (Table 1).

An interesting exception to the examples presented in this table is the case of sulphonamides and trimethoprim, which are completely synthetic antimicrobials with no natural analogs that inhibit two different steps (dihydropteroate synthase and dihydrofolate reductase) in the biosynthesis of the key metabolic intermediate, folic acid. With these antibiotics bacterial resistance occurs by the acquisition of genes encoding (target) enzymes that are refractory to the two inhibitors. Thus resistant strains possess mechanisms to by-pass both the inhibited steps in the biosynthetic pathway; there is presently no information on the origin of these alien genes.

Table 1. Resistance determinants with biochemical homologues in antibiotic-producing organisms

Antibiotic	Resistance mechanisms*
Penicillins Cephalosporins	ß-lactamases penicillin-binding proteins
Aminoglycosides	acetyltransferases phosphotransferases adenyltransferases
Chloramphenicol	acetyltransferases
Tetracyclines	efflux system ribosomal protection
Macrolides Streptogramins Lincosamines	ribosomal RNA methylation esterases phosphotransferases acetyltransferases
Phosphonates	phosphorylation glutathionylation (?)
Bleomycin	acetyltransferase immunity protein
Vancomycin	D-Ala-D-Lac ligase

*Multiple drug resistance (MDR) efflux systems are common to producing organisms and clinical isolates

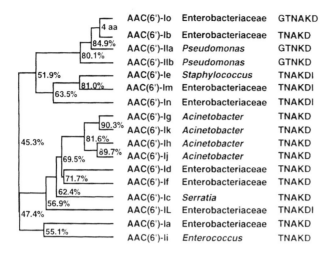

Figure 2. Dendogram showing a comparison of amino acid sequences of the aminoglycoside acetyltransferase (AAC6') family. The numbers represent % similarity in amino acid sequence between different proteins. Also indicated are the source bacterial species and in the right column, the antibiotic resistance spectrum associated with the different enzymes [G: gentamicin; T: tobramycin; N: netilmicin; A: amikacin; K: kanamycin; D: dibekacin; I: isepamicin]. (Figure kindly provided by G.H. Miller.)

Perhaps the best case for the role of heterologous sources as the origin of resistance genes comes from studies of aminoglycoside (AG) resistance. Three types of AG-modifying enzymes have been identified in clinical isolates of bacteria: *N*-acetyltransferases (AAC), *O*-phosphotransferases (APH), and *O*-adenyltransferases (AAD, ANT) (Davies and Wright, 1997). Largely due to the work of the group of Miller, Shaw, and Hare at the Schering-Plough Research Institute, the dynamics of the appearance of different AG enzymes relative to the use of the different AG antibiotics has been tracked world-wide (Miller, et al., 1997). As an example, resistant strains of the 6'-AG acetyltransferases (AAC6') have been analysed and a family of genes that originated in various geographical locations in response to local AG use has been identified. Surprisingly, this AAC6' family (Figure 2) could have been derived only from different (microbial) sources; it is not the result of a series of mutational alterations in a common precursor gene (as is found in the derivation of the extended-spectrum ß-lactamases, coming from one of several ancestors). The same pattern has been demonstrated for several other members of the AG-modifying enzymes (AAC3, APH3', etc.) (Shaw, et al., 1993). It is highly likely that AG-producing organisms contributed a significant number of these genes, since different AG-producing strains are known to elaborate different allelic forms of the same biochemical function. However, it should be pointed out that the producing strains may not have been the sole source of resistance determinants; there is convincing evidence that some of the AG-modifying enzymes are found in other bacterial species and may play a role in cell-wall synthesis (a housekeeping function).

Interestingly, many of the genes for AG-modifying enzymes are found as the components of integrons, and it can be concluded that they were initially inherited as gene cassettes, as is true for several antibiotic resistance genes.

The role of integrons as the major mechanism of acquisition and dissemination of resistance genes in many classes of gram-negative bacteria has been well-established by the work of Hall and Stokes (Recchia and Hall, 1997). Simply put, integrons are naturally-occurring gene expression structures possessing a site-specific integration mechanism for the insertion of open reading frames (gene cassettes) downstream of a strong constitutively-acting promoter (Lévesque, et al., 1995) (Figure 3). Tandem insertions of open reading frames permit the construction of multidrug-resistant elements that can apparently be shuffled to enhance expression of specific determinants.

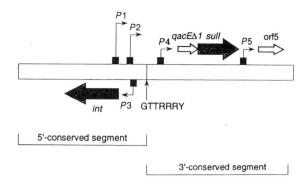

Figure 3. The structure of the elemental integron. The GTTRRRY sequence in the centre is the integration site. The *int* gene is transcribed in a leftward direction from promoter P (lower arrow) and *qac* and *sul* genes rightward from promoter P (upper arrow). Promoters P1 and P2 are responsible for transcription of the antibiotic resistance gene cassettes inserted at the integration site. Produced by permission of P. Roy (see Lévesque et al., 1995).

The integrons have been shown to be essential components of the resistance plasmids associated with the initial epidemic of antibiotic-resistant enterobacterial infections that took place in the early 1950s, which was the first description of the phenomenon of multidrug resistance in bacteria. The actual source of integrons and their associated integrases is unclear; they may well have been derived from temperate bacteriophages, but at present, the three integron integrases that have been identified appear to be quite distinct from the known phage integrases (Capy, et al., 1996). In addition, integrons do not seem to be present in enterobacterial pathogens isolated prior to the introduction of antibiotics for antimicrobial therapy. The "Murray Collection" of pathogenic enterobacteria dating back to 1916 has been screened for the presence of antibiotic-resistance genes and integrons, with negative results (Mazel and Davies, unpublished). Where did the integrons come from?

Although we do not have the answer to this question yet, the finding that the repeated nucleotide sequences typical of pathogenic *Vibrio* sp. (VCRs) are significantly related to integrons would suggest that this type of gene acquisition mechanism pre-dates the introduction of antibiotics. The studies of Mazel and colleagues (Mazel, et al., submitted) have demonstrated that the gene-VCR structure is a substrate for the integron integrases and can be inserted into the *att*I site of an integron. Furthermore, the gene-VCR clusters, which are large structures (super-integrons?) comprising scores of open-reading-frames with (likely) different functions, possess associated integrases which are related phylogenetically to those of the integron. Thus gene-cassette capture systems are common in bacteria, are likely to be ancient (a *V. metschnikovii* isolate from 1888, just 5 years after the isolation of *V. cholerae,* possesses a VCR cluster with accompanying integrase), and must have played roles in the acquisition of genes for pathogenicity and for antibiotic resistance. Might this gene-capture mechanism be responsible also for other acquired functions (such as biodegradation)? The implications of such accumulation mechanisms in the construction of pathogenicity islands (as well as resistance islets) should be readily apparent.

The general conclusion to be drawn is that bacteria have extraordinary genetic flexibility in terms of both mechanisms and functions. Bacterial genomes represent a large natural pool of diverse genetic information that can be accessed under appropriate selection pressures, using a variety of gene acquisition and dissemination mechanisms. Human application of toxic agents on massive scales activates these genetic systems to promote survival of the microbial population. As a result, each and every antibiotic will have a finite lifetime depending on the magnitude and nature of its use; the development of antibiotic resistance is inevitable. Appropriate regulation of antibiotic usage is therefore critical to the continued future of successful antimicrobial therapy, and certain obvious rules must be followed (Cohen, 1997). J. Lederberg has noted that microbes are formidable opponents in the conquest of the biosphere:

> Human intelligence, culture and technology have left all other plant and animal species out of the competition. ... But we have too many illusions that we can govern ... the microbes that remain our competitors of last resort for domination of the planet. In natural evolutionary competition, there is no guarantee that we will find ourselves the survivor(s). Joshua Lederberg 1994

Whether or not the consequences are *so* dire is a matter of opinion. However, there is no doubt that if medical science wishes to continue its success in the therapy of infectious diseases, a substantial re-evaluation of the use and abuse of antibiotics is needed.

REFERENCES

Benveniste, R and Davies, J, 1973, Aminoglycoside antibiotic-inactivating enzymes in actinomycetes similar to those present in clinical isolates of antibiotic-resistant bacteria. *Proc Natl Acad Sci USA* 70:2276–2280.

Capy, P, Vitalis, R, Langin, T, Higuet, D, and Bazin, C, 1996, Relationships between transposable elements based upon the integrase-transposase domains: Is there a common ancestor? *J Mol Evol* 42:359–368.

Ciba Foundation Symposium 207, 1997, *Antibiotic Resistance: Origins, Evolution, Selection and Spread*, John Wiley & Sons, Chichester.

Cohen, ML, 1997, Epidemiological factors influencing the emergence of antimicrobial resistance, in: *Antibiotic Resistance: Origins, Evolution, Selection and Spread*, John Wiley & Sons, Chichester (Ciba Foundation Symposium 207) pp. 223–237.

Davies, J, 1994, Inactivation of antibiotics and the dissemination of resistance genes. *Science* 264:375–382.

Davies, J and Wright, GD, 1997, Bacterial resistance to aminoglycoside antibiotics. *Trends Microbiol* 5:234–240.

Fleming, A, 1946, Chemotherapy: yesterday, today and tomorrow. The Linacre Lecture delivered at Cambridge on May 6, 1946, reprinted in *Fifty Years of Antimicrobials: Past Perspectives and Future Trends*, Soc. Gen. Microbiol. 53rd Symp. April 1995, Cambridge University Press, Cambridge England, pp 1–18.

Harington, C, 1957, in *Drug Resistance in Micro-Organisms. Mechanisms of Development*, Ciba Foundation Symposium, J. & A. Churchill, London, p. 3.

Leclercq, R and Courvalin, P, 1997, Resistance to glycopeptides in enterococci. *Clin Infect Dis* 24:545–556.

Lederberg, J, speech before the Irvington Institute for Medical Research, Bankers Trust Company, New York, February 8, 1994.

Lévesque, C, Piché, L, Larose, C, and Roy, PH, 1995, PCR mapping of integrons reveals several novel operons of resistance genes. *Antimicrob Agents Chemother* 39:185–191.

Levy, SB, 1992, *The Antibiotic Paradox: How Miracle Drugs Are Destroying the Miracle*, Plenum Press, New York.

Marshall, CG, Broadhead, G, Leskiw, BK, and Wright, GD, 1997, D-Ala-D-Ala ligases from glycopeptide antibiotic-producing organisms are highly homologous to the enterococcal vancomycin-resistance ligases VanA and VanB. *Proc Natl Acad Sci USA* 94:6480–6483.

Mazel, D, Dychinco, B. Webb, V A, and Davies, J, 1998, The *Vibrio cholerae* genome contains a new class of integron, submitted to *Science*.

Miller, GH, Sabatelli, FJ, Hare, RS, Glupczynski, Y, Mackey, P, Shlaes, D, Shimizu, K, Shaw, KJ, and the aminoglycoside resistance study groups, 1997, The most frequent aminoglycoside resistance mechanisms - changes with time and geographic area - a reflection of aminoglycoside usage patterns? *Clin Infect Dis* 24:S46–62.

Recchia, GD and Hall, RM, 1997, Origins of the mobile gene cassettes found in integrons. *Trends Microbiol* 5:389–384.

Shaw, KJ, Rather, PN, Hare, RS, and Miller, GH, 1993, Molecular genetics of aminoglycoside resistance genes and familial relationships of the aminoglycoside-modifying enzymes. *Microbiol Rev* 57:138–163.

Walsh, CT, Fisher, SL, Park, I-S, Prahalad, M, and Wu, Z, 1996, Bacterial resistance to vancomycin: five genes and one missing hydrogen bond tell the story. *Curr Biol* 3:21–28.

2

CLINICAL IMPACT OF ANTIBIOTIC RESISTANCE

Stephen A. Lerner

Division of Infectious Diseases, Department of Medicine
Department of Biochemistry and Molecular Biology
Wayne State University School of Medicine
Detroit, Michigan 48201

INTRODUCTION

The development of antimicrobial agents for clinical use has brought unquestionable benefits to individuals and to society. Infections that formerly were frequently fatal have become routinely curable. Furthermore, the availability of effective antibiotic therapy has facilitated the employment by physicians of potent immunosuppressive therapy in the control and treatment of other conditions such as cancer and transplant rejection, since resulting infections may be treated and are often suppressed or cured.

Despite these considerable benefits, the utilization of antimicrobial chemotherapy has also produced adverse consequences for individual patients. As with any medication, antibiotics can produce untoward side-effects, such as allergic reactions and impairment of organ function, as of the liver or kidneys. Unlike other medications, however, the use of antibiotics may also have adverse consequences outside the patient. Antibiotic treatment may lead to selection of resistance in the target organisms that cause infection and against which antibiotic therapy is directed. Thus, antibiotics ultimately lose their effectiveness as they are used over time, in contrast to other types of medication.

Occasionally, individual cells of an infecting strain of bacteria may acquire resistance to an antibiotic, either as a result of mutation or by acquisition of foreign genes from a resistant organism. In such a case, in the presence of the antibiotic the resistant cells will proliferate over their susceptible sibling cells, unless they are eliminated by host defenses of the treated patient. When such resistant cells proliferate, they not only exacerbate the patient's infection and complicate his/her treatment, but they may also produce adverse consequences for the wider society. Such resistant populations of pathogens that survive treatment may be shed into the environment, where they may infect other patients and complicate their therapy by limiting the antibiotic options. Over time, such antibiotic-re-

Resolving the Antibiotic Paradox, edited by Rosen and Mobashery.
Kluwer Academic / Plenum Publishers, New York, 1998.

sistant populations may become predominant in a localized environment, such as an intensive-care unit, a hospital, or a nursing home, or even in the broader community. Eventually, therefore, some antibiotics may thereby lose their utility. In response, physicians must update the antibiotic regimens that they use to treat various infections to keep ahead of the emergence and dissemination of resistance among pathogenic microorganisms. (I shall limit my comments to bacteria, but similar problems of resistance to therapeutic agents arise in fungi, viruses, and parasites as well.) Since bacteria that have developed or acquired resistance to an antibiotic are frequently resistant also to other antibiotics, the complexity of resistance patterns in bacteria may be quite confounding and may therefore require considerable ingenuity and innovation in the selection of antimicrobial therapeutic regimens from among limited choices. Thus, antibiotic costs include not only acquisition charges and adverse reactions to the drug, but also the costs resulting from resistance that is selected by antibiotic use.

Antibiotic therapy affects not merely the intended target pathogens, but also normal commensal, or colonizing, bacteria that are present in the patient. The elimination or reduction of this protective flora may permit the replacement by less virulent, but more antibiotic-resistant, organisms that may be of minor consequence in normal individuals but may produce serious infections in immunocompromised patients. Therefore, in such individuals antibiotic therapy is again a two-edged sword which permits the introduction of unwelcome intruders as it eliminates infectious pathogens that are causing disease. Novel antibiotic regimens are needed to treat infections caused by these antibiotic-resistant organisms which previously were considered to be of little consequence.

ANTIBIOTIC RESISTANCE OF CLINICAL IMPORTANCE

Presumed Resistance

Some types of antibacterial resistance have become so prevalent that the biology of the organism can be considered effectively altered, and one would rarely consider the use of the problematic antibiotic(s) unless susceptibility of the specific infecting bacterial strain had been documented. The prime example of a virtually complete loss of susceptibility is in *Staphylococcus aureus*. Although at the time of the introduction of penicillin G into clinical practice it had great effectiveness against *S. aureus*, very soon thereafter penicillin-resistant isolates of *S. aureus* began to appear. By the mid- to late-1950s, the vast majority of *S. aureus* isolates throughout the world were producing a ß-lactamase that inactivates penicillin G and thereby confers resistance to it (Medeiros, 1997). In response to this problem, semisynthetic penicillins that are poor substrates of this ß-lactamase, such as methicillin, oxacillin, and nafcillin, were developed in the 1960s for the treatment of such penicillin-resistant strains. (This subject is discussed in greater detail in the chapter by Bush and Mobashery.) These drugs are today the first-line anti-*S. aureus* agents in most settings, unless the local prevalence of methicillin-resistant *S. aureus* strains, which are resistant to all available ß-lactam drugs, mandates alternative presumptive therapy with vancomycin.

Penicillin resistance in *S. aureus* is the extreme example of presumed resistance, but resistance may be presumed in other situations as well. The approaches to the treatment of different infections caused by *Streptococcus pneumoniae* illustrate the balance between incidence of resistant infections and the urgency of effective initial therapy. Although the incidences of penicillin resistance and intermediate susceptibility are rising generally throughout the world (Austrian, 1994), in some communities they may still be relatively modest, 3–5% and 5–10%, respectively (Butler et al., 1996; Simor et al., 1996). The choice of therapy for various pneumococcal infections in such a community with relatively low incidence of resistance to penicillin (and some other agents as well) would depend on the severity of the infection. For instance, otitis media, which is usually caused by *S. pneumoniae*, would still likely be treated with a penicillin such as amoxicillin, since the drug is administered conveniently by mouth and is inexpensive. Therapy might fail occasionally because of resistance, although even untreated otitis media may in some cases resolve spontaneously. Nonetheless, the consequences of therapeutic failure would be slight, since the child can be brought back to the physician for evaluation and possible treatment with an alternative drug if the symptoms do not resolve. Similarly, for pneumococcal pneumonia that is sufficiently mild to warrant out-patient therapy (so-called "walking pneumonia"), the use of a penicillin may be justified if the patient is alerted to return for evaluation if symptoms do not improve within a specified time. If the degree of resistance to penicillin among resistant strains in the community is modest, penicillin may be used even for the treatment of more serious pneumococcal pneumonia if high doses are administered intravenously in the hospital. At the other extreme is the therapeutic approach to pneumococcal meningitis. Even infections caused by strains that are intermediately susceptible to penicillin may fail to respond optimally to penicillin therapy, since the penetration of penicillin into the cerebrospinal fluid is relatively poor. The consequences of delayed effective treatment are potentially disastrous, so one cannot rely on penicillin as initial therapy to treat pneumococcal meningitis that might be caused by intermediate or fully resistant strains. It has thus become standard practice to initiate therapy for suspected or documented pneumococcal meningitis with both vancomycin and a third-generation cephalosporin, even though such a regimen is expensive and exerts broad selective pressure. Once the susceptibility profile of the infecting strain is known, the treatment regimen is adjusted accordingly, e.g., to penicillin, if possible.

Urgent Problems of Resistance

Although there are many examples of clinically important antibiotic resistance that are proliferating and disseminating, several are of crucial importance because they are currently undergoing rapid evolution and spread and/or they leave little or no effective therapy against the target organisms.

Methicillin-Resistant Staphylococci. Following the introduction of methicillin in 1960 to overcome the ubiquitous problem of ß-lactamase-mediated resistance to penicillin (see above), very soon strains that were resistant to methicillin began to appear. From the late 1970s these methicillin-resistant *S. aureus* (MRSA) strains have spread throughout the world. The prevalence of methicillin resistance among hospital strains of *S. aureus* varies from only 1–2% to as high as 30–40% within Europe (Voss et al., 1994), and recently within the U.S. the nosocomial rates have been at least 35% (Centers for Disease Control and Prevention, 1997a). Although MRSA is especially a problem in tertiary-care hospitals, and especially in intensive-care units, it is now also prevalent in community hospitals and nursing homes (Jacoby and Archer, 1991). The prevalence of such resistance in nosocomial isolates of coagulase-negative staphylococci, such as *Staphylococcus epidermidis and Staphylococcus haemolyticus*, is even higher than in *S. aureus* (Jacoby and Archer, 1991). Methicillin-resistant staphylococci are resistant to *all* available ß-lactam antibiotics; vancomycin is the only antibiotic to which methicillin-resistant staphylococci have been, until very recently (see below), uniformly susceptible. Therefore, physicians have had to rely on this drug increasingly in recent years (Michel and Gutmann, 1997), adding to the selective pressure for vancomycin resistance in staphylococci and other organisms (see below). Although vancomycin has provided critically important presumptive and definitive therapy for methicillin-resistant staphylococci for which there was no alternative, it is at best an imperfect drug, less effective than the ß-lactams against methicillin-susceptible staphylococci (Levine et al., 1991). Therefore, vancomycin is considered a drug of last resort for staphylococcal infections.

Vancomycin (Multidrug)-Resistant Enterococci. Although the intrinsic virulence of enterococci is much less than that of *S. aureus*, over the past two decades they have become the second to third most commonly isolated organisms from hospital infections (Murray, 1997). Since enterococci are intrinsically resistant to most antibiotics, the available anti-enterococcal armamentarium at its best is quite restricted. The principal agents are ampicillin and vancomycin. Although these drugs, which interfere with cell-wall biosynthesis, are bactericidal against most other susceptible organisms, against most susceptible strains of enterococci they are merely bacteriostatic. For the optimal treatment of serious systemic infections caused by enterococci, such as endocarditis, a combined regimen of ampicillin or vancomycin plus an aminoglycoside, such as gentamicin or streptomycin, has been employed to produce a synergistic bactericidal effect. Over the past two decades increasing numbers of enterococci have acquired levels of resistance to aminoglycosides so high that they do not contribute to a synergistic effect and are thus not useful for the treatment of infections with such strains (Herman and Gerding, 1991). The utility of ampicillin in the treatment of enterococcal infections has been compromised over the past two decades by the relative increase in infections of *Enterococcus faecium*, a species that was formerly encountered much less commonly than the principal enterococcal species of man, *Enterococcus faecalis*. Since *E. faecium* is generally intrinsically resistant to ampicillin, consequently ampicillin has become increasingly less effective over time (Murray, 1997; Herman and Gerding, 1991). Furthermore, ß-lactamase-mediated resistance to ampicillin has been reported rarely; fortunately, it has not yet spread widely (Wells et al., 1992).

After three decades of clinical use of vancomycin, in 1988 the first examples of acquired resistance to this agent appeared, in clinical isolates of enterococci. Unfortunately, vancomycin resistance has entered predominantly *E. faecium*, so its overall incidence has increased as the proportion of this species has risen among enterococci. By 1993, CDC reported that 8% of all nosocomial enterococcal infections were caused by vancomycin-resistant strains, and 14% of those in intensive-care units (Centers for Disease Control and Prevention, 1993). The regular appearance of *E. faecium* strains which exhibit clinically significant resistance to ampicillin, vancomycin, and all of the aminoglycosides, and are thus not treatable with any available antibiotics is a cause of great concern and alarm. In response, the CDC has published guidelines aimed at preventing the spread and selection of vancomycin-resistant enterococci (Centers for Disease Control and Prevention, 1995). Fortunately, the pharmaceutical industry has directed its attention toward the development of new compounds with promise of efficacy against infections caused by these untreatable pathogens (Michel and Gutmann, 1997).

Vancomycin (Glycopeptide)-Intermediate S. Aureus (GISA). The emergence and dissemination of vancomycin resistance in enterococci raised the fear that this transmissible plasmid-borne resistance would enter *S. aureus*, since expression of vancomycin resistance in MRSA would produce a highly virulent human pathogen that is resistant to all available chemotherapy. In fact, experimental transfer of vancomycin-resistance genes from enterococci into MRSA in the laboratory was reported to result in vancomycin resistance (Noble et al., 1992). In addition, vancomycin-resistant subpopulations of *Staphylococcus haemolyticus* (Schwalbe et al., 1990) and *S. aureus* (Daum et al., 1992) were selected in the laboratory with increasing levels of glycopeptides such as vancomycin. Although infections caused by coagulase-negative staphylococci with reduced susceptibility to vancomycin had been recognized, (Garrett et al., 1997; Schwalbe et al., 1987), it was not until 1996 that the first clinical infection with vancomycin-intermediate (MIC 8μg/ml) *S. aureus* was recognized (Centers for Disease Control and Prevention, 1997a), and in 1997 the first isolate of a similar strain in the U.S. was reported (Centers for Disease Control and Prevention, 1997c). The mechanisms of this intermediate, or low-level, resistance to vancomycin are unknown but under investigation. It is not yet clear whether these isolates with diminished susceptibility to vancomycin herald outbreaks of even higher-level resistance. In response to the report of the Japanese isolate, CDC published guidelines to review and restrict the use of vancomycin, to screen carefully for other clinical isolates with diminished vancomycin susceptibility, and to prevent the spread of such strains if they should be identified in a patient (Centers for Disease Control and Prevention, 1997b). The development and approval of successful new antistaphylococcal drugs now assumes a greater urgency.

Broad Resistance to β-Lactams Due to Genetically Derepressed Class C Chromosomal β-Lactamases in Nosocomial Aerobic Gram-Negative Bacilli. With the introduction of expanded-spectrum cephalosporins into clinical therapy in the late 1970s and the 1980s, broad resistance to ß-lactams, including expanded-spectrum cephalosporins and aztreonam, but not carbapenems such as imipenem, was observed to emerge in nosocomial aerobic gram-negative bacilli, such as *Enterobacter* spp., *Pseudomonas aeruginosa*, *Serratia marcescens*, and *Citrobacter freundii* (Sanders and Sanders, 1986). This broad ß-lactam resistance was found to be due to mutational derepression of species-specific members of a family of related chromosomal class C ß-lactamases that are normally inducible and are active against a spectrum of substrates that parallels the spectrum of conferred resistance (Bush et al., 1995). Such resistance has been observed to emerge even during a patient's course of therapy (Chow et al., 1991). The prevalence of such resistance has risen to high levels that often force the presumption of resistance until it can be ruled out, especially in settings like intensive-care units, where such nosocomial species are common and broad-spectrum ß-lactams are utilized widely (Itokazu, 1996). Since resistance to possible alternative antibiotics is often present as well in such strains, we therefore encounter in these severely ill, debilitated patients pathogens for which no conventional antibiotic therapy is available, and this situation continues to worsen.

Mutational Evolution of Plasmid-Encoded Class A β-Lactamases. In the 1980s, as nosocomial gram-negative bacilli were developing broad resistance to extended-spectrum ß-lactams such as expanded-spectrum cephalosporins and the monobactam, aztreonam, as a result of increased production of intrinsic, chromosomally encoded class C ß-lactamases (see above), strains of *Escherichia coli* and *Klebsiella pneumoniae* began to appear with resistance to some or all of these agents, which are normally highly active against these species (Jacoby, 1997). Investigation of such resistant isolates has revealed that such resistance is usually due to the presence of mutant derivatives of plasmid-encoded class A ß-lactamases such as TEM or SHV. As a result of the mutations in these extended-spectrum ß-lactamases (ESBLs), the affinity for, and/or activity against, various of the extended-spectrum ß-lactams is enhanced, and thus resistance is conferred against these improved substrates (Bush et al., 1995; Medeiros, 1997). (Also see the chapter by Bush and Mobashery.) These resistant strains generally occur in outbreaks associated with hospitals, so their incidence and impact vary enormously among institutions (Itokazu, 1996) and the specific pattern of ß-lactam resistance depends upon the particular mutant derivative that is prevalent (Bush et al., 1995; Medeiros, 1997).

"Wild-type" class A ß-lactamases, such as TEM-1, TEM-2, and SHV-1, are readily inactivated by inhibitors like clavulanic acid, sulbactam, and tazobactam. Therefore, the therapeutic effectiveness of penicillins has been enhanced against resistant strains which bear such enzymes by administering them in combination with one of these inhibitors. However, single mutations at any of four sites in TEM and SHV ß-lactamases reduce the affinity of the resulting mutant enzymes for the inactivators and/or reduce the efficiency of inactivation, thereby restoring resistance to penicillins in the presence of the inactivator (Vakulenko, 1998). Thus, once again, selection of mutations threatens to overcome the clever strategy of reversing a prevalent mechanism of resistance by specific inhibition of the resistance mechanism. Fortunately, virtually all of the class A ESBLs from clinical isolates that have been tested at least retain their sensitivity to inactivation by clavulanic acid and the other ß-lactamase inhibitors (Medeiros, 1997).

Multidrug-Resistant Tuberculosis. The introduction of effective antimycobacterial treatment for tuberculosis was followed soon thereafter by emergence of resistance to individual agents that compromised therapy (Crofton and Mitchison, 1948; Canetti, 1965). Since the resistance to individual agents is drug-specific, the hallmark of treatment regimens has been the utilization of multiple drugs (a minimum of two drugs that are active against the infecting strain) to retard the emergence/selection of mutants that have developed resistance to a single drug (Cohn et al., 1959). Despite the rationale of this approach, resistance to each individual first- and second-line antimycobacterial agent has appeared in *Mycobacterium tuberculosis.* Such resistance is believed to be selected during treatment courses that are incomplete because of lack of adequate adherence to the prescribed multidrug regimen over a sufficient period of time to eradicate all of the organisms. As resistance to individual drugs was reported in clinical isolates of *M. tuberculosis,* the number of drugs recommended for treatment of tuberculosis was increased to maintain the principle of treatment with at least two active drugs. Nonetheless, accretion of resistances in individual strains progressed. By the early 1990s, outbreaks of multidrug-resistant tuberculosis (with *M. tuberculosis* strains resistant to at least isoniazid and rifampin) began to appear in patients with HIV infection (Dooley et al., 1992; Edlin at al., 1992; Frieden et al., 1993; Fischl et al., 1992; Monno et al., 1991), apparently by sequential selection of mutations conferring resistance to individual agents (Bifani et al., 1996). Multidrug resistance in *Mycobacterium tuberculosis* is often associated with a poor response to therapy, especially in HIV-infected patients (Frieden et al., 1993; Frieden et al., 1996; Pablos-Méndez et al., 1996), although the outcome can be improved considerably in HIV-infected (Salomon et al., 1995; Turett et al., 1995) and non-infected patients (Telzak et al., 1995) by prompt diagnosis and initiation of multidrug therapy, attention to adherence to treatment regimen, rapid reporting of drug susceptibilities in the infecting strain, and adjustment of the regimen accordingly. A recent report of the Global Project on Anti-Tuberculosis Drug Resistance Surveillance (Pablos-Méndez et al., 1998) examined prevalence of resistance to four first-line anti-tuberculosis drugs (isoniazid, rifampin, ethambutol, and streptomycin) in *M. tuberculosis* strains isolated in 28 countries around the world. Although the prevalence of resistance to any of these drugs was only 12.6% (median among countries) and 12.9% (in the U.S.), and the prevalence of resistance to more than one of the tested drugs was only 5.0% (median among countries) and 4.5% (in the U.S.), these figures were much higher for some other areas of the world.

The list of available first-line anti-tuberculosis agents is relatively short: isoniazid, rifampin, pyrazinamide, ethambutol, and streptomycin. In addition, kanamycin or amikacin may be useful as a replacement for streptomycin when they are active against streptomycin-resistant strains. There have been no new agents to add to this list in the past 25 years. Fluoroquinolones have utility for the treatment of multidrug-resistant tuberculosis (Alangaden and Lerner, 1997), but they should at this point still be considered second-line agents. Thus, the options for treatment of multidrug-resistant tuberculosis with *at least* two active agents (or more for security against selection of additional resistance) are relatively limited, especially in geographic regions in which resistance to isoniazid, rifampin, and other agents occurs together in strains, and prior to the determination of the definitive susceptibilities. For chemoprophylaxis of contacts of people with tuberculosis that is suspected to be multidrug-resistant or of individuals with recent conversion of the tuberculin skin test in a geographic region with a high prevalence of multidrug-resistant tuberculosis, the choice of drugs is complicated by the desire to administer a relatively benign drug that is likely to eradicate the incipient or latent infection. Clearly then, we need to extend the list of effective anti-tuberculosis drugs with agents that are active against strains that are resistant to the currently available drugs. Although the problem of multidrug-resistant tuberculosis is not yet out of control in the U.S., it is already a major problem in other areas of the world where both the prevalence of tuberculosis and of multidrug resistance are much higher. Concerted efforts of cooperation among international agencies, governments, and pharmaceutical companies are needed to address this increasing problem.

CONCLUSION

What can clinicians and the medical community do to retard the erosion of antibiotic effectiveness brought about by the selection and dissemination of antibiotic-resistant microorganisms? Over 12 million kg of antibiotics produced annually in the U.S. are used in man (Levy, 1998). (Almost as much is also used in animals, both for therapy and for growth promotion.) It is a truism that such massive exposure of bacteria to antibacterial antibiotics will accelerate the selection of resistant organisms. Therefore, it is incumbent upon the medical establishment and individual practitioners to utilize antibiotics prudently, in situations in which the likelihood of benefit is sufficient to justify such use. For initial therapy, when the identity and the susceptibility of the infecting organisms are generally not yet known, it might be desirable and acceptable to treat broadly against a wide spectrum of possible pathogens. However, once the situation has been clarified after several days, it is critical to reassess the therapy to determine whether it can be adjusted to focus more narrowly on the organisms that require treatment. Furthermore, although it is not central to this discussion, it should be mentioned that considerable attention and effort are directed toward control of spread of antibiotic-resistant organisms from infected patients and the environment to other patients.

The scientific and pharmaceutical communities also have important roles to play. First, greater understanding of novel mechanisms of resistance and how they arise and disseminate may provide greater insight into how to use these important drugs clinically to minimize selection and spread of resistance. Second, such knowledge may suggest pharmaceutical strategies to circumvent resistance and thereby to restore to renewed utility old antibiotics whose effectiveness had been seriously compromised. Third, we need continued efforts, such as those described in this book, employing novel approaches of antibiotic development directed toward clinically important organisms whose therapy is threatened or compromised by resistance. Last, we urge that when novel antibacterial compounds are developed, early studies should be directed to investigation of mechanisms of resistance that are already present in microorganisms and of resistance that can be selected *in vitro*, since such findings might herald novel resistance which might arise in targeted or other bacteria once the drug is used clinically.

REFERENCES

Alangaden, G.J. and Lerner, S.A., 1997, The clinical use of fluoroquinolones for the treatment of mycobacterial diseases, *Clin. Infect. Dis.* 25:1213.

Austrian, R., 1994, Confronting drug-resistant pneumococci, *Ann. Intern. Med.* 121:807.

Bifani, P.J., Plikaytis, B.B., Kapur, V., et al., 1996, Origin and interstate spread of a New York City multidrug-resistant *Mycobacterium tuberculosis* clone family, *J. Amer. Med. Assoc.* 275:452.

Bush, K., Jacoby, G.A., and Medeiros, A.A., 1995, A functional classification scheme for ß-lactamases and its correlation with molecular structure, *Antimicrob. Agents Chemother.* 39:1211.

Butler, J. C., Hofmann, J.H., Cetron, M.S., Elliott, J.A., Facklam, R.R., and Breiman, R.F., 1996, The continued emergence of drug-resistant *Streptococcus pneumoniae* in the United States: an update from the Centers for Disease Control and Prevention's Pneumococcal Sentinel Surveillance System, *J. Infect. Dis.* 174:986.

Canetti, G., 1965, Present aspects of bacterial resistance in tuberculosis, *Am. Rev. Resp. Dis.* 92:687.

Centers for Disease Control and Prevention, 1989–1993, 1993, Nosocomial enterococci resistant to vancomycin, *Morb. Mortal. Wkly. Rep.* 42:597.

Centers for Disease Control and Prevention, 1995, Recommendations for preventing the spread of vancomycin resistance. Recommendations of the Hospital Infection Control Practices Advisory Committee (HICPAC), *Morb. Mortal. Wkly. Rep.* 44:1.

Centers for Disease Control and Prevention, 1997a, Reduced susceptibility of *Staphylococcus aureus* to vancomycin – Japan, 1996, *Morb. Mortal. Wkly. Rep.* 46:624.

Centers for Disease Control and Prevention, 1997b, Interim guidelines for prevention and control of staphylococcal infection associated with reduced susceptibility to vancomycin, *Morb. Mortal. Wkly. Rep.* 46:626.

Centers for Disease Control and Prevention, 1997c, *Staphylococcus aureus* with reduced susceptibility to vancomycin – United States, 1997, *Morb. Mortal. Wkly. Rep.* 46:765.

Chow, J.W., Fine, M.J., Shlaes, D.M., et al., 1991, *Enterobacter* bacteremia: clinical features and emergence of antibiotic resistance during therapy, *Ann. Intern. Med.* 115:585.

Cohn, M.L., Middlebrook, G., and Russell, W.F., Jr., 1959, Combined drug treatment of tuberculosis. I. Prevention of emergence of mutant populations of tubercle bacilli resistant to both streptomycin and isoniazid *in vitro*, *J. Clin. Invest.* 38:1349.

Crofton, J. and Mitchison, D.A., 1948, Streptomycin resistance in pulmonary tuberculosis, *Br. Med. J.* 2:1009.

Daum, R.S., Gupta, S., Sabbagh, R., and Milewski, W.M., 1992, Characterization of *Staphylococcus aureus* isolates with decreased susceptibility to vancomycin and teicoplanin: isolation and purification of a constitutively produced protein associated with decreased susceptibility, *J. Infect. Dis.* 166:1066.

Dooley, S.W., Jarvis, W.R., Martone, W.J., and Snider, D.E., Jr., 1992, Multidrug-resistant tuberculosis, *Ann. Intern. Med.* 117:257.

Edlin, B.R., Tokars, J.I., Grieco, M.H., et al., 1992, An outbreak of multidrug-resistant tuberculosis among hospitalized patients with the acquired immunodeficiency syndrome, *N. Engl. J. Med.* 326:1514.

Fischl, M.A., Uttamchandani, R.B., Daikos, G.L., et al., 1992, An outbreak of tuberculosis caused by multiple-drug-resistant tubercle bacilli among patients with HIV infection, *Ann. Intern. Med.* 117:177.

Frieden, T.R., Sherman, L.F., Maw, K.L., et al., 1996, A multi-institutional outbreak of highly drug-resistant tuberculosis: epidemiology and clinical outcomes, *J. Am. Med. Assoc.* 276:1220.

Frieden, T.R., Sterling, T., Pablos-Méndez, A., et al., 1993, The emergence of drug-resistant tuberculosis in New York City, *N. Engl. J. Med.* 328:521.

Garrett, D.O., Jochimsen, E., Murfitt, K., et al, 1997, The impending apocalypse: the emergence of vancomycin resistance in Staphylococcus spp. (Abstr. S1), *Infect. Control Hosp. Epidemiol.* 18:P32.

Herman, D.J. and Gerding, D.N., 1991, Antimicrobial resistance among enterococci, *Antimicrob. Agents Chemother.* 35:1.

Itokazu, G.S., Quinn, J.P., Bell-Dixon, C., et al, 1996, Antimicrobial resistance rates among aerobic gram-negative bacilli recovered from patients in intensive care units: evaluation of a national postmarketing surveillance program, *Clin. Infect. Dis.* 23:779.

Jacoby, G.A., 1997, Extended-spectrum ß-lactamases and other enzymes providing resistance to oxyimino-ß-lactams, *Infect. Dis. Clin. N. Am.* 11:875.

Jacoby G.A. and Archer, G.L., 1991, New mechanisms of bacterial resistance to antimicrobial agents, *J. Infect. Dis.* 324:601.

Levine, D.P., Fromm, B.S., and Reddy, B.R., 1991, Slow response to vancomycin or vancomycin plus rifampin in methicillin resistant *Staphylococcus aureus* endocarditis, *Ann. Intern. Med.* 115:674.

Levy, S.B., 1998, Multidrug resistance --- a sign of the times, *N. Engl. J. Med.* 338:1376 .

Medeiros, A.A., 1997, Evolution and dissemination of ß-lactamases accelerated by generations of ß-lactam antibiotics, *Clin. Infect. Dis.* 24(Suppl 1):S19.

Michel, M. and Gutmann, L., 1997, Methicillin-resistant *Staphylococcus aureus* and vancomycin-resistant enterococci: therapeutic realities and possibilities, *Lancet* 349:1901 .

Monno, L., Angarano, G., Carbonara, S., et al., 1991, Emergence of drug-resistant *Mycobacterium tuberculosis* in HIV-infected patients, *Lancet* 337:852.

Murray, B.E., 1997, Vancomycin-resistant enterococci, *Am. J. Med.* 101:284 .

Noble, W.C., Virani, Z., and Cree, R.G., 1992, Co-transfer of vancomycin and other resistance genes from *Enterococcus faecalis* NCTC 12201 to *Staphylococcus aureus*, *FEMS Microbiol. Lett.* 72:195.

Pablos-Méndez, A., Sterling, T.R., and Frieden, T.R., 1996, The relationship between delayed or incomplete treatment and all-cause mortality in patients with tuberculosis, *J. Am. Med. Assoc.* 276:1223.

Pablos-Méndez, A., Raviglione, M.C., Laszlo, A., et al., 1998, Global surveillance for antituberculosis-drug resistance, *N. Engl. J. Med.* 338:1641.

Sanders, C.C. and Sanders, W.E., Jr, 1986, Type I beta-lactamase of gram-negative bacteria: interactions with beta-lactam antibiotics, *J. Infect. Dis.* 154:792 .

Salomon, N., Perlman, D.C., Friedmann, P., et al., 1995, Predictors and outcome of multidrug-resistant tuberculosis, *Clin. Infect. Dis.* 21:1245.

Schwalbe, R.S., Ritz, W.J., Verma, P.R., et al., 1990, Selection for vancomycin resistance in clinical isolates of *Staphylococcus haemolyticus, J. Infect. Dis.* 161:45.

Schwalbe, R.S., Stapleton, J.T., and Gilligan, P.H., 1987, Emergence of vancomycin resistance in coagulase-negative staphylococci, *N. Engl. J. Med.* 316:927.

Simor, A.E., Louie, M., Canadian Bacterial Surveillance Network, and Low, D.E., 1996, Canadian national survey of prevalence of antimicrobial resistance among clinical isolates of *Streptococcus pneumoniae, Antimicrob. Agents Chemother.* 40:2190.

Telzak, E.E., Sepkowitz, K., Alpert, P., et al., 1995, Multidrug-resistant tuberculosis in patients without HIV infection, *N. Engl.J. Med.* 333:907.

Turett, G.S., Telzak, E.E., Torian, L.V., et al., 1995, Improved outcomes for patients with multidrug-resistant tuberculosis, *Clin. Infect. Dis.* 21:1238.

Vakulenko, S.B., Geryk, B., Kotra, L.P., Mobashery, S., and Lerner, S.A., 1998, Selection and characterization of ß-lactam-ß-lactamase inactivator-resistant mutants following PCR mutagenesis of the TEM-1 ß-lactamase gene, *Antimicrob. Agents Chemother.* 42:in press.

Voss, A., Milatovic, D., Wallrauch-Schwarz, C., Rosdahl, V.T., and Braveny, I., 1994, Methicillin-resistant *Staphylococcus aureus* in Europe, *Eur. J. Clin. Microbiol. Infect. Dis.* 13:50.

Wells, V.D., Wong, E.S., Murray, B.E., et al., 1992, Infections due to beta-lactamase-producing, high-level gentamicin-resistant *Enterococcus faecalis*, *Ann. Intern. Med.* 116:285.

3

REVERSING TETRACYCLINE RESISTANCE

A Renaissance for the Tetracycline Family of Antibiotics

Stuart B. Levy and Mark Nelson

Center for Adaptation Genetics and Drug Resistance
Tufts University School of Medicine
Boston, Massachusetts 02111

The frequency of antibiotic resistance among common human and animal pathogens has continued to rise despite concerted efforts to improve antibiotic use and increase awareness of antibiotic resistance among providers and consumers of these valuable agents (1). Among hospital and community acquired infections, there are more than a dozen organisms whose multidrug resistance means that some individuals may contract infections for which there is only one drug with which to treat, or even in some instances, no drugs at all (Table 1). Among the latter organisms are the hospital acquired vancomycin-resistant Enterococcus, *Pseudomonas aeruginosa* and *Acinetobacter baumanii*. The methicillin-resistant *Staphylococcus aureus* strains which have recently emerged with chromosomally-specified decreased susceptibility to vancomycin are also potentially the ones that could eventually be untreatable. In the community, *Mycobacterium tuberculosis* is a major problem with the *Pneumococcus* not far behind, especially as cephalosporin resistance rises and the use of this life-saving drug is lost. Vancomycin is the only drug left, used with a cephalosporin, to treat meningitis caused by the very common invasive pneumococcus.

Approaches to the resistance problem have to include care and improvement in use. It is clear that the antibiotic resistance problem arises from the misuse and overuse of these therapeutic agents which select for the originally rare, but soon not so uncommon, traits which provide resistance to the antibiotics. Resistance is not confined to the bacterium in which it may first arise; most of the resistance determinants can be transferred to other bacteria on plasmids and transposons which can be exchanged by cell-to-cell contact, via free naked DNA lost from lysed cells, or via bacterial viruses, the bacteriophages. (Fig 1.) Thus, the genetic fluidity of the bacterial flora plus the selective ability of antibiotics have created an environment in which common genes are found in multiply diverse organisms inhabiting very different ecologic and geographic niches. The power of antibiotics has paradoxically been their downfall; antibiotics select for the survivors which then thwart their efficacy (2).

Resolving the Antibiotic Paradox, edited by Rosen and Mobashery.
Kluwer Academic / Plenum Publishers, New York, 1998.

Table 1. Major multiple antibiotic
resistant bacterial problems

Hospital	Community
Staphylococcus aureus	*Streptococcus pneumoniae*
Enterococcus faecium / E. faecalis	*Mycobacterium tuberculosis*
Klebsiella sp.	*Neisseria gonorrhoeae*
Enterobacter sp.	*Streptococcus pyogenes*
Pseudomonas aeruginosa	*Escherichia coli*
Acinetobacter baumanii	

While education and increased awareness are steady and ongoing approaches which must be encouraged and supported in order to resolve the resistance problem, certainly the finding of novel antimicrobials is an important way to control propagation and spread of the multidrug resistant strains which have emerged worldwide. One approach has been to look for new targets, and thereby discover structurally unrelated drugs which will not face previously selected resistance determinants in the environment. Another approach, being followed in our laboratory, is to take a well-respected, highly successful antibiotic which

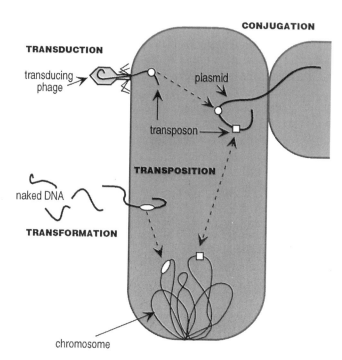

Figure 1. Gene exchange among bacteria. Bacteria have a number of mechanisms by which they transfer and acquire genes, including those for antibiotic resistance. By cell-to-cell contact, a closed circular extrachromosomal DNA molecule called a plasmid can be exchanged among different bacteria including those of distant genera (**conjugation**). Plasmids may bear resistance genes incorporated into the DNA as a transposon, a small, discrete unit of DNA which can move independently from one host DNA vehicle to another (**transposition**). Bacterial viruses or bacteriophages can deliver DNA bearing genes from other bacteria, including transposons, into a new bacterial host, where it can be incorporated into resident plasmids or into the chromosome (**transduction**). Naked DNA itself can be picked up by certain bacteria, e.g., *Hemophilus influenzae* or *Streptococcus pneumoniae* and be incorporated into the chromosome (**transformation**). Some of these DNAs may contain resistance genes, including transposons.

Table 2. Tetracycline resistance determinant class* with
principal bacterial hosts.

Efflux[+]		Ribosome protection[+]
Gram negative	Gram positive	
A *Pseudomonas*	K *Staphylococcus*	M *Enterococcus*
B *Escherichia coli*	*Streptococcus*	O *Campylobacter*
C *Salmonella*	L *Staphylococcus*	Q *Bacteroides*
D *Aeromonas*	*Streptococcus*	S *Listeria*
E *Aeromonas*	P$_A$ *Clostridium difficile*	T *Streptococcus*
G *Vibrio*		U *Enterococcus*
H *Pasteurella*		P$_B$ *Clostridium difficile*

* Major bacterial host for the determinant is listed.
[+] Resistance mechanism.

has lost its efficacy due to resistance and devote attention to its renaissance. We discovered some years ago the mechanism for tetracycline resistance among gram negative bacteria (3). That mechanism, an energy dependent drug efflux system, has been a paradigm for other efflux systems which have subsequently been described in our and other laboratories (4–6). A second mechanism for tetracycline resistance involves ribosomal protection, initially described by Vickers Burdett (7). These two kinds of mechanisms, embodied in almost twenty related but distinguishable determinants, represent the mechanistic approach to tetracycline resistance found in all resistant organisms (Table 2).

The tetracyclines are broad spectrum antibiotic agents discovered in 1948 which bind to the ribosome and inhibit protein synthesis. There are a number of tetracyclines currently in use, all introduced more than 20 years ago (Table 3). Their efficacy is currently limited to a few bacterial infections since most of the previous target organisms have emerged with resistance. Clinical uses, originally up to dozens of organisms, are now limited to largely the rickettsia, lyme disease, chlamydia and bacteria associated with acne.

Early studies in our laboratory examined the uptake of tetracyclines into resistant and susceptible bacteria. Of importance, using purified radioactively-labeled tetracycline, we saw a clear distinction in tetracycline accumulation between isogenic susceptible and resistant *E. coli*. The susceptible strain accumulated many-fold more drug than the resistant cell when energy was supplied, whereas both susceptible and resistant cells took up the same amount of drug when energy-depleted (3). These findings suggested that tetracycline was being actively extruded from the cell (Fig. 2).

With the development of an everted membrane vesicle assay, based on studies of calcium efflux by Barry Rosen (8), we could demonstrate an active efflux of tetracycline unequivocally (3). This was, in fact, the first demonstration of active efflux as a mechanism of resistance for a chemotherapeutic agent. With an energy source, the everted membrane vesicles actively took up the drug, whereas in the presence of inhibitors, or in the absence of energy, they did not. If an inhibitor were introduced during the assay, the drug came streaming out of the everted vesicles, proving that it was still in a soluble form, and not forming an insoluble precipitate (Fig. 3).

Tetracycline transport into the everted vesicles required energy. Studies in this laboratory (3), and in greater detail by Akihito Yamaguchi and his group (9, 10), have shown that this transport is magnesium dependent, and that it is, in fact, a tetracycline-magne-

Table 3. The tetracycline family of antibiotics

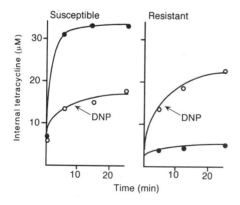

Compound	R_5	R_6a	R_6b	R_7
Chlortetracycline	H	CH_3	OH	Cl
Oxytetracycline	OH	CH_3	OH	H
Tetracycline	H	CH_3	OH	H
Demeclocycline	H	H	OH	Cl
Methacycline	OH	$=CH_2$	—	H
Doxycycline	OH	CH_3	H	H
Minocycline	H	H	H	$N(CH_3)_2$

sium complex (10) which is exchanged for a proton in what is an electroneutral exchange utilizing a pH gradient.

The prototype for the tetracycline efflux system studied in this laboratory has been that specified by transposon 10. Using *E. coli* minicells, we were able to identify the protein in the cell membrance, and called it Tet protein (11). The gene sequence revealed a protein structure of two domains separated by a large cytoplasmic loop. These domains, designated the alpha and beta domains, are both required for resistance and efflux. Previous studies showed that a single site mutation in either domain caused a loss of antibiotic resistance and of efflux. However, placing two polypeptides, each bearing a single mutation in either the alpha or beta domain, in the same cell allowed for an inter-complementation and restoration of at least part of the resistance phenotype and the efflux system (12, 13). These studies demonstrated an interaction between the alpha and beta domains. In subsequent studies, fusions of the alpha and beta domains of two similar and two distinct classes of tetracycline resistance determinants, those for classes A and C which are 78% identical, and B and C which are 45% identical, were prepared in order to help define domain function (14). Only those hybrids made from the Class A-Class C combination

Figure 2. Tetracycline accumulation by resistant and susceptible *E. coli* cells. Radioactively-labeled tetracycline was provided to *E. coli* with or without plasmid R222 bearing the tetracycline resistance determinant on transposon Tn*10*. In the presence of an energy source (glucose), the susceptible cell accumulated tetracycline above that which diffuses into the de-energized cell (+1 mM DNP). In contrast, the resistant cell, when incubated with glucose, kept the tetracycline out. (Adapted from ref. 3.)

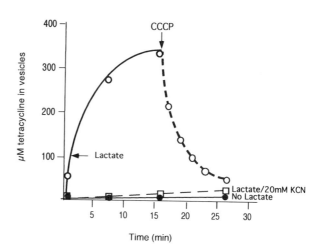

Figure 3. Tetracycline uptake by everted membrane vesicles. Everted vesicles were prepared from the *E. coli* ML308-225 strain bearing plasmid R222. Vesicles were incubated with radioactively labeled tetracycline in the presence of energy (lactate, open circles) or in the absence of energy (no lactate or lactate + 20 mM cyanide). Only vesicles energized by lactate accumulated tetracycline, which was released from the cells when the vesicles were treated with carbonyl cyanide *m*-chlorophenyl hydrazone (CCCP, 100 μM).

produced a resistance phenotype; it was intermediate between that of the two determinants alone (14). The Class B-Class C hybrids were inactive (Table 4). The conclusion from these studies was that there was an essential interaction between alpha and beta domains, and that these domains had evolved together to form the different efflux-mediated resistance determinants (see Table 2).

In complementary studies to understand and eventually crystallize this protein, we undertook a number of different ways to purify it to homogeneity. Initial studies used a beta-galactosidase fusion which allowed the purification of the protein, however in an inactive, denatured state (15). The purified Tet protein was used to produce antibodies against the protein which have been useful in ongoing studies today. Later attempts tried fusions to glutathione transferase and maltose binding protein, but without much success. More recently a polyhistidine fusion brought success. With the latter method, rapid purification of the protein in a native state was attained in a dodecymaltoside detergent (16). The purified Tet-his protein had the appropriate CD-spectrum analysis for a largely alpha-helical structure and appeared to bind tetracycline in the detergent (16). More recent reconstitution studies from this laboratory (17) and those of Yamaguchi (18) have shown that the protein by itself in a native state can transport tetracycline into proteoliposomes.

An important characteristic that we wished to examine was the association of the two domains of the protein and the possibility that the protein acted as a dimer in its transport of tetracycline. This idea came from the genetic complementation studies using mu-

Table 4. Effect of domain switching on tetracycline resistance

Tet protein	Tetracycline MIC (μg/ml)*
Tet A	182
Tet B	150
Tet C	54
Tet A/C	99
Tet B/C	1.5
Tet C/B	3.1
Tet B/C + Tet C/B	18

*Derivatives of *E. coli* BC32 tested by gradient plate method (14).

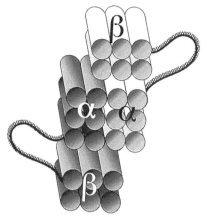

Figure 4. Proposed model for the Tet protein dimer in the membrane of the bacterial cell. This model is based on an α-α domain binding revealed by biochemical studies and an α-β interaction suggested by genetic studies.

tants of the Class B determinant (12, 13) and from studies of hybrid Tet protein described above (14). In fact, by binding Tet protein through a polyhistidine tail to a nickel column, we could show that there was a binding between the alpha domains of two polypeptides (19). Although the genetic data supported an alpha-beta interaction, such an interaction at the level of binding in these experiments was not detected. Thus this implied association was not discernible under the conditions used. Still, the data allowed a model which put the alpha domains of two proteins together, with each touching a beta domain (Fig. 4).

In an attempt to restore tetracycline efficacy, we proposed to develop tetracyclines which could block the tetracycline efflux protein and thereby let tetracycline enter the cell and reach its target, the ribosome. A group of tetracycline-like molecules were obtained commercially or from pharmaceutical companies; others were synthesized. In the everted membrane assay, those drugs which interfered with tetracycline transport were considered potential blockers of the efflux protein. As a control for this assay, we showed that the successful blockers did not interfere with the integrity of the energized vesicle using acridine orange (20) as a fluorescence monitor. Such a control was included to rule out the possibility that the compound's effect on tetracycline transport was not because it destroyed the proton-motive force across the membrane.

Through the tetracycline efflux blocker assay, a large group of compounds with inhibitory activity were identified (20, 21). Of these were those with substitutions at the C13 of ring C of methacycline, and substitutions at C5, in ring B of doxycycline or methacycline. By examining a large number of derivatives at the C13 position, a correlation could be made between the size and hydrophobicity of the constituent at the C13 position, which would be a preferred substituent for blocking of the efflux protein. These blocking studies revealed a hypothetical hydrophobic pocket in Tet protein with particular length and width dimensions and a corresponding lipopholicity which were involved in tetracycline's binding to the protein (Fig. 5).

The compounds were then tested against whole cells of *E. coli, Staphylococcus aureus* and *Enterococcus faecalis* bearing different tetracycline efflux determinants. In order to determine whether the approach could be extended to the other mechanism of resistance, namely that of ribosomal protection, we tested as well an enterococcus bearing the Class M ribosomal protection mechanism. These studies, with prototype blocking agents of the C13 class, and more recently the C5 class (unpublished), demonstrated that the drug not only worked as an everted vesicle blocker, but also in whole cells creating a synergistic inhibitory activity with doxycycline or tetracycline (Fig. 6).

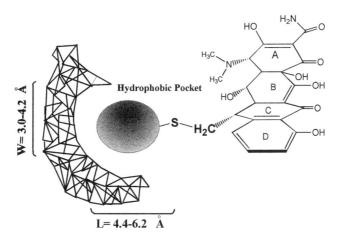

Figure 5. The putative hydrophobic drug pocket in Tet protein. By a series of chemical syntheses involving changes at the C13 site in methacycline, the length and width parameters of a hypothetical hydrophobic pocket in the Tet protein was revealed (20, 21).

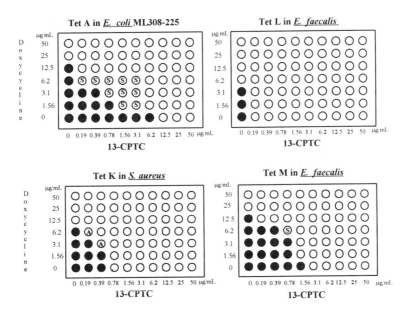

Figure 6. Susceptibility of bacteria bearing different tetracycline resistance determinants to the C13 analog 13-cyclopentyl tetracycline (13-CPTC). Drugs were tested alone and together in order to identify a synergistic effect (marked S) for those determinants in which the blocking agent 13-CPTC interfered with the function of the resistance mechanism and allowed doxycycline to inhibit cell growth. Synergy was noted in *E. coli* bearing the Class A efflux protein or *E. faecalis* bearing the Class M ribosomal protection mechanism. The drug alone was effective against *E. faecalis* bearing the TetL efflux protein. An additive effect (A) was noted for *S. aureus* bearing TetK.

Work along these lines continues with the identification of other resistance blocking agents which increased activities, some of which appear to have activity on their own.

As resistance to antibiotics mounts, the need for new antimicrobials is essential. While the identification of structurally novel compounds is certainly one route to answering the problem, the restoration of older, very successful drugs, such as we are doing with the tetracyclines, provides another approach and could lead to a needed renaissance of a family of antimicrobial agents which the practicing clinician knows well. The efficacy of the anti-resistance approach has precedence in the success of compounds like clavulanic acid which blocks beta-lactamases and allow earlier beta-lactam antibiotics to be effective, e.g., the combination of clavulanic acid with amoxycillin. Our studies demonstrate that resistance mediated by a membrane efflux protein or a ribosomal protection protein can also be successfully approached in this way with the potential of returning efficacy to an important class of clinical therapeutic agents.

ACKNOWLEDGMENTS

The work described was supported in part by grants from the National Institutes of Health and through Tufts University School of Medicine.

REFERENCES

1. S.B. Levy, The Challenge of Antibiotic Resistance, *Scientific American* 278:32–39 (1998).
2. S. B. Levy. *The Antibiotic Paradox: How Miracle Drugs Are Destroying the Miracle*, Plenum, New York (1992).
3. L.M.McMurry, R. Petrucci and S.B. Levy, Active efflux of tetracycline encoded by four genetically different tetracycline resistance determinants in *E. coli. Proc. Natl. Acad. Sci. USA* 77:3974–3977 (1980).
4. S.P. Cohen, D.C. Hooper, J.S. Wolfson, K.S. Souza, L.M. McMurry, and S.B. Levy, Endogenous active efflux of norfloxacin in susceptible *Escherichia coli. Antimicrob. Agents Chemother.* 32:1187–1191 (1988) .
5. S.B. Levy, Active efflux mechanisms for antimicrobial resistance. *Antimicrob. Agents Chemother.* 36:695–703 (1992).
6. H. Nikaido, Prevention of drug access to bacterial targets: permeability barriers and active efflux, *Science* 264:382–388 (1994).
7. V. Burdett, Streptococcal tetracycline resistance mediated at the level of protein synthesis, *J. Bact.* 165:564–569 (1986).
8. B.P. Rosen and J.S. McClees, Active transport of calcium in inverted membrane vesicles of *Escherichia coli. Proc. Natl. Acad. Sci. USA* 71:5042–5046 (1974).
9. M.A. Kaneko, Yamaguchi and T. Sawai, Energetics of tetracycline efflux system encoded by Tn10 in *Escherichia coli. FEBS Letters* 193:194–197 (1985).
10. A. Yamaguchi, T. Udagawa and T. Sawai, Transport of divalent cations with tetracycline as mediated by the transposon Tn10-encoded tetracycline resistance protein, *J. Biol. Chem.* 265:4809–4813 (1990).
11. S.B. Levy and L. McMurry, Detection of an inducible membrane protein associated with R-factor-mediated tetracycline resistance, *Biochem. Biophys. Res. Comm.* 56:1060–1068 (1974).
12. M.S. Curiale and S.B. Levy, Two complementation groups mediate tetracycline resistance determined by Tn*10. J. Bacteriol.* 151:209–215 (1982).
13. M.S. Curiale, L.M. McMurry and S.B. Levy, Intracistronic complementation of the tetracycline resistance membrane protein specified by Tn*10. J. Bacteriol.* 157:211–217 (1984).
14. R.A. Rubin and S.B. Levy, Interdomain hybrid Tet proteins confer tetracycline resistance only when derived from more closely related members of the *tet* gene family. *J. Bacteriol.* 172:2303–2312 (1990).
15. R.K. Hickman, L. M. McMurry and S. B. Levy, Overproduction and purification of the Tn*10*-specified inner membrane tetracycline resistance protein Tet using fusions to β-galactosidase, *Molec. Microbiol.* 4:1241–1251 (1990).

16. M.L. Aldema, L.M. McMurry, A.R. Walmsley and S.B. Levy, Purification of the Tn*10*-specified tetracycline efflux antiporter TetA in a native state as a polyhistidine fusion protein, *Molec. Microb.* 19:187–195 (1996).

17. C. Saraceni-Richards and S.B. Levy, *unpublished.*

18. Y. Someya, Y. Moriyama, M. Futai, T. Sawai and A. Yamaguchi, Reconstitution of the metal-tetracycline/H$^+$ antiporter of *Escherichia coli* in proteoliposomes including F_0F_1-ATPase, *FEBS Letters* 374:72–76 (1995).

19. L.M. McMurry and S.B. Levy, The N-terminal half of the Tn*10*-encoded tetracycline efflux protein TetA contains a functional dimerization domain, *J. Biol. Chem.* 276:22752–22757 (1995).

20. M.L. Nelson, B.H. Park, J.S. Andrews, V.A. Georgian, R.C. Thomas and S.B. Levy, Inhibition of the tetracycline efflux antiport protein by 13-thio-substituted 5-hydroxy-6-deoxy tetracyclines, *J. Med. Chem.* 36:370–377 (1993).

21. M.L. Nelson, B.H. Park and S.B. Levy, Molecular requirements for the inhibition of the tetracycline antiport protein and the effect of potent inhibitors on growth of tetracycline resistant bacteria, *J. Med. Chem.* 37:1355–1361 (1994).

AMINOGLYCOSIDE ANTIBIOTICS

Structures, Functions, and Resistance

Gerard D. Wright,[1] Albert M. Berghuis,[1] and Shahriar Mobashery[2]

[1]Department of Biochemistry
McMaster University
Hamilton, Ontario, Canada, L8N 3Z5
[2]Department of Chemistry
Wayne State University
Detroit, Michigan 48202

AMINOGLYCOSIDE DISCOVERY AND STRUCTURES

The aminoglycoside-aminocyclitol antibiotics (hereafter termed aminoglycosides) are a large family of water soluble, cationic molecules which exhibit broad antimicrobial spectra. While the moniker aminoglycoside refers to a vast array of structurally diverse compounds, they all share the incorporation of a six-membered aminocyclitol ring (Fig. 1). The aminoglycosides find use in the treatment of many bacterial infections caused by both Gram-positive and Gram-negative organisms, and are generally administered by injection or intravenously as a result of their relatively poor oral absorption (Edson and Terrell, 1991). Despite some problems of toxicity and bacterial resistance (described in detail below), these antibiotics continue to be a critically important component of our modern antimicrobial arsenal.

The discovery of the first two aminoglycoside antibiotics, streptomycin in 1944 (Schatz et al., 1944) and neomycin in 1949 (Waksman and Lechevalier, 1949), by Selman Waksman (for which he was awarded the Nobel Prize in Physiology and Medicine in 1952) presaged the identification and characterization of a series of clinically useful aminoglycosides over the next 40 years (Table 1). The importance of these initial findings was immediately apparent and its use in the treatment of tuberculosis was reported within one year of the discovery of streptomycin (Hinshaw and Feldman, 1945), and it remains a key component of modern anti-mycobacterial therapy (Musser, 1995).

Aminoglycosides fall into two general structural classes: those that incorporate a 2-deoxystreptamine ring, and those that do not (Table 2). The first group can be subdivided

Resolving the Antibiotic Paradox, edited by Rosen and Mobashery.
Kluwer Academic / Plenum Publishers, New York, 1998.

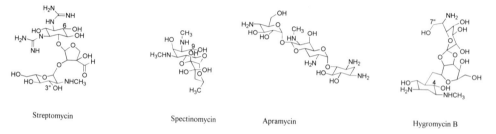

Antibiotic	R_1	R_2	R_3	R_4	R_5	R_6	R_7
Neomycin B	NH_2	OH	H		H	CH_2NH_2	H
Neomycin C	NH_2	OH	H		H	CH_2NH_2	H
Paromomycin	OH	OH	H		H	CH_2NH_2	H
Lividomycin A	OH	H	H		H	CH_2NH_2	mannose
Lividomycin B	OH	H	H		H	CH_2NH_2	H
Ribostamycin	NH_2	OH	H	H			
Butirosin	NH_2	OH		H			

Antibiotic	R_1	R_2	R_3	R_4	R_5	R_6	R_7	R_8	R_9	R_{10}
Kanamycin A	H	NH_2	OH	OH	OH	H	H	H	OH	CH_2OH
Kanamycin B	H	NH_2	OH	OH	NH_2	H	H	H	OH	CH_2OH
Tobramycin	H	NH_2	H	OH	NH_2	H	H	H	OH	CH_2OH
Dibekacin	H	NH_2	H	H	NH_2	H	H	H	OH	CH_2OH
Arbekacin	H	NH_2	H	H	NH_2		H	H	OH	CH_2OH
Amikacin	H	NH_2	OH	OH	OH		H	H	OH	CH_2OH
Gentamicin B	H	NH_2	OH	OH	OH	H	CH_3	OH	CH_3	H
Isepamicin	H	NH_2	OH	OH	OH		CH_3	OH	CH_3	H
Gentamicin C1	CH_3	$NHCH_3$	H	H	NH_2	H	CH_3	OH	CH_3	H
Gentamicin C1a	H	NH_2	H	H	NH_2	H	CH_3	OH	CH_3	H
Gentamicin C2	CH_3	NH_2	H	H	NH_2	H	CH_3	OH	CH_3	H
G418	CH_3	OH	OH	OH	NH_2	H	CH_3	OH	CH_3	H
Sisomicin*	H	NH_2	H	H	NH_2	H	CH_3	OH	CH_3	H
Netilmcin*	H	NH_2	H	H	NH_2	CH_2CH_3	CH_3	OH	CH_3	H

* Unsaturation in the 6-aminoglucose ring ($\Delta5'$-4')

Streptomycin   Spectinomycin   Apramycin   Hygromycin B

Figure 1. Structures of aminoglycoside antibiotics. Numbers indicate sites of common enzymatic modification.

Table 1. Aminoglycoside antibiotics and their sources

Aminoglycoside	Source	Reference
Streptomycin	*Streptomyces griseus*	(Schatz et al., 1944)
Spectinomycin	*Streptomyces spectabilis*	(Mason et al., 1961)
Neomycin	*Streptomyces fradiae*	(Waksman and Lechevalier, 1949)
Kanamycin	*Streptomyces kanamyceticus*	(Umezawa et al., 1957)
Gentamicin[1]	*Micromonospora purpurea*	(Weinstein et al., 1963)
Tobramycin	*Streptomyces tenebrarius*	(Higgins and Kastners, 1967)
Ribostamycin	*Streptomyces ribosidificus*	(Shomura et al., 1970)
Butirosin	*Bacillus circulans*	(Woo et al., 1971)
Sisomicin	*Micromonospora inyoesis*	(Weinstein et al., 1970)
Amikacin	Semisynthetic derivative of kanamycin B	(Kawaguchi et al., 1972)
Netilmicin	Semisynthetic derivative of sisomicin	(Kabins et al., 1976)
Isepamicin	Semisynthetic derivative of gentamicin B	(Nagabhushan et al., 1978)

[1]Convention has the suffix 'mycin' given to compounds derived from *Streptomyces* while the suffix 'micin' refers to compounds derived from other organisms.

into compounds derivatized at positions 4 and 5, or at positions 4 and 6 of the 2-deoxystreptamine ring(Fig. 1). Convention has the numbering of the 6-aminohexose ring linked to position 4 of the 2-deoxystreptamine designated by prime (') and the hexose or pentose ring linked to position 5 or 6, designated double prime ("). Many of these compounds are natural products produced primarily by bacteria of the group actinomycetes, but several are semisynthetic derivatives of naturally occurring compounds (Table 1, Fig. 1). There are no compounds in current clinical use which are derived from total synthesis.

Aminoglycosides are primarily used for the treatment of Gram-negative and Gram-positive bacterial infections, but some also find use in the treatment of amaeboid or protozoal infections (Berman and Fleckenstein, 1991); e.g., paromomycin for treatment of *Cryptosporidium parvum* infections (Fichtenbaum et al., 1994). Aminoglycosides have been used in other contexts as well. They have been shown to inhibit HIV-1 production by blocking the binding of the viral regulatory protein Rev to its response element (Wang et al., 1997; Werstuck et al., 1996; Zapp et al., 1993). In addition, aminoglycoside resistance genes are also extensively used as genetic markers for eukaryotic and prokaryotic molecular biology. For example, the use of the *neo* resistance cassette confers resistance to the aminoglycoside G-418, which is toxic to mammalian and bacterial cells.

Table 2. Representative aminoglycoside antibiotics

2-Deoxystreptamine aminoglycosides		Other aminoglycosides
4,5-disubstituted	4,6-disubstituted	
Neomycin	Kanamycin	Streptomycin
Ribostamycin	Amikacin	Spectinomycin
Butirosin	Gentamicin	Hygromycin
Lividomycin	Isepamicin	Apramycin
Paromomycin	Tobramycin	Fortimicin
	Netilmicin	
	Sisomicin	
	Dibekacin	

MODE OF ACTION OF AMINOGLYCOSIDE ANTIBIOTICS

One of the major benefits of the aminoglycosides is that with only a few exceptions such as spectinomycin, which is bacteriostatic, these antibiotics are bactericidal agents. The primary target for aminoglycosides appears to be the ribosome, as point mutations in ribosomal proteins and ribosomal RNA (rRNA), as well as methylation of specific bases of rRNA can confer high-level antibiotic resistance. Chemical footprinting studies have revealed that most aminoglycosides bind to the tRNA binding (A-site) region of the 16S rRNA of the 30S ribosomal subunit, but different bases are protected in the presence of different aminoglycosides (Moazed and Noller, 1987; Woodcock et al., 1991). Thus neomycin, paromomycin, gentamicin and kanamycin all protect A1408 and G1494 (*Escherichia coli* 16S rRNA numbering), and spectinomycin protects C1063 and G1064. In contrast, the non-A site directed compound streptomycin, strongly protects A913, A914 and A915.

The NMR structure of paromomycin bound to a 27-nucleotide portion of the 16S rRNA encompassing the conserved A site internal loop region, has recently been reported (Fig. 2; Fourmy et al., 1996). The antibiotic binds within the major grove and makes many contacts to the RNA, either through direct hydrogen bonds, or via intermediary water molecules. In particular, N7 of G1494 binds to the C3 amino group of the 2-deoxystreptamine ring, a common site of acetylation which results in aminoglycoside resistance (*vide infra*). Other common sites of aminoglycoside modification conferring antibiotic resistance e.g. 3'-OH and 6'-OH (which is often an amino group in other aminoglycosides), also make contacts with backbone phosphates of the rRNA.

While it is clear that aminoglycoside affinity for the ribosome is key to antibiotic action, the elucidation of the precise mechanism of cell death has been elusive. Aminoglycoside binding to ribosomes appears to be reversible, with dissociation constants in the µM-nM range, which would seemingly suggest the likelihood of a bacteriostatic effect. A key element in this process is the uptake of antibiotic into the cell. Aminoglycosides gain entry into the bacterial cell in a multiphasic fashion (reviewed in Davis, 1987; Hancock, 1981; Taber et al., 1987). The first step is energy independent and involves initial passage through the outer membrane and periplasmic space in Gram-negative organisms, and the cell wall assembly in Gram-positives, which is followed by binding of the cationic aminoglycoside to the exterior of the cell membrane by electrostatic interactions. An energy-dependent phase (EDP-I) then ensues, in which the positively charged molecules gain entry to the cytosol. A protein mediator for this process has remained elusive, though recent

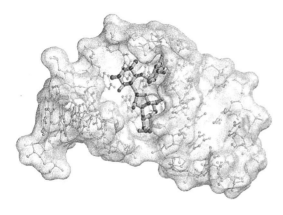

Figure 2. NMR structure of paromomycin bound to a 27-nucleotide portion of the 16S rRNA (Fourmy et al., 1996) (PDB code 1PBR).

work indicates that a single 47 kDa integral inner-membrane protein in *E. coli* binds with high affinity to aminoglycosides, and may prove to be the transporter protein for these antibacterial agents (Roestamadji and Mobashery; unpublished results). The process of import of the aminoglycoside into the cell requires energy derived from the transmembrane electrical potential ($\Delta\psi$) established by the bacterial electron transport system (Bryan and Kwan, 1983; Bryan and Van Den Elzen, 1977; Gilman and Saunders, 1986). Sensitivity of EDP-I to inhibitors of electron transport such as CN⁻, carbonyl cyanide-*m*-chlorophenyl-hydrazone (CCCP) and anaerobiosis, provide evidence for the requirement of a threshold $\Delta\psi$. This initial process results in modest uptake of the aminoglycoside in the cell. The next step, EDP-II, is rapid and also energy-dependent. This step may occur after aminoglycosides have bound initially to some sensitive ribosomes and accounts for the bulk of the *irreversible* accumulation of antibiotic in the bacterial cells prior to cell death. The entry of large concentrations of aminoglycoside into the cell has pleiotropic effects. These include mistranslation of mRNA to yield aberrant proteins (Gorini, 1974; Lando et al., 1973), depletion of polyribosomes (Luzzatto et al., 1969), loss of cell membrane integrity resulting in increased permeability and efflux of ions such as K^+ (Busse et al., 1992; Dubin and Davis, 1961; Hancock, 1961), inhibition of DNA replication (Tanaka et al., 1984), and blockade of the initiation of DNA replication by disruption of *oriC*-membrane interaction (Matsunaga et al., 1986).

Davis has shown that misread proteins can target the cell membrane (Davis et al., 1986) which lead him to propose a unifying theory for the bactericidal action of aminoglycosides (Davis, 1987; Fig. 3). This proposal suggests that a small amount of aminoglycoside antibiotic penetrates the cell during EDP-I and the initial phase of EDP-II and binds to susceptible ribosomes, which results in the misreading of mRNA and the formation of misfolded, non-functional proteins. These proteins can interact with the membrane resulting in loss of membrane integrity causing ion efflux and the formation of pores precipitating additional irreversible influx of antibiotic which saturates all ribosomes in an irreversible fashion, resulting in cell death.

Support for concentration-dependent interactions between ribosomes and aminoglycosides comes from titration of ribosomes with aminoglycosides (Le Goffic et al., 1979) and by photoaffinity labeling of *Escherichia coli* 70S ribosomes with an [³H]-azidobenzyl derivative of tobramycin (Tangy et al., 1983). The latter experiments showed labeling primarily of ribosomal proteins, principally L6, S4 and S5, rather than rRNA. At high concentrations of label (20 µM), such as those expected in EDP-II, mRNA misreading is prevalent and virtually all ribosomal proteins were labeled indicating a major, and possibly catastrophic, infiltration of the antibiotic into the ribosomal structure. In addition, Busse and colleagues have suggested that for bactericidal aminoglycoside antibiotics, the degradation products of the misfolded proteins can sequester aminoglycoside molecules within the cell, thus accounting for their irreversible uptake (Busse et al., 1992). Bacteriostatic aminoglycosides do not result in misreading of mRNA and thus do not cause membrane damage (Bakker, 1992).

While it is clear that a precise model which adequately reflects all the experimentally determined effects of aminoglycosides remains elusive, we can nevertheless say that the ribosome is the primary target for aminoglycoside antibiotics and that membrane damage appears to play a role, probably a central one, in cell death. Paradoxically, one report has shown that gentamicin covalently linked to bovine serum albumin, and thus incapable of penetrating the cell, exhibits protein synthesis inhibition, membrane damage, and bactericidal activities in *Pseudomonas aeruginosa* (Kadurugamuwa et al., 1993). Reconciliation

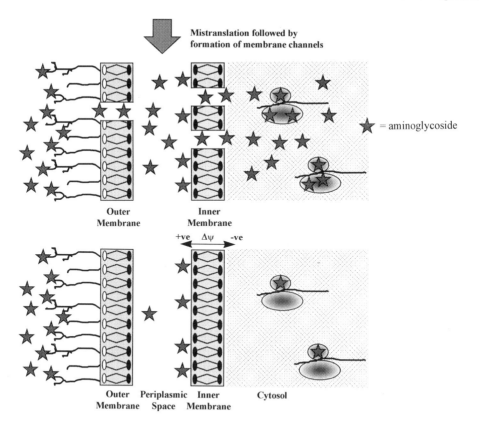

Figure 3.   Model for entry and bactericidal action of aminoglycoside antibiotics in Gram-negative bacterial cells.

of these results with the proposed models for aminoglycoside action is not straightforward and points to a need for additional research in this area.

AMINOGLYCOSIDE RESISTANCE

Resistance to aminoglycosides, like other antibiotics, can be intrinsic or acquired. Of these mechanisms of resistance, two general classes emerge, enzymatic and non-enzymatic. The latter are exclusively intrinsic in nature and, with the exception of a few cases such as streptomycin resistance in *Mycobacterium tuberculosis*, do not play a significant role in clinical resistance. On the other hand, enzymatic resistance, which is generally but not exclusively acquired, is the most prevalent means of aminoglycoside resistance in the clinic. The following sections detail the current knowledge of aminoglycoside resistance mechanisms.

Non-Enzymatic Resistance

As noted above, aminoglycoside entry into the bacterial cell requires an intact electron transport chain to establish a sufficient $\Delta\psi$ for antibiotic transport to occur, thus anaerobic bacteria are in essence intrinsically resistant to aminoglycosides (reviewed in Bryan, 1984; Schlessinger, 1988). Mutations which affect $\Delta\psi$ are also known to result in

Table 3. Aminoglycoside resistance by rRNA methylases

Organism	Gene	Reference
Micromonospora purpurea,		
Micromonospora rosea	*grm*	(Kelemen et al., 1991)
Micromonospora zionensis	*sgm*	(Kojic et al., 1992)
Micromonospora olivasterospora	*fmrO*	(Ohta and Hasegawa, 1993b)
Streptomyces tenjimariensis	*kamA (fmrT)*	(Ohta and Hasegawa, 1993a)
Streptomyces tenebrarius	*kamB*	(Skeggs et al., 1987)
Saccharopolyspora hirsuta	*kamC*	(Holmes et al., 1991)
Streptomyces tenebrarius	*kgmB*	(Holmes and Cundliffe, 1991)

aminoglycoside resistance (Miller et al., 1980), and an ATP synthase γ-subunit mutant which shows broad aminoglycoside resistance, may also fall into this category (Humbert and Altendorf, 1989). Another mechanism of aminoglycoside resistance by altered uptake of the drug is operational in some strains of *P. aeruginosa*, where overexpression of OprH saturates the aminoglycoside binding sites on the outer membrane lipopolysaccharide thus preventing the initial energy-independent phase of drug uptake (Young et al., 1992).

Point mutations in rRNA can also confer drug resistance, thus mutation of C1192 of the 16S rRNA results in spectinomycin resistance in *E. coli* (Sigmund et al., 1984). Streptomycin is a first line drug for the treatment of *M. tuberculosis* infection and in this organism, clinical resistance to the aminoglycoside is conferred exclusively by point mutations in the 16S rRNA and ribosomal protein S12 (reviewed in Musser, 1995).

Enzymatic Resistance: Ribosomal Modification

Target alteration is a common strategy for resistance to antibiotics. For example, resistance to thiostrepton, macrolide, lincosamide, and streptogramin antibiotics is frequently the result of methylation of specific bases of rRNA (Cundliffe, 1987; Leclercq and Courvalin, 1991). In many aminoglycoside producing organisms, methylation of the 16S rRNA provides high-level resistance to the antibiotics (Beauclerk and Cundliffe, 1987; Matkovic et al., 1984; Thompson et al., 1985) (Table 3). Methylation occurs at N7 of guanine and is S-adenosylmethionine dependent. This target modification results in high-level resistance to aminoglycosides (MIC > 500 μg/mL), yet unlike the *erm* genes which methylate the 23S rRNA and confer macrolide, lincosamide and streptogramin resistance, the 16S rRNA methylases have not been identified in aminoglycoside resistant clinical isolates thus far, and detailed analysis of the structures and mechanisms of these enzymes is lacking.

Enzymatic Resistance: Aminoglycoside Modification

Three distinct mechanisms of covalent modification of aminoglycosides have been observed: *O*-nucleotidyltransfer, *N*-acetyltransfer and *O*-phosphoryltransfer. These reactions are catalyzed by discrete classes of enzymes and are by far the most prevalent and clinically relevant mode of aminoglycoside resistance. The modified aminoglycosides have reduced predilection for the high-affinity sites on the bacterial ribosome, which results in a drug resistance phenotype. The enzyme and gene nomenclature presently used to describe aminoglycoside resistance was largely defined in an excellent review by Shaw and colleagues, which presented a thorough description of the genes identified in each class (Shaw et al., 1993). First, each enzyme is designated by class: ANT for nucleotidyl-transferases, AAC for acetyltransferases, and APH for phosphotransferases. The class is followed by a number in parentheses which describes the regiospecificity of group transfer and this is followed by a roman numeral designating a unique aminoglycoside resistance profile. Distinct genes which confer identical resistance phenotypes are further designated by a lower case letter. For example, *ant(6)-Ia* encodes a streptomycin nucleotidyltransferase which modifies position 6 of the drug; *aac(6')-Ic* encodes an acetyltransferase which modifies aminoglycosides at position 6', and has the same resistance profile as *aac(6')-Ia* or *aac(6')-Ib*, but is a unique protein.

The second-substrate requirements of all these enzymes, either ATP or acetyl-CoA, necessitate intracellular localization, and there is no compelling evidence for periplasmic localization of the enzymes in Gram-negative organisms. All these enzymes would appear therefore to be cytosolic.

The aminoglycoside resistance genes are generally found on mobile genetic elements such as transposons and plasmids, but some are chromosomal in origin. The genes found in clinically important Gram-negative organisms tend to be more diverse, while in Gram-positives, resistance is generally limited to *aac(6')-aph(2")* (Gent^R), encoding a unique bifunctional resistance enzyme, *aph(3')-IIIa* (Kan^R), and *ant(6)* (Strep^R). A recent survey of resistance patterns has shown that the usage of aminoglycosides in clinical settings over the past several years has resulted in a change in the prevalence of resistance mechanisms (Miller et al., 1997). The previously high prevalence of *ant(2")* (Gent^R, Tobr^R) in Gram-negative organisms has now given way to a more complex pattern in which *aac(6')-I* genes are combined with other resistance determinants such as *aac(3)* and *ant(2")* as a result of the introduction of newer aminoglycosides such as netlimicin. Thus the clinical use of aminoglycosides is under constant pressure from an evolving response by target organisms.

Aminoglycoside Nucleotidyltransferases (ANT)

Several *ant* genes have been cloned which confer resistance to a broad spectrum of aminoglycosides (Table 4). The enzymes catalyze the reaction:

$$NTP + aminoglycoside \rightarrow PPi + NMP\text{-}aminoglycoside$$

The enzymes in essence activate the aminoglycoside for modification via the α-phosphoryl of a nucleotide monophosphate (NMP) with concomitant loss of pyrophosphate (PPi). Since ATP is the most prevalent nucleotide triphosphate (NTP) in the cell, these enzymes are no doubt in fact adenyltransferases. ANT(2") is very common in Gram-negative organisms and is a major cause of clinical drug resistance (Miller et al., 1997), however several other ANTs are known and have been cloned from a variety of organisms (Fig. 4).

Ant(6). The streptomycin modifying enzyme ANT(6) has been partially purified from *Bacillus subtilis* Marburg 168 where it is encoded by a chromosomal gene (Kono et al., 1987) and the structure and regiospecificity of the adenylated product unambiguously assigned by ^{1}H and ^{13}C NMR (O'hara et al., 1988). The 53% identical enzyme encoded by pJH1 in *Enterococcus faecalis* (Ounissi and Courvalin, 1987) has not been fully characterized, although the enzyme purified from an *E. coli* overexpression system was found to readily adenylate streptomycin (Michealis constant (K_m) 22 µM), but spectinomycin was neither a substrate nor an inhibitor (D. Daigle, S. Clugston, T. Clarke, & G. Wright, unpublished).

Table 4. Aminoglycoside nucleotidyltransferases

Enzyme	Profile	Source	Phenotype[1]	Reference
ANT(6)	Ia	*Enterococcus faecalis*	Strep	(Ounissi and Courvalin, 1987)
	Ib[2]	*Bacillus subtilis*		(Ohmiya et al., 1989)
ANT(9)	Ia	*Staphylococcus aureus*	Spec	(Murphy, 1985)
	Ib	*Enterococcus faecalis*		(LeBlanc et al., 1991)
ANT(4')	Ia	*Staphylococcus aureus*	Kan, Tob, Amik, Neo	(Matsumura et al., 1984)
ANT(2")	Ia	*Enterobacteriaceae*	Kan, Gent, Tob	(Lee et al., 1987)
ANT(3")	Ia	*Enterobacteriaceae*	Strep, Spec	(Hollingshead and Vapnek, 1985)

[1] List is not necessarily complete, only reported phenotype given
[2] Chromosomal gene.
Abbreviations: Kan, kanamycin; Amik, amikacin; Tob, tobramycin; Neo, neomycin; Strep, streptomycin; Spec, spectinomycin.

Ant(3") and Ant(9). ANT(3") is a 34.6-kDa enzyme encoded by a gene which is widely distributed among several enterobacterial transposons (Hollingshead and Vapnek, 1985). The enzyme is reported to modify streptomycin at position 3" and spectinomycin at position 9. Two enzymes with only spectinomycin modification capacity are also known in Gram-positive cocci, ANT(9)-Ia from *Staphylococcus aureus* (Murphy, 1985) and ANT(9)-Ib from *E. faecalis* (LeBlanc et al., 1991). The *S. aureus* gene encodes a protein with a molecular mass of 28.9 kDa and a predicted pI of 8.0, the only aminoglycoside resistance protein thus far reported with a positive charge at neutral pH (in contrast, ANT(9')-Ib and ANT(3") have respective predicted pIs of 6.2 and 4.8). Protein sequence alignment shows that the two ANT(9) enzymes from Gram-positive organisms are 36% identical (57 % similar) and that ANT(3") is 28% identical to ANT(9)-Ia and 23% identical to ANT(9)-Ib (51% and 45% similarity, respectively). The molecular basis for the difference in substrate specificity between these enzymes is unknown. We note that streptomycin is neither a substrate nor an inhibitor of the purified ANT(9)-Ia (D. Daigle, G. Wright, unpublished), thus despite the sequence homology with ANT(3"), the staphylococcal enzyme does not recognize streptomycin. ANT(3") has an N-terminal extension of roughly 45 amino acids when compared to the ANT(9) enzymes and this may contribute to the ability to adenylate streptomycin, but no supporting evidence is currently available.

Ant(2"). ANT(2") confers resistance to gentamicin C and is among the most highly prevalent aminoglycoside modifying determinants in the *Enterobacteriaceae* (Miller et al., 1997). The enzyme has been purified from an *E. coli* construct and studied in some detail by Northop and colleagues (Gates and Northrop, 1988a-c; Van Pelt and Northrop, 1984).

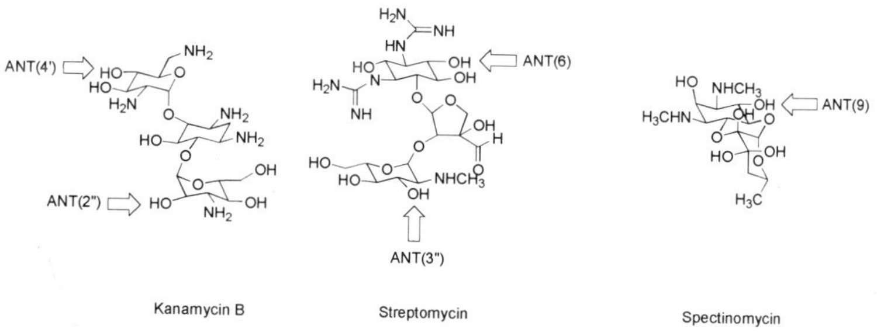

Figure 4. Regiospecificity of ANTs.

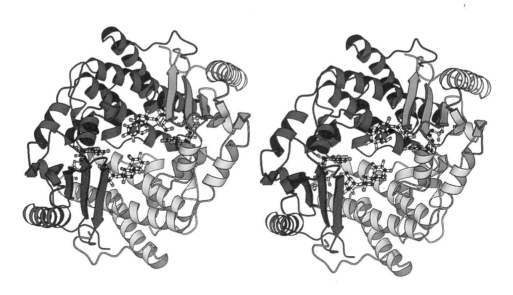

Figure 5.   Structure of ANT(4') dimer (Perdersen et al., 1995; PDB code 1KNY).

The 31.5-kDa enzyme shows a broad substrate specificity both for aminoglycosides and NTPs with K_m in the low to sub μM range (Gates and Northrop, 1988c). Steady-state kinetic measurements have revealed a Theorell-Chance kinetic mechanism, a special case of ordered BiBi where the reaction occurring in the ternary complex does not contribute to the overall rate of catalysis (Gates and Northrop, 1988a). In this case, Mg-ATP binds first followed by aminoglycoside. The release of adenylated aminoglycoside is rate-limiting and preceded by release of pyrophosphate (Gates and Northrop, 1988a,b). The regio- and stereochemistry of adenyltransfer have also been determined using (Sp)-[α-[17]O]dATP as substrate (Van Pelt et al., 1986,1990). The reaction occurs with inversion at the phosphoryl center, consistent with direct attack of the 2"-OH at the α-phosphate.

   Ant(4'). The three-dimensional structure of ANT(4') from *S. aureus* has been determined in the native state to 3.0 Å (Sakon et al., 1993), and bound to kanamycin and the non-hydrolyzable ATP analogue β-γ-methyleneadenosine 5'-triphosphate (AMPCPP) to 2.5 Å (Perdersen et al., 1995) (Fig. 5). The enzyme is a dimer with two distinct heterodimeric catalytic sites. One subunit provides the bulk of the ATP binding residues and the Mg^{2+} ligands and the other subunit provides Lys149 which contacts the α-phosphate, facilitating its transfer to the aminoglycoside. Both subunits contribute to aminoglycoside binding. Specifically, in the crystal structure, kanamycin forms hydrogen bonds to Glu67 from one subunit and Glu141 and Glu145 from the other subunit (Fig. 6). A further analysis of the aminoglycoside-binding pocket reveals that in addition to these negatively charged residues, several other acidic residues line the wall of the pocket (Glu67 from one subunit, and Asp95 and Glu142 from the other subunit). As a consequence, a highly negative patch is present on the surface of ANT(4'), which is undoubtedly responsible for attracting the positively charged aminoglycosides to its active site (Fig. 7).

   As noted above, the stereochemistry of phosphoryl transfer catalyzed by ANT(2") indicates an associative mechanism where the α-phosphate of ATP undergoes direct attack

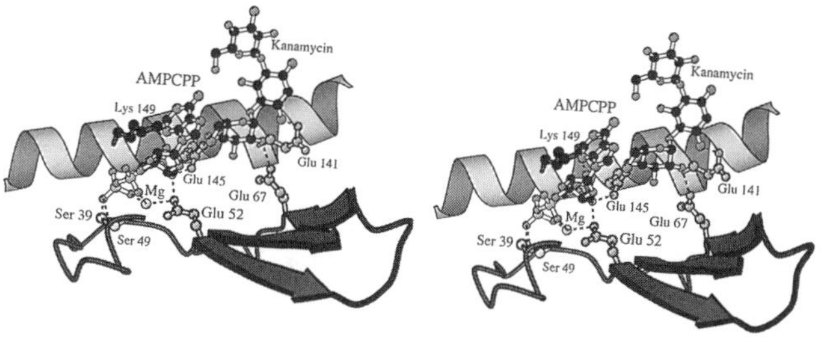

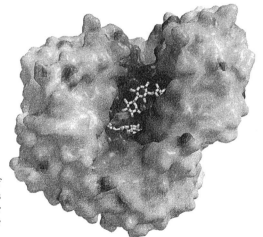

Figure 6. Close-up view of the active site of ANT(4'). Subunits I and II are colored dark and light gray, respectively.

by the nucleophilic hydroxyl group of the aminoglycoside. Based on this precedent, the molecular structure of the ANT(4') ternary complex has been analyzed. In the three-dimensional structure of the dead-end complex of ANT(4')•AMPCPP•kanamycin, kanamycin is positioned such that the 4'-OH approaches the α-phosphate of ATP in a direct line, though the nucleophilic hydroxyl is quite distant (5.0 Å) from the reactive phosphate (Perdersen et al., 1995). The view of the active site has permitted some speculation on the amino acid side chains which could contribute to adenyl transfer. With ATP sequestered in the subunit I binding site, Lys149 of subunit II is appropriately placed to polarize the α-phosphate, rendering it more electrophilic and thus aiding in catalysis by lowering the energy barrier. Glu145 of subunit II is positioned to act as a general base, deprotonating the 4'-OH and increasing its nucelophilicity (Fig. 8). These assignments need to be confirmed by additional studies including site-directed mutagenesis.

Figure 7. Negatively charged patch on the surface of ANT(4'). The surface of ANT(4')•AMPCPP dimer is shown with darker shading corresponding to greater negative charge. Also shown are the two positively charged kanamycin molecules bound to the enzyme.

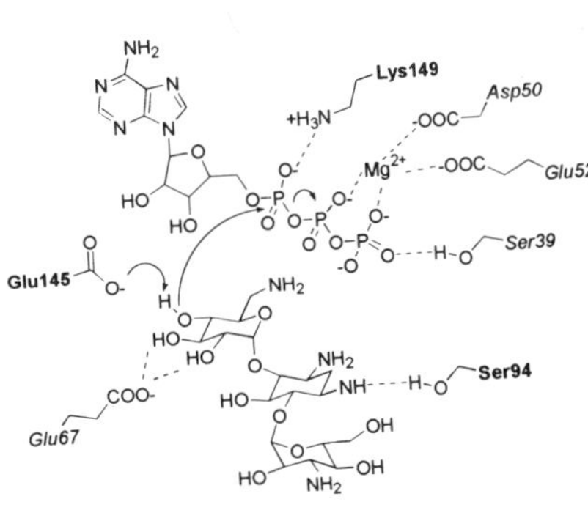

Figure 8. Proposed mechanism of the adenyl-transfer reaction catalyzed by ANT(4'). Amino acids contributed by the same subunit are differentiated by bold and italic lettering.

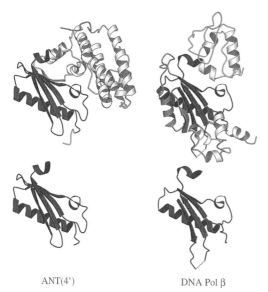

Figure 9. Comparison of ANT(4') and rat DNA polymerase β. Top left and right depicts the ANT(4') monomer and the 31-kD C-terminal domain of DNA polymerase (Sawaya et al., 1994; PDB code 1BPB), respectively. The homologous folding motif is colored in dark gray. The bottom figures highlight the homologous regions between ANT(4') and DNA polymerase β (Holm and Sander, 1995).

Holm and Sander have noted that part of the protein fold of ANT(4') is very similar to that of another NMP transferase, that for the rat DNA polymerase β (Holm and Sander, 1995; Fig. 9). Additionally, the sequence, GS(Xaa)10–12(DE)Xaa(DE) (where X is any amino acid), located in the N-terminus of ANT enzymes is conserved among a variety of NMP transferases (Holm and Sander, 1995). This sequence includes amino acids which are required for positioning of Mg^{2+}-ATP. The invariant Ser forms a hydrogen bond to the γ-phosphate of ATP and the conserved Asp and/or Glu residues coordinate the Mg^{2+} ion (Figs. 6 and 8). This suggests that the active site geometry, at least the nucleotide-binding portion, is conserved among ANT enzymes and other NMP transferases which share this motif.

The ANT enzymes are highly interesting, not only because of their importance in clinical aminoglycoside resistance, but also for their structure and mechanism which share similarities with other NMP transferases. The precise mechanism of NMP-transfer, however, remains to be conclusively determined. The solution of additional three-dimensional structures for ANTs, in addition to ANT(4'), along with detailed mechanistic studies which include site-directed mutagenesis are required for a thorough understanding of the enzymes.

Aminoglycoside Acetyltransferases (AAC)

Modification of aminoglycosides by acetylation is one of the most prevalent mechanisms of clinical aminoglycoside resistance (Miller et al., 1997; Shaw et al., 1993). The AAC enzymes catalyze the reaction:

$$\text{Acetyl-CoA} + \text{aminoglycoside} \rightarrow \text{CoASH} + N\text{-Acetyl-aminoglycoside}$$

The AAC family is highly diverse at the gene and protein level (Table 5), though the regiospecificity of aminoglycoside modification is limited to positions 1 and 3 of the 2-deoxystreptamine ring, and positions 6' and 2' of the 6-aminohexose ring (Fig. 10). The enzymes are generally in the size range of 15–22 kDa, though one enzyme, AAC(6')-Ie,

Table 5. Aminoglycoside acetyltransferases

Enzyme	Profile	Source	Phenotype[1]	Reference
AAC(2')	Ia[2]	*Providencia stuartii*	Gent, Tob, Amik	(Rather et al., 1993b)
	Ib-e[2]	*Mycobacteria*	Gent, Tob	(Ainsa et al., 1997)
	II	*Streptomyces kasugaaensis*	Gent, Arbek	(Hotta et al., 1996)
AAC(6')	Ia	*Citrobacter diversus*	Kan, Tob, Amik, Neo	(Tenover et al., 1988)
	Ib	*Enterobacteriaceae*	Kan, Tob, Amik, Neo	(Tran van Nhieu and Collatz, 1987)
	Ic[2]	*Serratia marcescens*	Kan, Tob, Amik, Neo	(Shaw et al., 1992b)
	Id	*Klebsiella* sp. *(Tn4000)*	Kan, Tob, Amik, Neo	(Schmidt et al., 1988)
	If	*Enterobacter cloacae*	Kan, Tob, Amik, Neo	(Terán et al., 1991)
	Ig,h,j,k	*Acinetobacter* sp.	Kan, Tob, Amik, Neo	(Lambert et al., 1994a, Rudant, 1994)
	Ii[2]	*Enterococcus faecium*	Kan, Tob, Amik, Neo	(Costa et al., 1993)
	Il	*Citrobacter freundii*	Kan, Tob, Amik, Neo	(Hannecart-Pokorni et al., 1997)
	Im	*Escherichia coli*	Kan, Tob, Amik, Neo	(Shaw, 1997)
	In	*Citrobacter freundii*	Kan, Tob, Amik, Neo	(Wu et al., 1997)
	Ie	*Enterococci*	Kan, Tob, Amik, Neo	(Ferretti et al., 1986)
		Staphylococci	Fort	(Rouch et al., 1987)
	II	*Pseudomonas aeruginosa*	Kan, Tob, Gent, Neo	(Shaw et al., 1989)
AAC(1)	I	*Escherichia coli*	Neo, Apra	(Lovering et al., 1987)
AAC(3)	Ia	*Enterobacteriaceae*	Gent, Fort	(Tenover et al., 1989) (Schwocho et al., 1995)
	Ib	*Pseudomonas aeruginosa*	Gent, Fort	
	IIa	*Enterobacteriaceae*	Gent, Tob, Dibek, Net, Siso	(Vliegenthart et al., 1989)
	IIb	*Serratia marcescens*	Gent, Tob, Dibek, Net, Siso	(Rather et al., 1992)
	IIc	*Escherichia coli*		(Vakulenko and Entina, 1990)
	IIIa	*Pseudomonas* spp.	Gent, Tob, Dibek	(Vliegenthart et al., 1991)
	IIIb	*Pseudomonas aeruginosa*		(Shaw et al., 1992a)
	IIIc	*Pseudomonas aeruginosa*		(Shaw and Leal, 1992)
	IV	*Salmonella* spp.	Gent, Tob, Dibek, Net, Apra	(Bräu et al., 1984)
	VI	*Enterobacter cloacae*	Gent, Tob, Siso, Net,	(Rather et al., 1993a)
	VII	*Streptomyces rimosus*		(Lopez-Cabrera, et al., 1989)
	VIII	*Streptomyces fradiae*	Gent, Kan, Neo, Paro, Livid	(Salauze et al., 1991)
	IX	*Micromonospora chalcea*	Gent, Kan, Neo, Paro, Livid	(Salauze et al., 1991)
	X	*Streptomyces griseus*	Gent, Kan, Neo, Paro, Livid	(Ishikawa and Hotta, 1991)

[1] List is not necessarily complete, only reported phenotype are given
[2] Chromosomal gene
Abbreviations: Kan, kanamycin; Tob, tobramycin; Dibek, dibekacin; Amik, amikacin; Isep, isepamicin; Arbek, arbekacin; Neo, neomycin; But, butirosin; Ribos, ribostamycin; Paro, paromomycin; Livid, lividomycin; Gent, gentamicin C; Net, netilmicin; Siso; sisomicin; Apr, apramycin; Fort, fortimicin.

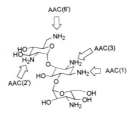

Kanamycin B

Figure 10. Regiospecificity of AACs.

forms the N-terminal region of a unique bifunctional enzyme which possesses APH(2")
activity as well (described below). Unlike the ANT and APH enzymes, there is no signature protein motif which is common to all members of the family and the amino acid sequences are generally quite diverse.

AAC(2'). The *aac(2')-I* genes are unusual in that they are integrated into the bacterial genome and not derived from an extrachromosomal element. The genes appear to be
universally present in *Providencia stuartii* (Rather et al., 1993b, Clarke et al., 1996) and
mycobacteria (Aínsa et al., 1997). The transcriptional activation of *aac(2')-Ia* from *P. stuartii* has been extensively studied by Rather's group. The gene is expressed at low levels
in wild-type cells, but mutants were isolated with substantially increased *aac(2')-Ia*
mRNA levels (Rather et al., 1993b). This predicted the existence of *trans* activating factors which control gene regulation. A search for regulators of *aac(2')-Ia* expression has resulted in the identification of five genes with the ability to influence gene expression:
aarA, aarB, aarC, aarD and *aarP*. AarA, B, C, and D are negative regulators of *aac(2')-Ia*
expression (Macinga and Rather, 1996; Rather and Orosz, 1994; Rather et al., 1993b,
1997b) while AarP is a MarA, SoxS homologue with a predicted helix-turn-helix motif
and *aac(2')-Ia* transcriptional activation activity (Macinga et al., 1995). Disruption of
aarP resulted in decreased levels of *aac(2')-Ia* mRNA while overexpression of AarP in *E.
coli* conferred a multiple antibiotic resistance (Mar) phenotype and activated *nfo*, a SoxS
target (Macinga et al., 1995). Recently, expression of *aac(2')-Ia* has been shown to be
negatively regulated by a cell-density-dependent extracellular factor, probably a peptide
(Rather et al., 1997a).

P. *stuartii*, like many bacteria, has *O*-acetylated peptidoglycan (Clarke, 1993). Mutants which over- or under-express *aac(2')-Ia* show changes in the levels of peptidoglycan
O-acetylation and cell morphology suggesting some contribution to cell wall biosynthesis
(Payie and Clarke, 1997; Payie et al., 1995,1996). AAC(2')-Ia is not restricted to acetyl-
CoA as an acyl donor and surprisingly can use *O*-acetyl peptidoglycan components to *N*-
acetylate gentamicin (Payie and Clarke, 1997). This observation, along with previous
results demonstrating a role for AAC(2')-Ia in cell morphology, suggests that this enzyme
may be involved in peptidoglycan biosynthesis or degradation, or perhaps lipopolysaccharide acetylation (Payie and Clarke, 1997). Thus the aminoglycoside-resistance phenotype
conferred by the chromosomally encoded AAC(2') may be a serendipitous secondary effect rather than a primary function.

AAC(6'). The AAC(6') family of aminoglycoside-modifying enzymes is highly diverse with two phenotypic subfamilies, I and II, all of which have predicted molecular
masses of 16–21 kDa. The AAC(6')-I enzymes confer resistance to amikacin, gentamicin
C1a and C2 but not gentamicin C1, while all the gentamicin C isoforms are modified by
the AAC(6')-II enzymes, but amikacin is not. The *aac(6')-Ib* and *aac(6')-IIa* genes are
74% identical and give rise to proteins with 76% sequence identity. Rather and colleagues,
through a series of domain exchange experiments between AAC(6')-Ib and AAC(6')-IIa
followed by the isolation and characterization of mutant enzymes, have found that a single
point mutation in AAC(6')-Ib, Leu119Ser, is sufficient to convert the resistance profile of
the enzyme to that of AAC(6')-IIa (Rather et al., 1992b). A clinical isolate of *Pseudomonas fluorescens*, which exhibited an AAC(6')-II phenotype (Amik^S, Gent^R) was found
to harbor an *aac(6')-Ib* gene with a single base mutation resulting in a protein with a corresponding Leu83Ser substitution (Lambert et al., 1994b). Thus, this position plays an important role in defining substrate specificity. A complete understanding of the role of this

position in substrate affinity awaits the determination of a high-resolution three-dimensional structure of one of these enzymes.

AAC(6')-Ib (also known as AAC(6')-IV) has been isolated from *E. coli* in two forms which behave differently on dye-ligand and size-exclusion chromatography, and show different activities (Radika and Northrop, 1984c). The more active form appears to be a tetramer based on gel-filtration chromatography. The less active form was non- covalently associated with an entity which possesses a chromophore at 260 nm, the loss of which resulted in conversion of the enzyme to the more active form. The nature of the chromophore is unknown, but could point to possible inhibitors of the enzyme. This enzyme has been well characterized in terms of aminoglycoside and acyl-CoA substrate specificity (Radika and Northop, 1984a). The enzyme accepts a broad range of both aminoglycoside and acyl-CoA substrates. The K_m values for aminoglycosides were quite low, generally in the submicromolar range and, like many aminoglycoside-modifying enzymes, AAC(6')-Ib exhibited significant aminoglycoside (but not acyl-CoA) substrate inhibition with K_i values $\geq 15 \times K_m$ (Radika and Northrop, 1984a), and the kinetic mechanism was determined to be rapid equilibrium random BiBi (Radika and Northrop, 1984b). In this mechanism, either the aminoglycoside or acetyl-CoA may bind first and the order of product release, CoASH or acetyl-aminoglycoside, is also random. In addition, the rates of dissociation of substrates and products are rapid compared to the acyl-transfer. Thus, the latter is largely rate-limiting. Amino acid residues which contribute to catalysis have not been determined.

Low-level resistance to many aminoglycosides in *Enterococcus faecium* is the result of the chromosomal *aac(6')-Ii* gene (Costa et al., 1993). Overexpression of AAC(6')-Ii in *E. coli* has permitted the rapid purification of this dimeric enzyme for biochemical studies and crystallization. Recently, crystals of AAC(6')-Ii grown in the presence of cofactor and/or kanamycin have been obtained (L.E. Wybenga and A.M. Berghuis; unpublished results). The quality of these protein crystals is sufficient to allow for a structure determination at atomic resolution. Crystals of AAC(6')-Ii grown in the presence of the co-substrate acetyl-CoA display a resolution limit of 2.2 Å (measured on the Cornell High-Energy Synchrotron Source F2 beamline), and crystals of the enzyme grown in the presence of kanamycin and CoASH show diffraction beyond 2.8 Å (measured on the Brookhaven National Laboratories National Synchrotron Light Source X8C beamline). Steady-state kinetic analysis has confirmed the broad aminoglycoside specificity of the enzyme predicted by the resistance profile, but revealed low specificity rate constants ($k_{cat}/K_m \sim 10^{3-4} \ \text{M}^{-1}\text{s}^{-1}$) (Wright and Ladak, 1997). This observation suggests it to be an enzyme which is not optimally evolved for aminoglycoside modification and may point to some other role in cell metabolism, although an *aac(6')-Ii* deletion mutant of *E. faecium* had no discernible phenotype other than loss of aminoglycoside resistance (Costa et al., 1993). The structures of isepamicin and butirosin bound to the enzyme have recently been determined by NMR techniques (DiGiammarino et al., 1997). These studies demonstrate that the enzyme binds 4,5- and 4,6-disubstituted aminoglycosides differently, as predicted by steady-state kinetic measurements (Wright and Ladak, 1997).

AAC(3). Members of the AAC(3) class of enzymes are distributed among many bacterial genera, including the aminoglycoside-producing actinomycetes (Table 5). These enzymes are larger than the AAC(6') proteins (approximately 30 kDa) and confer resistance to the gentamicins and many other clinically important aminoglycoside antibiotics. Unlike the AAC(6') class of modifying enzymes, the AAC(3) family is more homogenous with significant homology in their N-termini. Two AAC(3) enzymes have been purified and partially characterized, AAC(3)-I (Williams and Northrop, 1976) and AAC(3)-IV (Bräu and Piepersburg, 1985). The latter was shown to be a monomer by gel filtration methods and showed aminoglycoside K_m values from 11 μM for apramycin to 241 μM for kanamycin. The AAC(3)-I has been the most thoroughly studied enzyme of this class. Williams and Northrop have described the purification (Williams and Northrop, 1976), substrate specificity (Williams and Northrop, 1978b) and kinetic mechanism (Williams and Northrop, 1978a) of this enzyme. AAC(3)-I was shown to have aminoglycoside K_m values ranging from 0.3 μM (gentamicin C1) to 25.2 μM (gentamicin B), and only acetyl-CoA and propionyl-CoA could serve as acyl-donors (Williams and Northrop, 1978b). Specificity rate constants (($V_{max}/E_t)/K_m$) were quite high and, for the best substrates, gentamicin C1a and kanamycin B, were greater than 10^7 $M^{-1}s^{-1}$, approaching the rate of diffusion of small molecules in solution (10^{8-9} $M^{-1}s^{-1}$). The 4,5-disubstituted aminoglycosides such as neomycin, paromomycin and ribostamycin, as well as amikacin and kanamycin A were not substrates but competitive inhibitors of the substrate tobramycin. The kinetic mechanism was determined to be random BiBi, in rapid equilibrium with the good substrates gentamicin C1a and sisomicin, and non-rapid equilibrium with the relatively poor substrate tobramycin (Williams and Northrop, 1978a). This work has not yet been followed up by additional mechanistic or structural studies.

The AAC enzymes have emerged over the past decade as key aminoglycoside resistance elements in the clinic. Unfortunately, our understanding of the structure and mechanism of these diverse enzymes has not kept pace. Three-dimensional structures of representative AAC(6') and AAC(3) enzymes are particularly required. Given the general overall lack of amino acid sequence similarity among the AAC(6')s especially, several structures will no doubt be required in order to adequately compare enzymes. Similarly, the molecular mechanisms of acetyl transfer are not known. Therefore, much additional investigation is required.

Aminoglycoside Phosphoryltransferases (APH)

Modification of aminoglycosides by phosphorylation is catalyzed by a group of kinases termed APHs which catalyze the following reaction:

$$ATP + aminoglycoside \rightarrow ADP + Phospho\text{-}aminoglycoside$$

Enzymes are known which modify all classes of aminoglycosides (Table 6, Fig. 11). APH(3') are common and representatives are found in both Gram-negative and Gram-positive organisms, but APH(2") appears to be largely confined to Gram-positives at this time. APHs share amino acid sequence homology in the C-terminal regions of the enzymes of particular significance is the consensus sequence HGD(Xaa)3–6N(V/I) which mutagenesis studies and a three-dimensional structure have implicated in phosphoryl transfer.

Aph(3'). APH(3')s phosphorylate many 2-deoxystreptamine aminoglycosides, notably kanamycin and neomycin. At least seven distinct classes (I-VII) have been identified (Shaw et al., 1993). All are approximately 30 kDa in size and, with the exception of the type III and V classes, found in Gram-negative organisms.

The best studied aminoglycoside kinase is APH(3')-IIIa found primarily in Gram-positive cocci, although it has been detected in the Gram-negative organism *Campylobacter coli* (Papadopoulou and Courvalin, 1988; Taylor et al., 1988). It should be noted that this is a

Table 6. Aminoglycoside phosphotransferases

Enzyme	Profile	Source	Phenotype[1]	Reference
APH(3')	Ia	*Escherichia coli*	Kan, Neo, Ribos, Livid	(Oka et al., 1981)
	Ib	*Escherichia coli*		(Pansegrau et al., 1987)
	Ic	*Klebsiella pneumonia*		(Lee et al., 1991)
	II	*Escherichia coli*	Kan, Amik, Neo, But, Ribos	(Beck et al., 1982)
	III	*Enterococcus faecalis*	Kan, Amik, Isep, Neo, But,	(Trieu-Cuot and
		Staphylococcus aureus	Ribos, Livid	Courvalin, 1983) (Gray and Fitch, 1983)
	IV	*Bacillus cirulans*	Kan, Neo, But, Ribos	(Herbert et al., 1986)
	V a[2]	*Streptomyces fradiae*	Neo, Ribos	(Thompson and Gray, 1993)
	V b[2]	*Streptomyces ribosidificus*		
	V c[2]	*Micromonospora chalcea*		(Hoshiko et al., 1988); (Salauze and Davies, 1991)
	VI	*Acinetobacter baumanni*	Kan, Amik, Isep, Neo, But, Ribos	(Martin et al., 1988)
	VII	*Campylobacter jejuni*	Kan, Amik, Isep, Neo, But, Ribos, Livid	(Tenover et al., 1988)
APH(4)	Ia	*Escherichia coli*	Hygr	(Gritz and Davies, 1983)
APH(7")	Ia	*Streptomyces hygroscopicus*	Hygr	(Zalacain et al., 1986)
APH(2")	Ia	*Enterococcus faecalis*	Gent, Net, Siso, Kan, Amik, Isep, Neo, But	(Ferretti et al., 1986) (Rouch et al., 1987)
	Ic	*Staphylococcus aureus*	Ribos, Livid	(Chow et al., 1997)
		Enterococcus gallinarum		
APH(3")	Ia	*Streptomyces griseus*	Strep	(Heinzel et al., 1988)
	Ib	*Escherichia coli*		(Scholz et al., 1989)
APH(6)	Ia	*Streptomyces griseus*	Strep	(Distler et al., 1987)
	Ib	*Streptomyces glaucescens*		(Vögtli and Hütter, 1987)
	Ic	*Escherichia coli*		(Mazodier et al., 1985)
	Id	*Escherichia coli*		(Scholz et al., 1989)
	Ia	*Legionella pneumophila*	Spec	(Suter et al., 1997)
APH(9)	Ib	*Streptomyces flavopersicus*		(Lyutzkanova, et al., 1997)

[1] List is not necessarily complete, only reported phenotype are given.
[2] Chromosomal gene.
Abbreviations: Kan, kanamycin; Amik, amikacin; Isep, isepamicin; Neo, neomycin; But, butirosin; Ribos, ribostamycin; Livid, lividomycin; Gent, gentamicin C; Net, netilmicin; Siso; sisomicin; Hygr, hygromycin; Strep, streptomycin; Spec, spectinomycin.

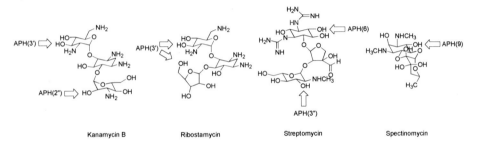

Kanamycin B   Ribostamycin   Streptomycin   Spectinomycin

Figure 11. Regiospecificity of APHs.

highly significant observation which demonstrates the potential of gene transfer between Gram-positive and -negative organisms. The *aph(3')-IIIa* gene has been cloned from *E. faecalis* (Trieu-Cuot and Courvalin, 1983) and *S. aureus* (Gray and Fitch, 1983) and the protein has been overexpressed and purified in *E. coli* (McKay et al., 1994b). The enzyme was purified as a mixture of monomer and dimer, the latter arising from two inter-molecular disulfide bonds, but both forms are kinetically indistinguishable in the steady state. APH(3')-IIIa has a broad substrate profile and will phosphorylate and confer resistance to a wide range of aminoglycosides. Specificity, rate constants for turnover are in the range of 10^4–10^5 $M^{-1}s^{-1}$, turnover numbers (k_{cat}) are uniformly in the range of 1.7–4.0 s^{-1} and the enzyme shows substrate inhibition at high concentrations of aminoglycosides (McKay et al., 1994b). Purification of modified aminoglycosides followed by analysis by mass spectrometry, ^1H, ^{13}C and ^{31}P NMR has confirmed the transfer of phosphate to the 3'-hydroxyl group of kanamycin (McKay et al., 1994b), amikacin, neomycin, and butirosin (Thompson et al., 1996b). Lividomycin A, which lacks the 3'-hydroxyl, is also a good substrate and was found to be phosphorylated at position 5" of the pentose (Thompson et al., 1996b). Similarly, butirosin and neomycin can also be phosphorylated at this position, in fact double-phosphorylation at positions 3' and 5" has been demonstrated (Thompson et al., 1996b). The kinetic mechanism of the enzyme has been determined to be Theorell-Chance (McKay and Wright, 1995). In this mechanism, ATP binds first followed by the aminoglycoside, the phosphoaminoglycoside and ADP are then released sequentially. The mechanism implies that the rate of phosphoryl transfer does not contribute to the steady-state rate and that product release should be rate-limiting. This was confirmed by solvent isotope and viscosity effect experiments, which showed that ADP release was solely rate-limiting (McKay and Wright, 1996), which also accounted for similarity in k_{cat} values, despite the wide variation in the aminoglycoside structures.

The chemical mechanism of phosphoryl transfer in APHs has been the subject of some speculation, in particular, the presence of an invariant His residue in the conserved N-terminal regions of APH(3')s had been suggested to act as a phosphate accepting residue, relaying the phosphoryl group from the γ-position of ATP to the aminoglycoside hydroxyl (Martin et al., 1988). The equivalent His residue in APH(3')-IIIa, His188, was converted to an Ala and similarly, the three additional His residues in the enzyme were also individually mutated to Ala (Thompson et al., 1996a). All His→Ala mutant enzymes were fully active, indicating that they did not play a central role in phosphate transfer. However, much of the His188Ala protein was improperly folded as assessed by the observation that the vast majority of the mutant enzyme was insoluble, thus the conservation of this residue is doubtless due to selective pressure for the maintenance of protein structure rather than a direct role in phosphoryl transfer. In addition, positional isotope exchange experiments using γ-[^{18}O]-ATP were inconsistent with transfer of the phosphate to the enzyme during catalysis (Thompson et al., 1996a), thus all the evidence to date indicates that the mechanism of phosphoryl transfer is direct attack of the aminoglycoside hydroxyl on the γ-phosphate of ATP.

Affinity labeling of APH(3')-IIIa was accomplished using fluorosulfonylbenzoyl adenosine (FSBA; McKay et al., 1994a). FSBA was an irreversible inactivator of the enzyme which could be protected by the addition of ATP, consistent with targeting of the reagent to the nucleotide binding site. This reagent labeled two Lys residues, Lys33 and Lys44, the latter of which is conserved in all APH(3')s. Construction of Lys→Ala mutants confirmed the importance of Lys44 but not Lys33 in ATP binding (Hon et al., 1997).

The prediction that Lys44 was important to ATP binding was confirmed with the determination of the X-ray crystal structure of APH(3')-IIIa with ADP bound in the nucleotide-binding pocket to 2.2 Å (Hon et al., 1997). The structure revealed two APH(3')-IIIa•ADP monomers connected covalently through two intermolecular disulfide

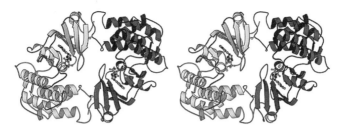

Figure 12. Three-dimensional structure of the APH(3')-IIIa dimer. The two monomers, which are shaded differently are connected through two disulfide bridges, in a head-to-tail-tail-to-head fashion. the two bound ADP molecules are also depicted.

bonds (Fig. 12). However, the interface between the two monomers did not contain extensive interactions. Furthermore, the active sites on the two monomers were separated by more than 20 Å. These observations suggested that dimer formation is not required for enzyme activity, unlike the situation described earlier for ANT(4') (Perdersen et al., 1995). The suggestion that APH(3')-IIIa is active as a monomer is in agreement with steady-state kinetic experiments which revealed no difference between APH(3')-IIIa dimer and monomer species (McKay et al., 1994b). Therefore, the remainder of this discussion will focus on the monomer structure of APH(3')-IIIa.

The APH(3')-IIIa monomer consists of two lobes connected by a tethering segment. The N-terminal lobe is composed of a five stranded anti-parallel β-sheet and two α-helices, the C-terminal lobe incorporates six helices and four short β-strands. The cleft between the two lobes forms the nucleotide-binding pocket, which harbors in this structure one ADP molecule coordinated to two magnesium ions (see Fig. 13). The specific arrangement of different secondary structure elements into a three-dimensional fold found in

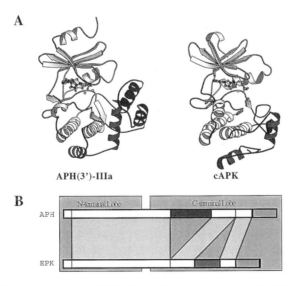

Figure 13. Structural similarity between APH(3')-IIIa and eukaryotic protein kinases. A) The structure of APH(3')-IIIa and the catalytic subunit of cyclic-AMP-dependent protein kinase (cAPK; Knighten et al., 1995; PDB code 1ATP). Regions that differ are shown in darker-shaded colors. B) A linear presentation of the enzymes, highlighting the structurally homologous sequences and the location of the inserts.

APH(3')-IIIa shows strong similarities to the classical eukaryotic protein kinase fold (e.g. Hubbard et al., 1994; Knighton et al., 1991; Owen et al., 1995; Taylor et al., 1992; Xu et al., 1996; Zhang et al., 1994). Specifically, the N-terminal domain and the core of the C-terminal domain, which combine to form the nucleotide-binding pocket, are essentially identical in the two types of structures. To illustrate this, in the N-terminal lobe, defined as residues 16–93, nearly 75% of the residues in APH(3')-IIIa are structurally identical to corresponding residues in the catalytic subunit of the cyclic-AMP-dependent protein kinase (cAPK) with an r.m.s. deviation for main-chain atoms of less than 2 Å. For the core of the C-terminal lobe, which is comprised of residues 108–125 and 187–233, this r.m.s. deviation is again less than 2 Å in comparison to cAPK (Fig. 13).

The availability of the three-dimensional structure for APH(3')-IIIa, the sequences of several related APH enzymes, the structures of several eukaryotic protein kinases, and additional sequences of serine/threonine and tyrosine protein kinases, allows for a structure-guided sequence alignment. Analysis of such an alignment will identify conserved residues, which in turn may provide insight into structure-function relationships for APH enzymes. In Fig. 14 and Table 7 such a sequence alignment and analysis are shown.

A few points from the structure-based sequence alignment analysis should be highlighted. The major differences between APHs and eukaryotic protein kinases are confined to the C-terminal lobe. Specifically, two regions can be identified which are fundamentally distinct between the two enzyme classes. First, the C-terminal end of the C-terminal lobe (from residue 233 onwards in both APH(3')-IIIa and cAPK) is folded differently in APH(3')-IIIa and protein kinases. Secondly, with respect to each other, both APHs and

Table 7. Role of strictly conserved residues in aminoglycoside phosphotransferases

Residue	Enzyme class[1]	Role	Interactions observed in APH(3')-IIIa
Gly 25	APH(3') APH	role unknown	—
Ser 27	APH(3')	nucleotide binding	Ser27 OH - ADP O2B
Lys 44	APH(3') APH EPK	nucleotide binding	Lys44 NZ - ADP
Glu 60	APH(3') APH EPK	nucleotide binding	Glu60 OE1& OE2 - Lys44 NZ
Trp 66	APH(3')	stability	side-chain packs against residue 130
Leu 67	APH(3')	stability	side-chain packs against residue 73
Pro 74	APH(3')	role unknown	—
Cys 130	APH(3')	stability	side-chain packs against residues 66 and 213
Pro 131	APH(3')	role unknown	—
Asp 153	APH(3')	substrate binding	electrostatic & H-bond (modeled)
His 188	APH(3') APH	stability	His188 NE2 - 207 O (H-bond)
Gly 189	APH(3')	stability	Gly189 CA packs agains side-chain of residue 219
Asp 190	APH(3') APH EPK	catalysis	Asp190 OD1 - antibiotic 3'/5'' OH (modeled)
Asn 195	APH(3') APH EPK	nucleotide binding	Asn195 OD1 - Mg^{2+}
Asp 208	APH(3') APH EPK	nucleotide binding	Asp208 OD1 & OD2 - Mg^{2+}
Arg 211	APH(3')	substrate binding	H-bond (modeled)
Gly 213	APH(3')	stability	Gly213 CA packs against residues 63 and 130
Ala 215	APH(3')	stability	Ala215 CB packs against side-chain of residue 219
Asp 216	APH(3')	stability	Asp219 OD1 - 183 N; Asp219 OD2 - 218 N
Asp 220	APH(3') EPK	stability	Asp220 OD1 - 188 N; Asp220 OD2 - H$_2$O - 191 O
Leu 260	APH(3')	stability	side-chain packs against residues 136, 140, and 143
Asp 261	APH(3')	substrate binding	electrostatic & H-bond (modeled)
Glu 262	APH(3')	substrate binding	electrostatic & H-bond (modeled)

[1]The extent of the conserved nature of the residue is indicated by whether it is only conserved in the APH(3') sub-family, or wether it is conserved in all aminoglycoside phosphorylating enzymes (APH), or if the residue is also conserved in eukaryotic protein kinase enzymes (EPK).

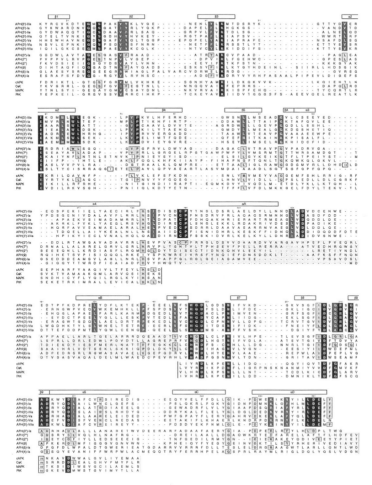

Figure 14. Protein sequence alignment of APHs and protein kinases. Boxed residues with white letters are either absolutely conserved (black background) or functionally conserved (grey background) within the APH(3') sub-family, the APH family or the protein kinase family of enzymes. Boxed residues which have a light-grey background are either absolutely or functionally conserved in another (sub-family, or are frequently (>75%) in more than one (sub-)family. Some inserts are shown as boxes with the number indicating the position of residues inserted at that location. Sequences which have a lightshaded background display no sequence homology to APH(3')-IIIa, and would likely display a different fold. Abbreviations: cAPH, cyclic-AMP-dependent protein kinase; CsK, casein kinases; MAPK, MAP kinase ERK2, PhK, phosphorylase kinase.

protein kinases possess an insert. In APHs an insert is located in-between helix α4 and strand β6, in eukaryotic protein kinases an insert is positioned just before helix α5 (Figs. 13 and 14). Although the conformation and location in the sequence differs between APHs and Ser/Thr/Tyr protein kinases, the positioning of these segments in the three-dimensional structure is similar. Both inserts are located in front of the nucleotide-binding pocket, ideally positioned to interact with substrates. In fact, it is well established that in eukaryotic protein kinases the insert is responsible for substrate specificity (Johnson et al., 1996), and in many cases this insert also corresponds to the activation segments; i.e., it contains the sites of phosphorylation which transform the kinase from an inactive to an ac-

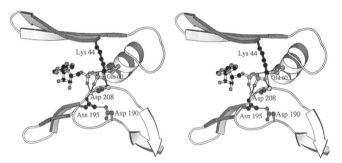

Figure 15. Close up of the active site of APH(3')-IIIa showing the five strictly conserved residues.

tive enzyme. Based on modeling studies (*vide infra*) it is likely that the APH insert is also involved in modulating substrate specificity.

Among APHs and eukaryotic protein kinases there are only five strictly conserved residues: Lys44, Glu60, Asp190, Asn195 and Asp208 (APH(3')-IIIa numbering). These five residues are all directly or indirectly involved in binding of the nucleotide, reflecting the structural similarity about the ATP-binding pocket between APHs and protein kinases (Fig. 15). Of these conserved residues, Asp190 is of particular interest, since this residue has been shown to be critical for catalysis in protein kinases (Cole et al., 1995; Madhusudan et al., 1994; Zhou and Adams, 1997). The importance of the active site Asp residue in protein kinases led to mutagenesis experiments in which Asp190 was converted to Ala in APH(3')-IIIa (Hon et al., 1997). The Asp190Ala enzyme was catalytically inactive, supporting a critical role for this residue and, based on precedent in protein kinases studies, it may be the active-site base required for deprotonation of the substrate hydroxyl group (Fig. 16). Thus, protein kinases and APH(3')-IIIa, and by inference all APHs, share a similar chemical mechanism for phosphoryl transfer.

Somewhat surprisingly, only two additional residues (beside the five residues discussed above) are conserved among all aminoglycoside phosphotransferases, namely Gly25 and His188. His188, as mentioned before, was previously postulated to be involved in catalysis, but mutagenesis studies have shown the residue to be important for protein stability (Thompson et al., 1996a). The reason for the conserved nature of residue 25 is unclear from the three-dimensional structure of APH(3')-IIIa and additional studies will be required to elucidate its role.

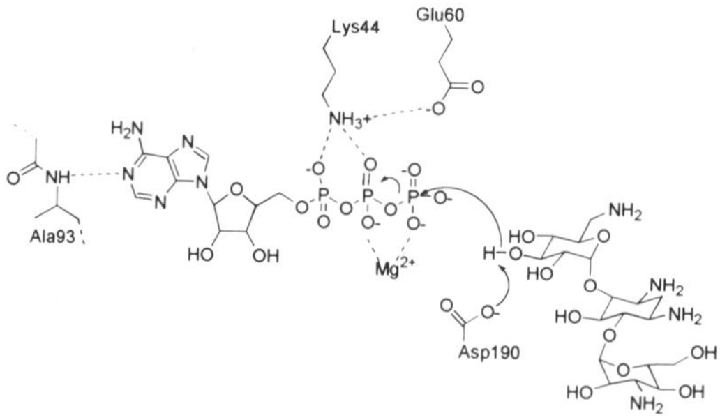

Figure 16. Proposed chemical mechanism of APH(3')-IIIa.

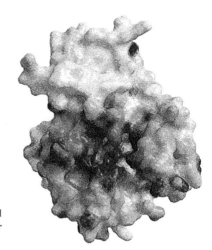

Figure 17. The negatively charged patch on the surface of APH (3')-IIIa. The surface of APH (3')-IIIa is shown. **ADP monomer** with darker shading corresponding to greater negative charge.

A structure of an aminoglycoside•APH(3')-IIIa complex is of particular interest for understanding the mechanism of aminoglycoside modification by this enzyme. Unfortunately, such a structure has so far remained elusive. The absence of this structural information does not, however, imply that nothing is known about the APH(3')-IIIa•aminoglycoside complex. Based on the required proximity of an aminoglycoside to Asp190 and the γ-phosphate group of ATP for catalysis, a limited area on the surface of APH(3')-IIIa was identified where antibiotic binding site was predicted to be located. This putative antibiotic binding site also corresponds exactly to a surface region with excessive negative charge, so as to provide favorable interactions with the positively charged antibiotics, analogous to what was seen for ANT(4') (Fig 17). In APH(3')-IIIa the putative antibiotic binding site is lined with nine acidic residues (Asp104, Asp153, Asp155, Glu157, Asp190, Glu230, Asp231, Asp261, and Glu262) and only three basic residues (Arg139, Arg211, and Arg219); most of these residues are functionally highly conserved in the APH(3') family of enzymes (Fig. 14). Studies on modified aminoglycosides which have a reduced positive charge have shown the critical importance of electrostatics in binding of several aminoglycoside phosphorylating enzymes (discussed below; McKay et al., 1996; Roestamadji et al., 1995a). Note that several of the residues implicated in aminoglycoside binding are located on the "APH insert", suggesting that this region of the enzyme is involved in determining substrate specificity.

In addition to the location of the antibiotic-binding site, structural information is also available for aminoglycosides when bound to APH(3')-IIIa. The conformations of both amikacin (a 4,6-disubstituted aminoglycoside) and butirosin A (a 4,5-disubstituted aminoglycoside) complexed to this enzyme have been examined by NMR (Cox et al., 1996; Cox and Serpersu, 1997). The NMR analysis of amikacin suggests that the two torsion angles of the glycosidic linkage between the primed ring and the 2-deoxy streptamine ring of the aminoglycoside can take on a variety of values. This implies that amikacin can be in several conformations when bound to APH(3')-IIIa. Presumably not all of the bound conformations are productive in terms of phosphoryl transfer, which might account for the significantly lower k_{cat}/K_m for this substrate (McKay et al., 1994b).

The conformation of butirosin A when bound to APH(3')-IIIa reveals that the primed and double-primed rings are in a stacking arrangement with both the 3'-OH and 5"-OH in close proximity to the γ-phosphate group of ATP. This is intriguing in that APH(3')-IIIa can phosphorylate both of these hydroxyl groups. Furthermore, it was assumed that phosphorylation of 3' and 5" hydroxyl groups by APH(3')-IIIa implied two distinct binding modes for butirosin. However, the NMR structure suggests that only one conformation of butirosin is present when bound to the enzyme and that this conformation allows either hydroxyl group to undergo phosphorylation.

The cumulative information on aminoglycoside binding to APH(3')-IIIa is extensive and can be used to model the antibiotic•enzyme•ATP ternary complex. Efforts to achieve this objective are currently in progress (J.D.W. Swartzenhauer and A.M. Berghuis; unpublished results). However, it is clear that these modeling studies require additional mutagenesis studies in order to test specific interactions which are predicted between enzyme and substrate.

APH(3')-I is the most common APH expressed by Gram-negative bacteria. APH(3')-Ia has been purified to homogeneity from *E. coli* using a neomycin-Sepharose affinity column (Siregar et al., 1995). Analogous to APH(3')-IIIa, the protein can exist as a dithiothreitol sensitive dimer or as a monomer. Kinetic parameters for a series of aminoglycosides and ATP have been determined and substrates give specificity rate constants, k_{cat}/K_m of 10^6–10^8 M^{-1}s^{-1}, indicating a highly evolved and efficient catalyst (Siregar et al., 1995). Aminoglycosides yielding k_{cat}/K_m of 10^6 M^{-1}s^{-1} also showed lower MIC values (≤ 8 μg/mL) while substrates with k_{cat}/K_m of 10^{7-8} M^{-1}s^{-1} gave rise to MICs of >1024 μg/mL. This parallels studies with other aminoglycoside-resistance enzymes, notably APH(3')-IIIa (McKay et al., 1994b), ANT(2") (Bongaerts and Molendijk, 1984; Dettertogh and Lerner, 1985), and AAC(6')-Ib (Radika and Northrop, 1984d). The biological significance of these observations is that aminoglycoside-modifying enzymes are optimally effective at low concentrations (sub K_m) of antibiotic, a scenario which is ideally suited to a detoxifying mechanism. Steady-state kinetic analysis of APH(3')-Ia is consistent with a rapid equilibrium random mechanism and the regiospecificity of phosphoryltransfer to the 3'-hydroxyl of kanamycin was confirmed by ^{1}H, ^{13}C and ^{31}P NMR (Siregar et al., 1995). These efforts indicate that a similar direct-displacement mechanism for the γ-phosphoryl group of ATP to the aminoglycoside hydroxyl moiety is also possible in this case, such as indicated for the APH(3')-IIIa, though the details of the mechanisms are slightly different.

In the absence of aminoglycosides, ATP is hydrolyzed with the following kinetic parameters by APH(3')-Ia: $K_m = 49 \pm 1$ μM, $k_{cat} = 0.023 \pm 0.002$ s^{-1}, $k_{cat}/K_m = 6.0$ x 10^2 M^{-1}s^{-1} (Roestamadji et al., 1995a). The K_m values for ATP for the ATPase activity are in the same range as those for the phosphotransferase activity in phosphorylation of aminoglycosides. This observation indicates that binding of aminoglycoside does not influence the affinity of the enzyme for ATP. In light of the fact that the concentration of ATP in bacteria is typically 3.0–3.3 mM (Bochner and Ames, 1982; Findly et al., 1983), saturation is seen for this activity at any given time. Since APHs are expressed constitutively, it would appear that APH(3')s are constantly hydrolyzing ATP *in vivo* in the absence of any aminoglycoside [APH(3')-IIIa though, does not have significant ATPase activity]. However, the value for k_{cat} is attenuated by as much as 4000-fold for the ATP hydrolase activity, hence the ATPase activity is not competitive with phosphorylation of aminoglycosides. Therefore, the enzyme phosphorylates amino- glycosides when these drugs are present, and it phosphorylates water ("ATPase" activity) when aminoglycosides are absent.

The APH(3')-Ia and the closely related APH(3')-Ic have also been respectively isolated from *E. coli* and *Klebsiella pneumoniae* and partially characterized (Lee et al., 1991). Enzymes were purified over neomycin-Sepharose and steady-state kinetic constants determined for several aminoglycosides and ATP. The K_m values were significantly higher than those determined by Siregar et al. (Siregar et al., 1995), but this is most likely due to the use of the less reliable phosphocellulose binding assay rather than the more robust and accurate spectrophotometric continuous determination of ADP by coupling its release to pyruvate kinase and lactate dehydrogenase. Nevertheless, it is clear from these studies that APH(3')-Ia and Ic are closely related enzymes.

Overexpression of APH(3')-Ia has been implicated in resistance to tobramycin, an aminoglycoside which lacks a 3'-hydroxyl group (Menard et al., 1993). It has been suggested that while tobramycin is definitely not a substrate for APH(3')-I, it can be bound by the enzyme and thus overexpression effectively can act as a sequestering mechanism which results in low-level resistance. However, two facts have yet to be reconciled with this proposal. First, the dissociation constant from APH(3') is at best 0.1 μM, thus the ribosome has comparable or higher affinity for the antibiotic with more than one binding site (Le Goffic et al., 1979), and second, the concentration of tobramycin binding sites provided by APH(3') relative to the binding sites on ribosomes per cell needs to be considered. Should this mechanism prove valid, this augurs poorly for future development of novel aminoglycosides designed to avoid enzymic modification.

APH(3')-II differs from APH(3')-I in its ability to confer resistance to butirosin and lividomycin. The enzyme has been purified from *E. coli* and its substrate specificity determined (Siregar et al., 1994). Specificity rate constants, k_{cat}/K_m, were on the order of 10^{4-7} $M^{-1}s^{-1}$ and a mutant enzyme, Glu182Asp, which had previously been reported (Yenofsky et al., 1990), has also been purified and characterized (Siregar et al., 1994). The K_m for ATP for this mutant was increased nine-fold over the wild-type enzyme implicating this residue in ATP binding. Comparison with the APH(3')-IIIa three-dimensional structure shows that Glu182 is actually quite distant from the ATP-binding site, and thus the change in K_m is unexpected.

APH(3')-II is derived from transposon Tn5 (Beck et al., 1982) and has been the subject of several site-directed mutagenesis experiments which were performed before the availability of the three-dimensional structure of APH(3')-IIIa to guide the efforts (Blázquez et al., 1991; Kocabiyik and Perlin, 1992a,b, 1994). Most of these studies were confined to the conserved C-terminal region and demonstrated the importance of His188 and Asp190 among other residues. One mutant in the N-terminal region, Val36Met, resulted in a 20-fold decrease in kanamycin resistance, though the enzyme was not purified. Val36 corresponds to Val31 in APH(3')-IIIa, which is located in the β-2 strand with the isopropyl side-chain lining the wall of the nucleotide-binding pocket, directly positioned above the ribose and α-phosphate group. Based on the structure, it is evident that a larger side chain (like a Met) would be predicted to prevent binding of ATP to the enzyme.

Electrostatic effects (e.g., hydrogen bonding and ion pairing) are believed to be significant for interactions of the resistance proteins and aminoglycosides. These interactions, even at sites remote from the seat of the enzymic reaction within the expanded active-site region may have a stabilizing effect on the structure for the transition state for the reaction that the enzyme catalyzes. Based on these observations, we expected that the ammonium/amine functions in aminoglycosides should make relatively strong interactions with the active sites of the resistance enzymes. The exact nature of these interactions remains unknown at the present. However, we decided to prepare a series of individually deaminated analogues of aminoglycosides to evaluate the importance of these interactions with the active sites of APH(3')s. Toward that goal, several compounds were synthesized (Fig. 18). Compounds **1–4** are based on the structure of neamine and compounds **5–7** are based on the structure of kanamycin A, both of which are excellent substrates for APH(3')s. In essence, this was "mutagenesis" on the substrate, instead of the enzyme.

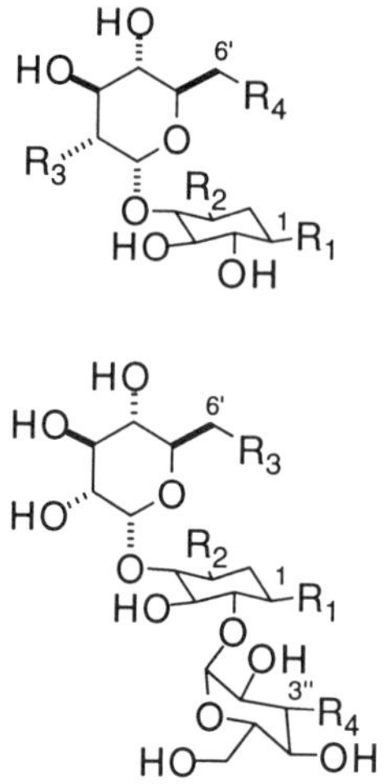

1 $R_1 = H, R_2 = R_3 = R_4 = \overset{+}{N}H_3$

2 $R_2 = H, R_1 = R_3 = R_4 = \overset{+}{N}H_3$

3 $R_3 = H, R_1 = R_2 = R_4 = \overset{+}{N}H_3$

4 $R_4 = H, R_1 = R_2 = R_3 = \overset{+}{N}H_3$

5 $R_1 = H, R_2 = R_3 = R_4 = \overset{+}{N}H_3$

6 $R_3 = H, R_1 = R_2 = R_4 = \overset{+}{N}H_3$

7 $R_4 = H, R_1 = R_2 = R_3 = \overset{+}{N}H_3$

Figure 18. Deaminated aminoglycosides prepared for study of ionic interactions with APH(3')s. Derivatives of neamine **1–4** and kanamycin A **5–7** were prepared.

Turnover of compounds **1–7** was studied with purified APH(3')-Ia, APH(3')-IIa and APH(3')-IIIa. Compounds **1–7** were all extremely poor substrates for both APH(3')-Ia and APH(3')-IIa (Roestamadji et al., 1995a). This was an unexpected finding, which argued for the critical importance of electrostatic interactions with the amino-acid residues in the active site in the course of turnover. In general, the K_m values increased modestly compared to the corresponding values for the parent compounds (neamine and kanamycin A). Insofar as K_m may approximate K_s, this indicated that binding of the compounds to the enzyme active sites had not been affected much. The most significant effects were manifested on k_{cat} values. These values decreased significantly by as much as 6 x 10^6-fold. Our results indicate that the binding energies of the enzyme to the transition-state species are within the high range of 6–11 kcal/mol. To our knowledge, these examples are the strongest interactions recorded between an ammonium/amine moiety and a counterpart in an enzyme active site.

Surprisingly, when surveyed against APH(3')-IIIa, an enzyme with broader substrate specificity and lower k_{cat}/K_m than APH(3')-Ia or -IIa, many of these deaminated compounds were relatively good substrates (McKay et al., 1996). Thus these enzymes, which perform similar functions and show significant amino acid sequence homology, interact with these compounds in dramatically different ways, an observation which provides a cautionary note for the development of broad specificity inhibitors of APHs based on aminoglycoside structure.

APH(3')-IV has been cloned from the butirosin producer *Bacillus circulans* (Herbert et al., 1986). The protein has been overexpressed in *E. coli* and purified using neomycin-Sepharose affinity chromatography. The regiospecificity of phosphate transfer to position 3' of ribostamycin was confirmed by ^{1}H and ^{13}C NMR (Sarwar and Akhtar, 1990). The APH(3')-V enzymes have been cloned from aminoglycoside producing actinomycetes such as the neomycin producers *Streptomyces fradiae* (Thompson and Gray, 1993) and *Micromonospora chalcea* (Salauze and Davies, 1991). The *aph(3')-Va* gene from *S. fradiae* is notable due to the lack of a 5'-leader sequence or ribosome binding site (Jones et al., 1992). The *aph(3')-VI* gene is found primarily in *Acinetobacter* spp. (Martin et al.,

1988) and the encoded protein is 54% similar to APH(3')-IIIa, but lacks the capacity to confer resistance to the 3'-deoxyaminoglycoside lividomycin A. APH(3')-IV from *Campylobacter jejuni* shows the highest similarity to APH(3')-IIIa (59%) and has a similar resistance phenotype differing only in resistance to amikacin (Tenover et al., 1988).

The findings reported in this section have significant implications for evolution of APH(3')s. At the present, it is not known from what primordial activity APH(3')s have evolved. In response to the challenge of aminoglycosides, the survival needs of bacteria would have favored selection of mutants in a primordial enzyme/protein such that it would have eventually acquired the new aminoglycoside-modifying (phosphorylating) activity. It would appear from our data with the deaminated compounds that evolution may have been geared in selection of mutations that would have recognized the amines of aminoglycosides as important determinants for this new activity. This is intuitively reasonable in light of the fact that the presence of amines in sugars is not so common, and would have permitted the ready specialization of these enzymes in the course of evolution.

Aph(2"). Gentamicin resistance in the Gram-positive cocci is almost exclusively the result of a bifunctional enzyme consisting of two domains with AAC(6')-Ie and APH(2")-Ia activities (Hodel-Christian and Murray, 1991; Kaufhold et al., 1992; Thal et al., 1993). The gene has been cloned from both *S. aureus* (Rouch et al., 1987) and *E. faecalis* (Ferretti et al., 1986) where it is located on plasmid pIP800 or Tn*4001*, respectively. The predicted protein sequence indicated two distinct domains consisting of AAC(6') in the N-terminus and APH(2") in the C-terminus, a prediction that has been confirmed by truncated gene constructs (Ferretti et al., 1986) and overexpression and purification of the individual domains from *E. coli* constructs (D. Daigle and G. Wright; unpublished results). The enzyme has been purified from *S. aureus* and *S. epidermidis* (Ubukata et al., 1984) as well as from expressing constructs in *E. coli* (Azucena et al., 1997) and *B. subtilis* (D. Daigle and G. Wright; unpublished results). The kinetic mechanisms of both activities have been determined to be random rapid equilibrium (Martel et al., 1983). The individually acetylated and phosphorylated aminoglycosides kanamycin (Azucena et al., 1997) and arbekacin (Kondo et al., 1993) have been purified and characterized by ^{1}H and ^{13}C NMR as well as doubly modified products, supporting unequivocally the predicted regiospecificity of group transfer as well as demonstrating that both phosphoryl and acetyl transfer can occur on one aminoglycoside molecule. It is perhaps this fact which is responsible for the very high MIC values (>1,000 mg/mL) regularly determined from clinical isolates. The purified enzyme shows a very broad capacity for aminoglycoside phosphorylation and acetylation with virtually all the 2-deoxystreptamine antibiotics serving as substrates. Among the substrates studied by Azucena et al. (1997) for this enzyme, all showed considerably better ability to undergo phosphorylation than acetylation. Consistent with these determinations, kanamycin A was shown to undergo phosphorylation exclusively in *in vivo* experiments (Azucena et al., 1997).

In addition, the AAC(6')-Ie acetylates fortimicin, a unique feature of this AAC(6'), though this is not a substrate for the APH(2") (Shaw et al., 1993; D. Daigle and G. Wright; unpublished results). The AAC(6') activity is not confined to *N*-acetylation, and the 6'-hydroxyl aminoglycosides, paromomycin and lividomycin A, are in fact substrates with k_{cat}/K_m of 10^3 M^{-1}s^{-1}, lower than 6'-amino compounds (k_{cat}/K_m of 10^{4-5} M^{-1}s^{-1}), but significant nonetheless (D. Daigle and G. Wright; unpublished results). The acetylated products are highly susceptible to base hydrolysis, consistent with 6'-*O*-acetylation which is an activity which is so far unique to this enzyme.

Initially, AAC(6')-APH(2") was thought to be found only in Gram-positive organisms. However, Kettner et al. (1991) have recently detected this enzyme in Gram-negative bacteria as well. This alarming report demonstrates the ability of a plasmid-encoded Gram-positive gene to be transferred and expressed in Gram-negative bacteria, whereby the resistance phenotype is disseminated to other less-related bacterial strains. The fact that this bifunctional enzyme is devastatingly effective at aminoglycoside modification heightens the importance of this observation.

A recently isolated gene from *Enterococcus gallinarum* encodes a protein with high homology (53% similar) to the N-terminus of the bifunctional AAC(6')-APH(2") enzyme and has a resistance profile consistent with APH(2") (Chow et al., 1997). This observation along with the recent isolation of the *aac(6')-Im* gene from *E. coli* (Shaw, 1997) which encodes an AAC(6')-Ie homologue, supports the proposal (Ferretti et al., 1986) that the bifunctional enzyme has arisen as a consequence of a gene fusion event.

Aph(4) and Aph(7"). Resistance to the aminoglycoside hygromycin B is frequently used as a marker for eukaryotic and bacterial cell culture studies. The gene responsible for this resistance is *aph(4)*, which was originally cloned from an *E. coli* isolate (Gritz and Davies, 1983). The gene encodes a protein of predicted mass of 39 kDa and the site of hygromycin phosphorylation has been determined by ^{1}H and ^{13}C NMR (Rao et al., 1983).

The hygromycin producer *Streptomyces hygroscopicus* also produces a phosphorylating enzyme, but the site of modification is the 7"-hydroxyl (Pardo et al., 1985). The gene encoding the enzyme has been cloned (Zalacain et al., 1986), expressed in *E. coli* (Zalacain et al., 1987a), and the protein purified to homogeneity over a hygromycin-Sepharose column (Zalacain et al., 1987b). The K_m for ATP was determined to be 36.4 μM and for hygromycin 0.56 μM. The protein migrates as a 41-kDa monomer by gel filtration (Pardo et al., 1985).

Aph(3") and Aph(6). APH(3") and APH(6)s are streptomycin selective kinases. The tandem genes, *strA-strB*, respectively, encode APH(3")-Ib and APH(6')-Id (Shaw et al., 1993). The *strA-strB* cassette is found on Gram-negative broad host range plasmids such as RSF1010 (Scholz et al., 1989) and transposons and is widely distributed in the environment (Sundin and Bender, 1996).

Similarly, the streptomycin-producing organism *Streptomyces griseus*, also encodes both an APH(3") and APH(6) (Distler et al., 1987; Heinzel et al., 1988). The *aphD* gene encodes the APH(6) enzyme and is clustered with aminoglycoside biosynthesis genes in *S. griseus* (Distler et al., 1987) and in *Streptomyces glaucescens* (Vögtli and Hütter, 1987) which also produces streptomycin. On the other hand, the *aphE* gene encodes the APH(3"), which is not associated with streptomycin biosynthetic genes.

Aph(9). A spectinomycin phosphotransferase gene has been cloned from *Legionella pneumophila*, the bacterium responsible for Legionnaire's disease (Suter et al., 1997). Initial enzyme assays have shown that the enzyme is specific to spectinomycin. This has been confirmed with purified enzyme from an *E. coli* overexpression construct (P. Thompson, D.W. Hughes, N.P. Cianciotto, & G. Wright; unpublished results). Spectinomycin is an excellent substrate with k_{cat}/K_m of 10^6 M^{-1}s^{-1}, other aminoglycosides such as streptomycin and kanamycin were neither substrates or inhibitors. Purification of the phospho-spectinomycin, followed by ^{1}H, ^{13}C and ^{31}P NMR have shown that the hydroxyl group at position 9 is the site of phosphoryl transfer, thus we propose that the enzyme should be designated APH(9)-Ia.

A gene encoding a spectinomycin specific APH, *spcN*, has also been cloned from the spectinomycin producer *Streptomyces flavopersicus* (Lyutzkanova et al., 1997). The predicted amino-acid sequence is not similar to APH(9) from *L. pneumophila*. The site of phosphorylation was predicted to be at either one or both hydroxyls at positions 7 or 9, though based on the precedents of adenylation and phosphorylation of position 9 noted above, it is likely that this enzyme is also an APH(9).

Inhibition of Aminoglycoside-Modifying Enzymes

Inhibition studies of aminoglycoside-modifying enzymes can be divided into two groups, those which are aminoglycoside-based inhibitors, and non-aminoglycoside inhibitors. Inhibition of many modifying enzymes by aminoglycosides is well established. Thus, tobramycin and dibekacin, 3'-deoxy aminoglycosides, are competitive inhibitors of kanamycin modification by APH(3') with K_{is} < 1 µM (McKay and Wright, 1995). Similarly, paromomycin and lividomycin A, both 6'-hydroxy aminoglycosides, are competitive inhibitors of kanamycin 6'-N-acetyltransfer catalyzed by AAC(6')-Ii with K_{is} of 1.06 µM and 0.50 µM, respectively (Wright and Ladak, 1997). 6'-Methyl-derivatives of kanamycin have also been shown to be effective antibiotics against strains bearing *aac(6')* genes (Umezawa et al., 1972). Inhibition of modifying enzymes by aminoglycosides generally has the potential added benefit that the inhibitors themselves may function as antibiotics.

Williams and Northrop prepared 3-*N*-chloroacetyl-CoA by incubation of β-chloroacetyl-CoA, gentamicin C1a and AAC(3)-I (Williams and Northrop, 1979). The chloroacetylated aminoglycoside was reacted *in situ* with CoASH to form a bisubstrate analogue which was purified, partially characterized, and used in inhibition studies of AAC(3)-I (Fig. 19A). This compound was a time-dependent enzyme inhibitor with a $t_{1/2}$ for the regain of activity of 34 min and a K_I of 0.5–2 nM, but could not reverse antibiotic resistance in an *E. coli* strain bearing the *aac(3)-I* gene, probably due to difficulty in transport across cell membranes. However, this study did demonstrate the feasibility and potential of the use of compounds with multisubstrate character as potent inhibitors of aminoglycoside-modifying enzymes.

A series of four regiospecifically synthesized *N*-bromoacetylated neamine derivatives have been prepared recently. All these compounds served both as substrates and affinity inactivators for APH(3')-IIa (Roestamadji and Mobashery; unpublished results). The sites of protein modifications were identified by mass-spectroscopic analyses of the proteolytic fragments in an effort to map the active site.

Mechanism-based inactivation of APH(3')-I and APH(3')-II by synthetic aminoglycoside analogues has been reported (Roestamadji et al., 1995b). Two compounds were synthesized, **8** and **9** (Fig. 20A), with a nitro group at position 2'. Phosphoryl transfer to the 3'-hydroxyl results in the positioning of a phosphate group β to the 2'-nitro group. This compound can readily undergo elimination of phosphate generating an electrophilic nitroalkene in the active site of the enzyme (Fig. 19B). This highly reactive compound is then postulated to alkylate susceptible amino acid side chains resulting in irreversible enzyme inactivation. Unfortunately, these compounds have not been found to be effective in reversing antibiotic resistance, but they provide the necessary precedent for the synthesis of additional analogues which may be more effective in this regard.

The similarity between APH(3') and protein kinases prompted a survey of known protein kinase inhibitors as potential inhibitors of APHs (Daigle et al., 1997). The indole carbazole, staurosporine, a potent inhibitor of protein kinase C, as well as erbstatin and tyrphostin analogues, which are known inhibitors of tyrosine protein kinases, did not in-

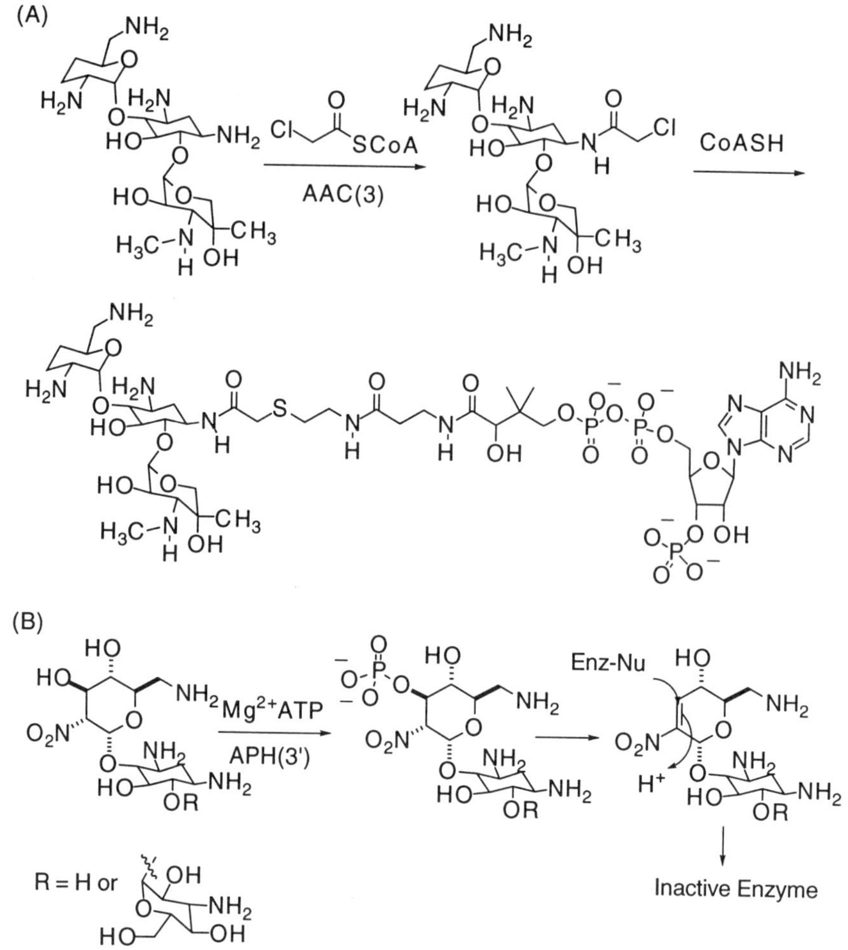

Figure 19. Inhibition of aminoglycoside-modifying enzymes. (A) Synthesis of bifunctional inhibitor of AAC(3). (B) Mechanism-based inactivation of APH(3') by 2'-deamino-2'-nitro aminoglycosides.

hibit APH(3')-IIIa or AAC(6')-APH(2") (Daigle et al., 1997; G. McKay, D. Daigle and G. Wright, unpublished results). On the other hand, the protein kinase inhibiting flavanoids, genestein and quercetin (Fig. 20B), were inhibitors of APH(3'), but not AAC(6')-APH(2") (Daigle et al., 1997). The most potent dual protein kinase/APH inhibitors were the isoquinolinesulfonamides of the H and CKI series (Fig. 20B). Several of these compounds gave K_i values below 100 µM for both APH(3')-IIIa and AAC(6')-APH(2") (Daigle et al., 1997). Inhibition was competitive with ATP and non-competitive against kanamycin. None of the compounds tested were able to reverse aminoglycoside resistance in bacterial cells harboring either the *aph(3')-IIIa* or *aac(6')-aph(2")* genes. However, this initial study augurs well for the synthesis of potent APH-directed compounds which incorporate the isoquinolinesulfonamide nucleus. The fact that many pharmaceutical companies have been active in the synthesis of protein kinase inhibitors suggests that among these, potent inhibitors of APHs already exist.

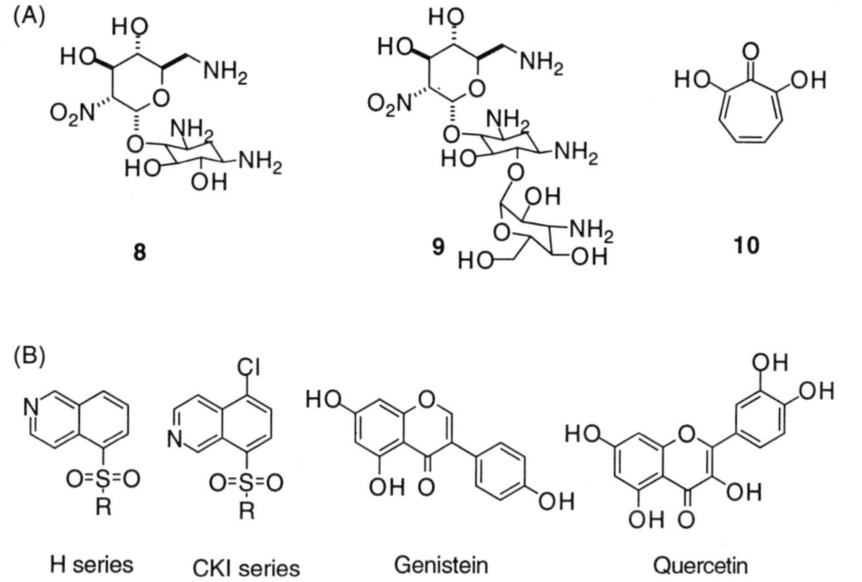

Figure 20. Inhibitors of aminoglycoside-modifying enzymes. (A) Compounds which inhibit aminoglycoside-modifying enzymes exclusively. (B) Protein kinase inhibitors which inhibit APHs.

7-Hydroxytropolone (compound **10**, Fig. 20A), a natural product produced by *Streptomyces neyagawaensis*, has been shown to be an inhibitor of ANT(2") (Allen et al., 1982). Inhibition was competitive with ATP (K_i = 10 μM), and either non- or un-competitive with respect to tobramycin. Several analogues of the lead compound were also found to have inhibitory activity, though only one of these, 4-isopropyl-7-hydroxytropolone, was comparable in potency to 7-hydroxytropolone. This compound did reverse tobramycin resistance in *E. coli* harboring the *ant(2")* gene, but not in cells with other aminoglycoside-modifying enzymes. This study provides valuable proof of concept for the use of inhibitors of aminoglycoside-modifying enzymes as a means of combating antibiotic resistance, in much the same fashion as β-lactamase inhibitors are clinically used to rescue the usefulness of β-lactam antibiotics (Sutherland, 1991).

Origin of Aminoglycoside-Modifying Enzymes

The variety and widespread dissemination of aminoglycoside resistance genes suggests that they have arisen from several different sources. Some genes are probably fortuitously resistance determinants; e.g., the chromosomal *aac(2')* from *P. stuartii* and *Mycobacteria* (Table 5), however, the majority of resistance genes are found on mobile genetic elements and undoubtedly have evolved specifically for the detoxification of aminoglycosides. A likely source for these genes are the aminoglycoside-producing organisms, a hypothesis put forth some 25 years ago by Benveniste and Davies who noted the similarities between aminoglycoside resistance enzymes expressed by clinical isolates and those found in antibiotic-producing organisms (Benveniste and Davies, 1973). Indeed, several *aac(3)* and *aph* genes have been cloned and sequenced from aminoglycoside-producing bacteria in the interim (Tables 5 and 6). Thus, these organisms are probably the reservoir for these genes where they are associated with self-resistance, although some of the genes are not clustered within the biosynthetic gene cluster; e.g., *aac(3)-VIII* from *S. fradiae* (Thompson et al., 1980) and their origins are therefore cryptic.

The origin of other resistance genes such as the members of the *aac(6')* and *ant* families is less obvious in that no aminoglycoside producer has yet been shown to harbor either of them. There are a few known chromosomal *aac(6')*s e.g. *aac(6')-Ic* and *Ii*, and it is possible that the other *aac(6')* genes have evolved from similar chromosomal elements. The fact that purified AAC(6')-Ii is a relatively poor aminoglycoside acetyltransferase (Wright and Ladak, 1997) suggests another function for this enzyme, and should one be found, it may point to a common origin for these enzymes. Protein sequence analysis has shown modest similarities between AACs and other bacterial acetyltransferases such as Rim I, Rim J, Rim L, CysE and LacA, and one (or several) of these may be an ancestor (Piepersberg et al., 1988,1991).

The ANTs, as noted above, share a common protein fold with enzymes which catalyze nucleotidyltransfer, and thus such genes may be the origin of *ant*s.

The three-dimensional structure of APH(3')-IIIa (Hon et al., 1997) has dramatically expanded on the observations (Brenner, 1987; Martin et al., 1988), most extensively described by Piepersberg's group (Heinzel et al., 1988), that APHs and protein kinases share regions of amino acids sequence similarity (Fig. 13 and 14). The fact that APH(3')-IIIa and protein kinases share a similar chemical mechanism and sensitivity to inhibitors suggests a close evolutionary link between these classes of enzymes. APHs also demonstrate measurable serine protein kinase activity (D. Daigle, G. McKay, G. Wright; unpublished results). Purified APH(3')-IIIa and AAC(6')-APH(2") were shown to phosphorylate several common protein kinase substrates including myelin basic protein and protamine. Actinomycetes and other bacteria encode Ser/Thr protein kinases (reviewed in Kennelly and Potts, 1996; Zhang, 1996), thus these are a potential source of APHs.

SIDE EFFECTS OF AMINOGLYCOSIDE ANTIBIOTICS

From the outset of their use as antibacterial agents, it has been known that aminoglycosides are associated with significant oto and nephrotoxicity (e.g., Hinshaw and Feldman, 1945). The severity of these effects is dependent on the nature of the aminoglycoside structure, and thus less toxic compounds are clinically used in place of for example, neomycin, which shows significant toxicity. In addition, monitoring of serum levels of aminoglycosides and once daily dosing has decreased the incidences of hearing loss as a result of aminoglycoside therapy. The details of the molecular mechanisms of the ototoxic side effects remains elusive despite much activity in the area.

Aminoglycosides are eliminated from the body virtually exclusively by glomerular filtration, thus the kidney is exposed to high levels of these antibiotics (Ali, 1995). The suggestion that a P-450-derived metabolite may be involved in toxicity (Crann et al., 1992) in both the kidney and the ear remains controversial (Sanders et al., 1993). Aminoglycosides are taken up by tubule cells on the brush border of the glomerulus and accumulate in lysosomes (Nassberger et al., 1990). Several studies have demonstrated pleiotropic effects of aminoglycosides, gentamicin in particular, on renal tissue; these include increased production of hydrogen peroxide, increase in the rate of phospholipidosis, inhibition of Na^+/K^+-ATPase, injury to organelles such as mitochondria and lysosomes, increase in thromboxane A2 and inhibition of protein synthesis (reviewed in Ali, 1995). A unifying feature in most of these effects, which parallels the findings in bacteria, is membrane damage.

Ototoxicity appears to be the result of specific toxicity to the outer hair cells (reviewed in Schacht, 1993). It has been proposed that a mechanism of toxicity is related to aminoglycoside affinity for phosphatidylinositol-4,5-bisphosphate and inhibition of ornithine decarboxylase (reviewed in Schacht, 1993) though it is not clear how these effects may result in the specificity of toxic effects. Hypersensitivity to aminoglycoside induced ototoxicity has also been shown to be associated with a A→G transition in the mitochondrial 12S rRNA of susceptible individuals (Cortopassi and Hutchin, 1994; Hutchin and Cortopassi, 1994). A model has been proposed in which this mutation results in mistranslation of mitochondrially encoded proteins such as complex I, which results in an increase in superoxide production and oxidative damage resulting in apoptosis (Cortopassi and Hutchin, 1994; Hutchin and Cortopassi, 1994). Aminoglycosides are also known to activate phospholipase C and this activity may also contribute to toxicity (Morris & Mensa-Wilmot, 1997).

Priuska and Schacht (1995) have shown recently that gentamicin has the ability to chelate iron ions and the complex can promote formation of free radicals effectively. These radicals are believed to be involved in adventitious reactions, which lead to adverse oto and renal toxicity. The same group showed subsequently that free-radical scavengers and iron chelators can prevent ototoxicity in experiments performed in guinea pigs, indicating the clinical promise for combination therapy of aminoglycosides in conjunction with these agents to overcome the toxicity of these versatile antibacterials (Song and Schacht, 1996).

CONCLUSIONS AND FUTURE DIRECTIONS

The rise of resistance to the aminoglycosides over the past several decades and the development of newer broad spectrum antibacterial agents has resulted in the marginalization of these potent antibiotics. The vast array of resistance enzymes and the mobilization of their corresponding genes would appear to prohibit significant new uses for these drugs. However, since there are only three general mechanisms of resistance: adenylation, acetylation and phosphorylation, and given the importance of discovering new antibiotics in the face of the growing crisis of antibiotic resistance, the aminoglycosides should be seriously reconsidered as antibiotics of choice. The development and clinical implementation of inhibitory compounds targeted to modifying enzymes which could rescue the use of aminoglycosides is not unreasonable. The recent advances in the knowledge of the molecular mechanisms and structure of aminoglycoside resistance enzymes has provided the basis for rational inhibitor design and has already resulted in modest success. Continued efforts in this area will provide additional knowledge which is critical for the development of new antibacterial agents and may result in a new era of wide spread use of these potent bactericidal agents.

ACKNOWLEDGMENTS

The work described from the authors' laboratories was funded by the Medical Research Council of Canada (A.M.B. and G.D.W.) and by the National Institutes of Health (S.M.). We thank members of the Wright laboratory and Lakshmi Kotra of the Mobashery laboratory for critical reading of the manuscript.

REFERENCES

Aínsa, J.A., Pérez, E., Pelicic, V., Berthet, F.X., Gicquel, B. and Martin, C., 1997, Aminoglycoside 2'-N-acetyl-transferase genes are universally present in mycobacteria: characterization of the *aac(2')-Ic* gene from *Mycobacterium tuberculosis* and the *aac(2')-Id* gene from *Mycobacterium smegmatis*, *Mol. Microbiol.* 24:431–441.

Ali, B.H., 1995, Gentamicin nephrotoxicity in humans and animals: some recent research, *Gen. Pharmacol.* 26:1477–1487.

Allen, N.E., Jr., W.E.A., Jr., J.N.H. and Kirst, H.A., 1982, 7-Hydroxytropolone: An inhibitor of aminoglycoside-2"-O-adenyltransferase, *Antimicrob. Agents Chemother.* 22:824–831.

Azucena, E., Grapsas, I. and Mobashery, S., 1997, Properties of a bifunctional bacterial antibiotic resistance enzyme that catalyzes ATP-dependent 2"-phosphorylation and acetyl-CoA-dependent 6'-acetylation of aminoglycosides, *J. Am. Chem. Soc.* 119:2317–2318.

Bakker, E.P., 1992, Aminoglycoside and aminocyclitol antibiotics: hygromycin B is an atypical bactericidal compound that exerts effects on cells of *Escherichia coli* characteristic for bacteriostatic aminocyclitols, *J. Gen. Microbiol.* 138:563–569.

Beauclerk, A.A. and Cundliffe, E., 1987, Sites of action of two ribosomal RNA methylases responsible for resistance to aminoglycosides, *J. Mol. Biol.* 93:661–671.

Beck, E., Ludwig, G., Auerswald, E.A., Reiss, B. and Schaller, H., 1982, Nucleotide sequence and exact localization of the neomycin phosphotransferase gene from transposon Tn5, *Gene.* 19:327–336.

Benveniste, R. and Davies, J., 1973, Aminoglycoside antibiotic-inactivating enzymes in actinomycetes similar to those present in clinical isolates of antibiotic-resistant bacteria, *Proc. Natl. Acad. Sci. U S A.* 70:2276–2280.

Berman, J.D. and Fleckenstein, L., 1991, Pharmacokinetic justification of antiprotozoal therapy. A US perspective, *Clin. Pharmacokinet.* 21:479–493.

Blázquez, J., Davies, J. and Moreno, F., 1991, Mutations in the *aphA-2* gene of transposon Tn5 mapping within the regions highly conserved in aminoglycoside-phosphotransferases strongly reduce aminoglycoside resistance, *Mol. Microbiol.* 5:1511–1518.

Bochner, B.R. and Ames, B.N., 1982, Complete analysis of cellular nucleotides by two-dimensional thin layer chromatography, *J. Biol. Chem.* 257:9759–9769.

Bongaerts, G.P.A. and Molendijk, L., 1984, Relation between aminoglycoside 2"-O-nucleotidyltransferase activity and aminoglycoside resistance, *Antimicrob. Agents Chemother.* 25:234–237.

Bräu, B. and Piepersburg, W., 1985, Purification and characterization of a plasmid-encoded aminoglycoside-(3)-N-acetyltransferase IV from *Escherichia coli*, *FEBS Letts.* 185:43–46.

Bräu, B., Pilz, U. and Piepersberg, W., 1984, Genes for gentamicin-(3)-N-acetyltransferases III and IV: I. Nucleotide sequence of the AAC(3)-IV gene and possible involvement of an IS140 element in its expression, *Mol. Gen. Genet.* 193:179–187.

Brenner, S., 1987, Phosphotransferase sequence homology, *Nature.* 329:21.

Bryan, L.E. (1984), Aminoglycoside resistance, in *Antimicrobial Drug Resistance* (L. E. Bryan, Ed.) pp 241–277, Academic Press, Orlando.

Bryan, L.E. and Kwan, S., 1983, Roles of ribosomal binding, membrane potential, and electron transport in bacterial uptake of streptomycin and gentamicin., *Antimicrob. Agents Chemother.* 23:835–845.

Bryan, L.E. and Van Den Elzen, H.M., 1977, Effects of membrane-energy mutations and cations on streptomycin and gentamicin accumulation by bacteria: a model for entry of streptomycin and gentamicin in susceptible and resistant bacteria, *Antimicrob. Agents Chemother.* 12:163–177.

Busse, H.-J., Wöstmann, C. and Bakker, E.P., 1992, The bactericidal action of streptomycin: membrane permeabilization caused by the insertion of mistranslated proteins into the cytoplasmic membrane of *Escherichia coli* and subsequent caging of the antibiotic inside the cells due to degradation of these proteins, *J. Gen. Microbiol.* 138:551–561.

Chow, J.W., Zervos, M.J., Lerner, S.A., Thal, L.A., Donabedian, S.M., Jaworski, D.D., Tsai, S., Shaw, K.J. and Clewell, D.B., 1997, A novel gentamicin resistance gene in *Enterococcus*, *Antimicrob. Agents Chemother.* 41:511–514.

Clarke, A.J., 1993, Extent of peptidoglycan O acetylation in the tribe Proteeae, *J. Bacteriol.* 175:4550–4553.

Clarke, A.J., Francis, D. and Keenleyside, W.J., 1996, The prevalence of gentamicin 2'-N-acetyltransferase in the Proteeae and its role in the O-acetylation of peptidoglycan, *FEMS Microbiol. Lett* 145:201–207.

Cole, P.A., Grace, M.R., Phillips, R.S., Burn, P. and Walsh, C.T., 1995, The role of the catalytic base in the protein tyrosine kinase Csk, *J. Biol. Chem.* 270:22105–22108.

Cortopassi, G. and Hutchin, T., 1994, A molecular and cellular hypothesis for aminoglycoside-induced deafness, *Hear. Res.* 78:27–30.

Costa, Y., Galimand, M., Leclercq, R., Duval, J. and Courvalin, P., 1993, Characterization of the chromosomal *aac(6')-Ii* gene specific for *Enterococcus faecium*, *Antimicrob. Agents Chemother.* 37:1896–1903.

Cox, J.R., McKay, G.A., Wright, G.D. and Serpesu, E.H., 1996, Arrangement of substrates at the active site of an aminoglycoside antibiotic 3'-phosphotransferase as determined by NMR, *J. Am. Chem. Soc.* 118:1295–1301.

Cox, J.R. and Serpersu, E.H., 1997, Biologically important conformations of aminoglycoside antibiotics bound to an aminoglycoside 3'-phosphotransferase as determined by transferred nuclear Overhauser effect spectroscopy, *Biochemistry.* 36:2353–2359.

Crann, S.A., Huang, M.Y., McLaren, J.D. and Schacht, J., 1992, Formation of a toxic metabolite from gentamicin by a hepatic cytosolic fraction, *Biochem. Pharmacol.* 43:1835–1839.

Cundliffe, E., 1987, On the nature of antibiotic binding sites in ribosomes, *Biochimie.* 69:863–869.

Daigle, D.M., McKay, G.A. and Wright, G.D., 1997, Inhibition of aminoglycoside antibiotic resistance enzymes by protein kinase inhibitors, *J. Biol. Chem.* 272: 24755–24758.

Davis, B.D., 1987, Mechanism of action of aminoglycosides, *Microbiol. Rev.* 51:341–350.

Davis, B.D., Chen, L.L. and Tai, P.C., 1986, Misread protein creates membrane channels: an essential step in the bactericidal action of aminoglycosides, *Proc. Natl. Acad. Sci. U S A.* 83:6164–6168.

DeHertogh, D.A. and Lerner, S.A., 1985, Correlation of aminoglycoside resistance with K_ms and V_{max}/K_m ratios of enzymatic modification of aminoglycosides by 2"-O-nucleotidyltransferase, *Antimicrob. Agents Chemother.* 27:670–671.

DiGiammarino, E.L., Draker, K.a., Wright, G.D. and Serpesu, E.H., 1997, Solution studies of isepamicin and conformational comparisons between isepamicin and butirosin A when bound to an aminoglycoside 6-N-acetyltransferase determined by NMR spectroscopy, *Biochemistry,* in press.

Distler, J., Braun, C., Ebert, A. and Piepersberg, W., 1987, Gene cluster for streptomycin biosynthesis in *Streptomyces griseus*: analysis of a central region including the major resistance gene, *Mol. Gen. Genet.* 208:204–210.

Dubin, D.T. and Davis, B.D., 1961, The effect of streptomycin on potassium flux in *Escherichia coli*, *Biochim. Biophys. Acta.* 52:400–402.

Edson, R.S. and Terrell, C.L., 1991, The aminoglycosides, *Mayo. Clin. Proc.* 66:1158–1164.

Ferretti, J.J., Gilmore, K.S. and Courvalin, P., 1986, Nucleotide sequence analysis of the gene specifying the bifunctional 6'-aminoglycoside acetyltransferase 2"-aminoglycoside phosphotransferase enzyme in *Streptococcus faecalis* and identification and cloning of gene regions specifying the two activities, *J. Bacteriol.* 167:631–638.

Fichtenbaum, C.J., Ritechie, D.J. and Powderly, W.G., 1994, Use of paromomycin for treatment of cryptosporidiosis in patients with AIDS, *Clin. Infect. Dis.* 16:298–300.

Findly, R.C., Gillies, R.J. and Shulman, R.G., 1983, In vivo phosphorus-31 nuclear magnetic resonance reveals lowered ATP during heat shock of *Tetrahymena*, *Science.* 219:1223–1225.

Fourmy, D., Recht, M.I., Blanchard, S.C. and Puglisi, J.D., 1996, Structure of the A site of *Escherichia coli* 16S ribosomal RNA complexed with an aminoglycoside antibiotic, *Science.* 274:1367–1371.

Gates, C.A. and Northrop, D.B., 1988a, Alternative substrate and inhibition kinetics of aminoglycoside nucleotidyltransferase 2"-I in support of a Theorell-Chance kinetic mechanism, *Biochemistry.* 27:3826–3833.

Gates, C.A. and Northrop, D.B., 1988b, Determination of the rate-limiting segment of aminoglycoside nucleotidyltransferase 2"-I by pH- and viscosity-dependent kinetics, *Biochemistry.* 27:3834–3842.

Gates, C.A. and Northrop, D.B., 1988c, Substrate specificities and structure-activity relationships for the nucleotidylation of antibiotics catalyzed by aminoglycoside nucleotidytransferase 2"-I, *Biochemistry.* 27:3820–3825.

Gilman, S. and Saunders, V.A., 1986, Accumulation of gentamicin by *Staphylococcus aureus*: the role of the transmembrane electrical potential, *J. Antimicrob. Chemother.*(17):37–44.

Gorini, L. (1974), Streptomycin and misreading of the genetic code, in *Ribosomes* (M. Nomura, A. Tissères and P. Lengyel, Eds.) pp 791–803, Cold Spring Harbor Laboratory, Cold Spring Harbor, NY.

Gray, G.S. and Fitch, W.M., 1983, Evolution of antibiotic resistance genes: The DNA sequence of a kanamycin resistance gene from *Staphylococcus aureus*, *Mol. Biol. Evol.* 1:57–66.

Gritz, L. and Davies, J., 1983, Plasmid-encoded hygromycin B resistance: the sequence of hygromycin B phosphotransferase gene and its expression in *Escherichia coli* and *Saccharomyces cerevisiae*, *Gene.* 25:179–188.

Hancock, R., 1961, Early effects of streptomycin on *Bacillus megaterium*, *J. Bacteriol.* 88:633–639.

Hancock, R.E., 1981, Aminoglycoside uptake and mode of action-with special reference to streptomycin and gentamicin. I. Antagonists and mutants, *J. Antimicrob. Chemother.* 8:249–276.

Hannecart-Pokorni, E., Depuydt, F., de Wit, L., van Bossuyt, E., Content, J. and Vanhoof, R., 1997, Characterization of the 6'-N-aminoglycoside acetyltransferase gene *aac(6')-II* associated with a *sulI*-type integron, *Antimicrob. Agents Chemother.* 41:314–318.

Heinzel, P., Werbitzky, O., Distler, J. and Piepersberg, W., 1988, A second streptomycin resistance gene from *Streptomyces griseus* codes for streptomycin-3"-phosphotransferase. Relationships between antibiotic and protein kinases, *Arch. Microbiol.* 150:184–192.

Herbert, C.J., Sarwar, M., Ner, S.S., I.G., G. and Akhtar, M., 1986, Sequence and interspecies transfer of an aminoglycoside phosphotransferase gene (APH) of *Bacillus circulans*. Self-defence mechanism in antibiotic-producing organisms, *Biochem. J.* 233:383–393.

Higgins, C.E. and Kastners, R.E., 1967, Nebramycin, a new broad-spectrum antibiotic complex. II. Description of *Streptomyces tenebrarius*, *Antimicrob. Agetns Chemother.* 7:324–331.

Hinshaw, H.C. and Feldman, W.H., 1945, Streptomycin in treatment of clinical tuberculosis: preliminary report, *Mayo Clin.* 20:313–318.

Hodel-Christian, S.L. and Murray, B.E., 1991, Characterization of the gentamicin resistance transposon Tn*5281* from *Enterococcus faecalis* and comparison to staphylococcal transposons Tn*4001* and Tn*4031*, *Antimicrob. Agents Chemother.* 35:1147–1152.

Hollingshead, S. and Vapnek, D., 1985, Nucleotide sequence analysis of a gene encoding a streptomycin/spectinomycin adenyltransferase, *Plasmid.* 13:17–30.

Holm, L. and Sander, C., 1995, DNA polymerase β belongs to an ancient nucleotidyltransferase superfamily, *Trends Biol. Chem.* 20:345–347.

Holmes, D.J. and Cundliffe, E., 1991, Analysis of a ribosomal RNA methylase gene from *Streptomyces tenebrarius* which confers resistance to gentamicin, *Mol. Gen. Genet.* 229:229–237.

Holmes, D.J., Drocourt, D., Tiraby, G. and Cundliffe, E., 1991, Cloning of an aminoglycoside-resistance-encoding gene, *kamC*, from *Saccharopolyspora hirsuta*: comparison with *kamB* from *Streptomyces tenebrarius*, *Gene.* 102:19–26.

Hon, W.C., McKay, G.A., Thompson, P.R., Sweet, R.M., Yang, D.S.C., Wright, G.D. and Berghuis, A.M., 1997, Structure of an enzyme required for aminoglycoside resistance reveals homology to eukariotic protein kinases, *Cell.* 89:887–895.

Hoshiko, S., Nojiri, C., Matsunaga, K., Katsumata, K., Satoh, E. and Nagaoka, K., 1988, Nucleotide sequence of the ribostamycin phosphotransferase gene and of its control region in *Streptomyces ribosidificus*, *Gene.* 68:285–296.

Hotta, K., Zhu, C.B., Ogata, T., Sunada, A., Ishikawa, J., Mizuno, S., Ikeda, Y. and Kondo, S., 1996, Enzymatic 2'-N-acetylation of arbekacin and antibiotic activity of its product, *J. Antibiot.* 49:458–464.

Hubbard, S.R., Wei, L., Ellis, L. and Hendrickson, W.A., 1994, Crystal structure of the tyrosine kinase domain of the human insulin receptor, *Nature.* 372:746–754.

Humbert, R. and Altendorf, K., 1989, Defective gamma subunit of ATP synthase (F1F0) from *Escherichia coli* leads to resistance to aminoglycoside antibiotics, *J. Bacteriol.* 171:1435–1444.

Hutchin, T. and Cortopassi, G., 1994, Proposed molecular and cellular mechanism for aminoglycoside ototoxicity, *Antimicrob. Agents Chemother.* 38:2517–2520.

Ishikawa, J. and Hotta, K., 1991, Nucleotide sequence and transcriptional start point of the *kan* gene encoding an aminoglycoside 3-N-acetyltransferase from *Streptomyces griseus* SS-1198PR, *Gene.* 108:127–132.

Johnson, L.N., Noble, M.E. and Owen, D.J., 1996, Active and inactive protein kinases: structural basis for regulation, *Cell.* 85:149–158.

Jones, R.L.D., Jaskula, J.C. and Janssen, G.R., 1992, *In vivo* translational start site selection on leaderless mRNA transcribed from the *Streptomyces fradiae aph* gene, *J. Bacteriol.* 174:4753–4760.

Kabins, S.A., Nathan, C. and Cohen, S., 1976, *In vitro* comparison of netilmicin, a semisynthetic derivative of sisomicin, and four other aminoglycoside antibiotics, *Antimicrob. Agents Chemother.* 10:139–145.

Kadurugamuwa, J.L., Clarke, A.J. and Beveridge, T.J., 1993, Surface action of gentamicin on *Pseudomonas aeruginosa*, *J. Bacteriol.* 174:5798–5805.

Kaufhold, A., Podbielski, A., Horaud, T. and Ferrieri, P., 1992, Identical genes confer high-level resistance to gentamicin upon *Enterococcus faecalis, Enterococccus faecium*, and *Streptococcus agalactiae, Antimicrob. Agents Chemother.* 36:1215–1218.

Kawaguchi, H., Naito, T., Nakagowa, S. and Fuijawa, K., 1972, BBK8, a new semisynthetic aminoglycoside antibiotic, *J. Antibiot.* 25:695.

Kelemen, G.H., Cundliffe, E. and Financsek, I., 1991, Cloning and characterization of gentamicin-resistance genes from *Micromonospora purpurea* and *Micromonospora rosea*, *Gene.* 98:53–60.

Kennelly, P.J. and Potts, M., 1996, Fancy meeting you here! a fresh look at "prokaryotic" protein phosphorylation, *J. Bacteriol.* 178:4759–4764.

Kettner, M., Macickova, T. and Kremery, V.J. (1991), in *Antimicrobial Chemotherapy in Immunocompromised Host, International Congress of Chemotherapy* pp 273–275, Berlin.

Knighton, D.R., Zheng, J.H., Ten Eyck, L.F., Ashford, V.A., Xuong, N.H., Taylor, S.S. and Sowadski, J.M., 1991, Crystal structure of the catalytic subunit of cyclic adenosine monophosphate-dependent protein kinase, *Science*. 253:407–14.

Kocabiyik, S. and Perlin, M.H., 1992a, Altered substrate specificity by substitutions at Tyr218 in bacterial aminoglycoside 3'-phosphotransferase, *FEMS Microbiol. Lett.* 93:199–202.

Kocabiyik, S. and Perlin, M.H., 1992b, Site-specific mutations of conserved C-terminal residues in aminoglycoside 3'-phosphotransferase II: Phenotypic and structural analysis of mutant enzymes, *Biochem. Biophys. Res. Commun.* 185:925–931.

Kocabiyik, S. and Perlin, M.H., 1994, Amino acid substitutions within the analogous nucleotide binding loop (P-loop) of aminoglycoside 3'-phosphotransferase-II, *Int. J. Biochem.* 26:61–66.

Kojic, M., Topisirovic, L. and Vasiljevic, B., 1992, Cloning and characterization of an aminoglycoside resistance determinant from *Micromonospora zionensis, J. Bacteriol.* 174:7868–7872.

Kondo, S., Tamura, A., Gomi, S., Ikeda, Y., Takeuchi, T. and Mitsuhashi, S., 1993, Structures of enzymatically modified products of arbekacin by methicillin-resistant *Staphylococcus aureus, J. Antibiot.* 46:310–315.

Kono, M., Ohmiya, K., Kanda, T., Noguchi, N. and O'hara, K., 1987, Purification and characterization of chromosomal streptomycin adenyltransferase from derivatives of *Bacillus subtilis* Marburg 168, *FEMS Microbiol. Letts.* 40:223–228.

Lambert, T., Gerbaud, G. and Courvalin, P., 1994a, Characterization of the chromosomal *aac(6')-Ij* gene of *Acinetobacter sp. 13* and the *aac(6')-Ih* plasmid gene of *Acinetobacter baumannii, Antimicrob. Agents Chemother.* 38:1883–1889.

Lambert, T., Ploy, M.-C. and Courvalin, P., 1994b, A spontaneous point mutation in the *aac(6')-Ib'* gene results in altered substrate specificity of aminoglycoside 6'-N-acetyltransferase of a *Pseudomonas fluorescens* strain, *FEMS Microbiol. Lett.* 115:297–304.

Lando, D., Cousin, M.A. and Privat de Garilhe, M., 1973, Misreading, a fundamental aspect of the mechanism of action of several aminoglycosides, *Biochemistry.* 12:4528–4533.

Le Goffic, F., Capmau, M.L., Tangy, F. and Baillarge, M., 1979, Mechanism of action of aminoglycoside antibiotics. Binding studies of tobramycin and its 6'-N-acetyl derivative to the bacterial ribosome and its subunits, *Eur. J. Biochem.* 102:73–81.

LeBlanc, D.J., Lee, L.N. and Inamine, J.M., 1991, Cloning and nucleotide base sequence analysis of a spectinomycin adenyltransferase AAD(9) determinant from *Enterococccus faecalis, Antimicrob. Agents Chemother.* 35:1804–1810.

Leclercq, R. and Courvalin, P., 1991, Bacterial resistance to macrolide, lincosamide, and streptogramin antibiotics by target modification, *Antimicrob. Agents Chemother.* 35:1267–1272.

Lee, K.-Y., Hopkins, J.D. and Syvanen, M., 1991, Evolved neomycin phosphotransferase from an isolate of *Klebsiella pneumonia, Mol. Microbiol.* 5:2039–2046.

Lee, S.C., Cleary, P.P. and Gerding, D.N., 1987, More than one DNA sequence encodes the 2"'-O-adenylyltransferase phenotype, *Antimicrob. Agents Chemother.* 31:667–670.

Lopez-Cabrera, M., Perez-Gonzalez, J.A., Heinzel, P., Piepersberg, W. and Jimenez, A., 1989, Isolation and nucleotide sequencing of an aminocyclitol acetyltransferase gene from *Streptomyces rimosus forma paromomycinus, J. Bacteriol.* 171:321–328.

Lovering, A.M., White, L.O. and Reeves, D.S., 1987, AAC(1): a new aminoglycoside-acetylating enzyme modifying the Cl amino group of apramycin, *J. Antimicrob. Chemother.* 20:803–813.

Luzzatto, L., Apirion, D. and Schlessinger, D., 1969, Polyribosome depletion and blockage of the ribosome cycle by streptomycin in *Escherichia coli, J. Mol. Biol.* 42:315–335.

Lyutzkanova, D., Distler, J. and Altenbuchner, J., 1997, A spectinomycin resistance determinant from the spectinomycin producer *Streptomyces flavopersicus, Microbiology.* 143:2135–2143.

Macinga, D.R., Parojcic, M.M. and Rather, P.N., 1995, Identification and analysis of *aarP*, a transcriptional activator of the 2'-N-acetyltransferase in *Providencia stuartii, J. Bacteriol.* 177:3407–3413.

Macinga, D.R. and Rather, P.N., 1996, *aarD*, a *Providencia stuartii* homologue of *cydD*: role in 2'-N-acetyltransferase expression, cell morphology and growth in the presence of an extracellular factor, *Mol. Microbiol.* 19:511–520.

Madhusudan, Trafny, E.A., Xuong, N.-H., Adams, J.A., Ten Eyck, L.F., Taylor, S.S. and Sowadski, J.M., 1994, cAMP-dependent protein kinase: Crystallographic insights into substrate recognition and phosphotransfer, *Prot. Sci.* 3:176–187.

Martel, A., Masson, M., Moreau, N. and Goffic, F.L., 1983, Kinetic studies of aminoglycoside acetyltransferase and phosphotransferase from *Staphylococcus aureus* RPAL, *Eur. J. Biochem.* 133:515–521.

Martin, P., Jullien, E. and Courvalin, P., 1988, Nucleotide sequence of *Acinetobacter baumannii aphA-6* gene: evolutionary and functional implications of sequence homologies with nucleotide-binding proteins, kinases and other aminoglycoside-modifying enzymes, *Mol. Microbiol.* 2:615–625.

Mason, D.J., Dietz, A. and Smith, R.M., 1961, Actinospectacin a new antibiotic.I. Discovery and biological properties, *Antibiot. Chemother.* 11:118–122.

Matkovic, B., Piendl, W. and Bock, A., 1984, Ribosomal resistance as a widespread self-defence in aminoglycoside-producing *Micromonospora* species, *FEMS Microbiol. Letts.* 24:273–276.

Matsumura, M., Katakura, Y., Imanaka, T. and Aiba, S., 1984, Enzymatic and nucleotide sequence studies of a kanamycin-inactivating enzyme encoded by a plasmid from thermophilic bacilli in comparison with that encoded by plasmid pUB110, *J. Bacteriol.* 160:413–420.

Matsunaga, K., Yamaki, H., Nishimura, T. and Tanaka, N., 1986, Inhibition of DNA replication initiation by aminoglycoside antibiotics, *Antimicrob. Agents Chemother.* 30:468–474.

Mazodier, P., Cossart, P., Giraud, E. and Gasser, F., 1985, Completion of the nucleotide sequence of the central region of Tn5 confirms the presence of three resistance genes, *Nucleic Acids Res.* 13:195–205.

McKay, G.A. and Wright, G.D., 1996, Catalytic mechanism of enterococcal kanamycin kinase (APH(3')-IIIa): Viscosity, thio, and solvent isotope effects support a Theorell-Chance mechanism, *Biochemistry.* 35:8680–8685.

McKay, G.A., Robinson, R.A., Lane, W.S. and Wright, G.D., 1994a, Active-site labeling of an aminoglycoside antibiotic phosphotransferase (APH(3')-IIIa), *Biochemistry.* 33:14115–14120.

McKay, G.A., Roestamadji, J., Mobashery, S. and Wright, G.D., 1996, Recognition of aminoglycoside antibiotics by enterococcal-staphylococcal aminoglycoside 3'-phosphotransferase type IIIa: Role of substrate amino groups, *Antimicrob. Agents Chemother.* 40:2648–2650.

McKay, G.A., Thompson, P.R. and Wright, G.D., 1994b, Broad spectrum aminoglycoside phosphotransferase type III from *Enterococcus*: Overexpression, purification, and substrate specificity, *Biochemistry.* 33:6936–6944.

McKay, G.A. and Wright, G.D., 1995, Kinetic mechanism of aminoglycoside phosphotransferase type IIIa: Evidence for a Theorell-Chance mechanism, *J. Biol. Chem.* 270:24686–24692.

Menard, R., Molinas, C., Arthur, M., Duval, J., Courvalin, P. and Leclerq, R., 1993, Overproducion of 3'-aminoglycoside phosphotransferase type I confers resistance to tobramycin in *Escherichia coli*, *Antimicrob. Agents Chemother.* 37:78–83.

Miller, G.H., Sabatelli, F.J., Hare, R.S., Glupczynski, Y., Mackey, P., Shlaes, D., Shimizu, K., Shaw, K.J. and Aminoglycoside Resistance Study Groups, 1997, The most frequent aminoglycoside resistance mechanisms--changes with time and geographic area: a reflection of aminoglycoside usage patterns?, *Clin. Infect. Dis.* 24:S46-S62.

Miller, M.H., Edberg, S.C., Mandel, L.J., Behar, C.F. and Steigbigel, N.H., 1980, Gentamicin uptake in wild-type and aminoglycoside-resistant small-colony mutants of *Staphylococcus aureus*, *Antimicrob. Agents Chemother.* 18:722–729.

Moazed, D. and Noller, H.F., 1987, Interaction of antibiotics with functional sites in 16S ribosomal RNA, *Nature.* 27:389–394.

Morris, J.C. and Mensa-Wilmot, K., 1997, Role of 2,6-dideoxy-2,6-diaminoglucose in activation of a eukaryotic phospholipase C by aminoglycoside antibiotics, *J. Biol. Chem.* 272:29554–29559.

Murphy, E., 1985, Nucleotide sequence of a spectinomycin adenyltransferase AAD(9) determinant from *Staphylococcus aureus* and its relationship to AAD(3")(9), *Mol. Gen. Genet.* 200:33–39.

Musser, J.M., 1995, Antimicrobial agent resistance in mycobacteria: molecular genetic insights, *Clin. Microbiol. Rev.* 8:496–514.

Nagabhushan, T.L., Cooper, A.B., Tsai, H., Daniels, P.J. and Miller, G.H., 1978, The syntheses and biological properties of 1-N-(S-4-amino-2-hydroxybutyryl)-gentamicin B and 1-N-(S-3-amino-2-hydroxypropionyl)-gentamicin B, *J. Antibiot.* 31:681–687.

Nassberger, L., Bergstrand, A. and DePierre, J.W., 1990, Intracellular distribution of gentamicin within the rat kidney cortex: a cell fractionation study, *Exp. Mol. Pathol.* 52:212–220.

O'hara, K., Ohmiya, K. and Kono, M., 1988, Structure of adenylylated streptomycin synthesized enzymatically by *Bacillus subtilis*, *Antimicrob. Agents Chemother.* 32:949–950.

Ohmiya, K., Tanaka, T., Noguchi, N., O'Hara, K. and Kono, M., 1989, Nucleotide sequence of the chromosomal gene coding for the aminoglycoside 6-adenylyltransferase from *Bacillus subtilis* Marburg 168, *Gene.* 78:377–378.

Ohta, T. and Hasegawa, M., 1993a, Analysis of the nucleotide sequence of *fmrT* encoding the self-defense gene of the istamycin producer, *Streptomyces tenjimariensis* ATCC 31602; comparison with the squences of *kamB* of *Streptomyces tenebrarius* NCIB 11028 and *kamC* of iCL102, *J. Antibiot.* 46:511–517.

Ohta, T. and Hasegawa, M., 1993b, Analysis of the self-defense gene (*fmrO*) of a fortimicin A (astromicin) producer, *Micromonospora olivasterospora*: comparison with other aminoglycoside-resistance-encoding genes, *Gene*. 127:63–69.

Oka, A., Sugisaki, H. and Takanami, M., 1981, Nucleotide sequence of the kanamycin resistance transposon Tn*903*, *J. Mol. Biol*. 147:217–226.

Ounissi, H. and Courvalin, P. (1987), Nucleotide sequences of streptococcal genes, in *Streptococcal Genetics* (J. J. Ferretti and R. Curtiss III, Eds.) pp 275, American Society for Microbiology, Washington, D.C.

Owen, D.J., Noble, M.E., Garman, E.F., Papageorgiou, A.C. and Johnson, L.N., 1995, Two structures of the catalytic domain of phosphorylase kinase: an active protein kinase complexed with substrate analogue and product, *Structure*. 3:467–482.

Pansegrau, W., Miele, L., Lurz, R. and Lanka, E., 1987, Nucleotide sequence of the kanamycin resistance determinant of plasmid RP4:Homology to other aminoglycoside 3'-phosphotransferases, *Plasmid*. 18:193–204.

Papadopoulou, B. and Courvalin, P., 1988, Dispersal in *Campylobacter spp.* of *aphA-3*, a kanamycin resistance determinant from gram-positive cocci, *Antimicrob. Agents Chemother*. 32:945–948.

Pardo, J.M., Malpartida, F., Rico, M. and Jimenez, A., 1985, Biochemical basis of resistance to hygromycin B in *Streptomyces hygroscopicus*--the producing organism, *J. Gen. Microbiol*. 131:1289–1298.

Payie, K.G. and Clarke, A.J., 1997, Characterization of gentamicin 2'-N-acetyltransferase from *Providencia stuartii*: its use of peptidoglycan metabolites for acetylation of both aminoglycosides and peptidoglycan, *J. Bacteriol*. 179:4106–4114.

Payie, K.G., Rather, P.N. and Clarke, A.J., 1995, Contribution of gentamicin 2'-N-acetyltransferase to the O-acetylation of peptidoglycan in *Providencia stuartii*, *J. Bacteriol*. 177:4303–4310.

Payie, K.G., Strating, H. and Clarke, A.J., 1996, The role of O-acetylation in the metabolism of peptidoglycan in *Providencia stuartii*, *Microb. Drug Resist*. 2:135–140.

Perdersen, L.C., Benning, M.M. and Holden, H.M., 1995, Structural investigation of the antibiotic and ATP-binding sites in kanamycin nucleotidyltransferase, *Biochemsitry*. 34:13305–13311.

Piepersberg, W., Distler, J., Heinzel, P. and Perez-Gonzalez, J.-A., 1988, Antibiotic resistance by modification: many resistance genes could be derived from cellular control genes in actinomycetes.-A hypothesis, *Actinomycetol*. 2:83–98.

Piepersberg, W., Heinzel, P., Mansouri, K., Mönnighoff, U. and Pissowotzki, K. (1991), Evolution of antibiotic resistance and production genes in streptomycetes, in *Genetics and product formation in Streptomyces* (S. Baumberg, H. Krügel and D. Novack, Eds.), pp. 161–170, Plenum Press, New York.

Priuska, E.M. and Schacht, J., 1995, Formation of free radicals by gentamycin and iron and evidence for an iron/gentamicin complex, *Biochem. Pharmacol*. 50:1749.

Radika, K. and Northop, D.B., 1984a, Substrate specificities and structure-activity relationships for acylation of antibiotics catalyzed by kanamycin acetyltransferase, *Biochemistry*. 23:5118–5122.

Radika, K. and Northrop, D.B., 1984b, The kinetic mechanism of kanamycin acetyltransferase derived from the use of alternative antibiotics and coenzymes, *J. Biol. Chem*. 259:12543–12546.

Radika, K. and Northrop, D., 1984c, Purification of two forms of kanamycin acetyltransferase from *Escherichia coli*, *Arch. Biochem. Biophys*. 233:272–285.

Radika, K. and Northrop, D.B., 1984d, Correlation of antibiotic resistance with V_{max}/K_m ratio of enzymatic modification of aminoglycosides by kanamycin acetyl-transferase, *Antimicrob. Agents Chemother*. 25:479–482.

Rao, R.N., Allen, N.E., Hobbs, J.N.J., Alborn, W.E.J., Kirst, H.A. and Paschal, J.W., 1983, Genetic and enzymatic basis of hygromycin B resistance in *Escherichia coli*, *Antimicrob. Agents Chemother*. 24:689–695.

Rather, P.N., Mann, P.A., Mierzwa, R., Hare, R.S., Miller, G.H. and Shaw, K.J., 1993a, Analysis of the *aac(3)-VIa* gene encoding a novel 3-N-acetyltransferase, *Antimicrob. Agents Chemother*. 37:2074–2079.

Rather, P.N., Mierzwa, R., Hare, R., Miller, G. and Shaw, K., 1992a, Cloning and DNA sequence analysis of an *aac(3)-Vb* gene from *Serratia marcescens*, *Antimicrob. Agents Chemother*. 36:2222–2227.

Rather, P.N., Munayyer, H., Mann, P.A., Hare, R.S., Miller, G.H. and Shaw, K.J., 1992b, Genetic analysis of bacterial acetyltransferases: Identification of amino acids determining the specificities of the aminoglycoside 6'-N-acetyltransferase Ib and IIa proteins, *J. Bacteriol*. 175:3196–3203.

Rather, P.N. and Orosz, E., 1994, Characterization of *aarA*, a pleiotrophic negative regulator of the 2'-N-acetyltransferase in *Providencia stuartii*, *J. Bacteriol*. 176:5140–5144.

Rather, P.N., Orosz, E., Shaw, K.J., Hare, R. and Miller, G., 1993b, Characterization and transcriptional regulation of the 2'-N-acetyltransferase gene from *Providencia stuartii*, *J. Bacteriol*. 175:6492–6498.

Rather, P.N., Parojcic, M.M. and Paradise, M.R., 1997a, An extracellular factor regulating expression of the chromosomal aminoglycoside 2'-N-acetyltransferase of *Providencia stuartii*, *Antimicrob. Agents Chemother*. 41:1749–1754.

Rather, P.N., Solinsky, K., A., Paradise, M.R. and Parojcic, M.M., 1997b, *aarC*, an essential gene involved in density-dependent regulation of the 2'-N-acetyltransferase in *Providencia stuartii*, *J. Bacteriol.* 179:2267–2273.

Roestamadji, J., Grapsas, I. and Mobashery, S., 1995a, Loss of individual electrostatic interactions between aminoglycoside antibiotics and resistance enzymes as an effective means to overcoming bacterial drug resistance, *J. Am. Chem. Soc.* 117:11060–11069.

Roestamadji, J., Grapsas, I. and Mobashery, S., 1995b, Mechanism-based inactivation of bacterial aminoglycoside 3'-phosphotransferases, *J. Am. Chem. Soc.* 117:80–84.

Rouch, D.A., Byrne, M.E., Kong, Y.C. and Skurray, R.A., 1987, The *aacA-aphD* gentamicin and kanamycin resistance determinant of Tn*4001* from *Staphylococcus aureus*: Expression and nucleotide sequence analysis, *J. Gen. Microbiol.* 133:3039–3052.

Sakon, J., Liao, H.H., Kanikula, A.M., Benning, M.M., Rayment, I. and Holden, H.M., 1993, Molecular structure of kanamycin nucleotidyl transferase determind to 3Å resolution, *Biochemistry.* 32:11977–11984.

Salauze, D. and Davies, J., 1991a, Isolation and characterization of and aminoglycoside phosphotransferase from neomycin-producing *Micromonospora chalcea*: Comparison with that of *Streptomyces fradiae* and other producers of 4,6-disubstituted 3-deoxystreptamine antibiotics, *J. Antibiot.* 44:1432–1443.

Salauze, D., Perez-Gonzalez, J.-A., Piepersberg, W. and Davies, J., 1991b, Characterization of aminoglycoside acetyltransferase-encoding genes of neomycin-producing *Micromonospora chalcea* and *Streptomyces fradiae*, *Gene.* 101:143–148.

Sanders, T.W.J., Reinhard, M.K., Jollow, D.J. and Hottendorf, G.H., 1993, Lack of *in vivo* evidence of a cytochrome P450 metabolite participating in aminoglycoside nephrotoxicity, *Biochem. Pharmacol.* 45:780–782.

Sarwar, M. and Akhtar, M., 1990, Cloning of aminoglycoside phosphotransferase (APH) gene from antibiotic-producing strain of *Bacillus circulans* into a high-expression vector, pKK223–3. Purification, properties and location of the enzyme, *Biochem. J.* 268:671–677.

Sawaya, M.R., Pelletier, H., Kumar, A., Wilson, S.H. and Kraut, J., 1994, Crystal structure of rat DNA polymerase β: evidence for a common polymerase mechanism, *Science.* 264:1930–1935.

Schacht, J., 1993, Biochemical basis of aminoglycoside ototoxicity, *Otolaryngol. Clin. North. Am.* 26:845–856.

Schatz, A., Bugie, E. and Waksman, S.A., 1944, Streptomycin, a substance exibiting antibiotic activity against Gram-positive and Gram-negative bacteria, *Proc. Soc. Exp. Biol. Med.* 55(66–69).

Schlessinger, D., 1988, Failure of aminoglycoside antibiotics to kill anaerobic, low-pH, and resistant cultures, *Clin. Microbiol. Rev.* 1:54–59.

Schmidt, F.R., Nucken, E.J. and Henschke, R.B., 1988, Nucleotide sequence analysis of 2''-aminoglycoside nucleotidyl-transferase ANT(2'') from Tn*4000*: its relationship with AAD(3'') and impact on Tn*21* evolution, *Mol. Microbiol.* 2:709–717.

Scholz, P., Haring, V., Wittmann-Liebold, B., Ashman, K., Bagdasarian, M. and Scherzinger, E., 1989, Complete nucleotide sequence and gene organization of the broad-host-range plasmid RSF1010, *Gene.* 75(271–288).

Schwocho, L.R., Schaffner, C.P., Miller, G.H., Hare, R.S. and Shaw, K.J., 1995, Cloning and characterization of a 3-N-aminoglycoside acetyltransferase gene, *aac(3)-Ib*, from *Pseudomonas aeruginosa*, *Antimicrob. Agents Chemother.* 39:1790–1796.

Shaw, K.J., 1997, Personal communication.

Shaw, K.J., Cramer, C.A., Rizzo, M., Mierzwa, R., Gewain, K., Miller, G.H. and Hare, R.S., 1989, Isolation, characterization, and DNA sequence analysis of an AAC(6')-II gene from *Pseudomonas aeruginosa*, *Antimicrob. Agents Chemother.* 33:2052–2062.

Shaw, K.J., Gomez-Lus, S. and Shannon, K.W., 1992a, unpublished sequence, GenBank accession no. L06160 .

Shaw, K.J. and Leal, I., 1992, unpublished sequence GenBank accession no. L06161 .

Shaw, K.J., Rather, P.N., Sabatelli, F.J., Mann, P., Munayyer, H., Mierzwa, R., Petrikkos, G.L., Hare, R.S., Miller, G.H., Bennett, P. and Downey, P., 1992b, Characterization of the chromosomal *aac(6')-Ic* gene from *Serratia marcescens*, *Antimicrob. Agents Chemother.* 36:1447–1455.

Shaw, K.J., Rather, P.N., Hare, R.S. and Miller, G.H., 1993, Molecular genetics of aminoglycoside resistance genes and familial relationships of the aminoglycoside-modifying enzymes, *Microbiol. Rev.* 57:138–163.

Shomura, T., Ezaki, N., Tsuruoka, T., Niwa, T., Akita, E. and Niida, T., 1970, Studies on antibiotic SF-733, a new antibiotic. I. Taxonomy, isolation and characterization, *J. Antibiot.* 23:155–161.

Sigmund, C.D., Ettayebi, M. and Morgan, E.A., 1984, Antibiotic resistance mutations in 16S and 23S ribosomal RNA genes of *Escherichia coli*, *Nucleic Acids Res.* 12:4653–4663.

Siregar, J.J., Lerner, S.A. and Mobashery, S., 1994, Purification and characterization of aminoglycoside 3'-phosphotransferase Type IIa and kinetic comparison with a new mutant enzyme, *Antimicrob. Agents Chemother.* 38:641–647.

Siregar, J.J., Miroshnikov, K. and Mobashery, S., 1995, Purification, characterization, and investigation of the mechanism of aminoglycoside 3'-phosphotransferase Type Ia, *Biochemistry* 34:12681–12688.

Skeggs, P.A., Holmes, D.J. and Cundliffe, E., 1987, Cloning of aminoglycoside-resistance determinants from *Streptomyces tenebrarius* and comparison with related genes from other actinomycetes, *J. Gen. Microbiol.* 133:915–923.

Song, B.B. and Schacht, J., 1996, Variable efficacy of radical scavengers and iron chelators to attenuate gentamicin ototoxicity in guinea pig *in vivo*, *Hearing Res.* 94:87.

Sundin, G.W. and Bender, C.L., 1996, Dissemination of the *strA-strB* streptomycin-resistance genes among commensal and pathogenic bacteria from humans, animals, and plants, *Mol. Ecol.* 5:133–143.

Suter, T.M., Viswanathan, V.K. and Cianciotto, N.P., 1997, Isolation of a gene encoding a novel spectinomycin phosphotransferase from *Legionella pneumophila*, *Antimicrob. Agents Chemother.* 41:1385–1388.

Sutherland, R., 1991, β-Lactamase inhibitors and reversal of antibiotic resistance, *Trends Pharmacol. Sci.* 12:227–232.

Taber, H.W., Mueller, J.P., Miller, P.F. and Arrow, A.S., 1987, Bacterial uptake of aminoglycoside antibiotics, *Microbiol. Rev.* 51:439–457.

Tanaka, N., Matsunaga, K., Yamaki, H. and Nishimura, T., 1984, Inhibition of initiation of DNA synthesis by aminoglycoside antibiotics, *Biochem. Biophys. Res. Commun.* 122:460–465.

Tangy, F., Capmau, M.-L. and Le Goffic, F., 1983, Photo-induced labelling of *Escherichia coli* ribosomes by a tobramycin analog, *Eur. J. Biochem.* 131:581–587.

Taylor, D.E., Yan, W., Ng, L.K., Manavathu, E.K. and Courvalin, P., 1988, Genetic characterization of kanamycin resistance in *Campylobacter coli*, *Ann. Inst. Pasteur Microbiol.* 139:665–676.

Taylor, S.S., Knighton, D.R., Zheng, J., Ten Eyck, L.F. and Sowadski, J.M., 1992, Structural framework for the protein kinase family, *Annu. Rev. Cell Biol.* 8:429–62.

Tenover, F.C., Filpula, D., Phillips, K.L. and Plorde, J.J., 1988, Cloning and sequencing of a gene encoding an aminoglycoside 6'-*N*-acetyltransferase from an R factor of *Citrobacter diversus*, *J. Bacteriol.* 170:471–473.

Tenover, F.C., Gilbert, T. and O'Hara, P., 1988, Nucleotide sequence of a novel kanamycin resistance gene, *aphA-7*, from *Campylobacter jejuni* and comparison to other kanamycin phosphotransferase genes, *Plasmid.* 22:52–58.

Tenover, F.C., Phillips, K.L., Gilbert, T., Lockhart, P., O'Hara, P.J. and Plorde, J.J., 1989, Development of a DNA probe from the deoxyribonucleotide sequence of a 3-N-aminoglycoside acetyltransferase [AAC(3)-I] resistance gene, *Antimicrob. Agents Chemother.* 33:551–559.

Terán, F.J., Suárez, J.E. and Mendoza, M.C., 1991, Cloning, sequencing, and use as a molecular probe of a gene encoding an aminoglycoside 6'-*N*-acetyltransferase of broad substrate profile, *Antimicrob. Agents Chemother.* 35:714–719.

Thal, L.A., Chow, J.W., Patterson, J.E., Perri, M.B., Donabedian, S., Clewell, D.B. and Zervos, M.J., 1993, Molecular characterization of highly gentamicin-resistant *Enterococcus faecalis* isolates lacking high-level streptomycin resistance, *Antimicrob. Agents Chemother.* 37:134–137.

Thompson, C.J. and Gray, G.S., 1993, Nucleotide sequence of a streptomycete aminoglycoside phosphotransferase gene and its relationship to phosphotransferases encoded by resistance plasmids, *Proc. Natl. Acad. Sci. U S A.* 80:5190–5194.

Thompson, C.J., Ward, J.M. and Hopwood, D.A., 1980, DNA cloning in *Streptomyces*: resistance genes from antibiotic-producing species, *Nature.* 286:525–527.

Thompson, J., Skeggs, P.A. and Cundliffe, E., 1985, Methylation of 16S ribosomal RNA and resistance to the aminoglycoside antibiotics gentamicin and kanamycin determined by DNA from the gentamicin-producer, *Micromonospora purpurea*, *Mol. Gen. Genet.* 201:168–173.

Thompson, P.R., Hughes, D.W. and Wright, G.D., 1996a, Mechanism of aminoglycoside 3'-phosphotransferase type IIIa: His188 is not a phosphate-accepting-residue, *Chem. Biol.* 3:747–755.

Thompson, P.R., Hughes, D.W. and Wright, G.D., 1996b, Regiospecificity of aminoglycoside phosphotransferase from *Enterococci* and *Staphylococci* (APH(3')-IIIa), *Biochemistry.* 35:8686–8695.

Tran van Nhieu, G. and Collatz, E., 1987, Primary structure of an aminoglycoside 6'-N-acetyltransferase AAC(6')-4, fused in vivo with the signal peptide of the Tn3-encoded $-lactamase, *J. Bacteriol.* 169:5708–5714.

Trieu-Cuot, P. and Courvalin, P., 1983, Nucleotide sequence of the *Streptococcus faecalis* plasmid gene encoding the 3'5''-aminoglycoside phosphotransferase type III, *Gene.* 23:331–341.

Ubukata, K., Yamashita, N., Gotoh, A. and Konno, M., 1984, Purification and characterization of aminoglycoside-modifying enzymes from *Staphylococcus aureus* and *Staphylococcus epidermidis*, *Antimicrob. Agents Chemother.* 25:754–759.

Umezawa, H., Nishimura, Y., Tsuchiya, T. and Umezawa, S., 1972, Syntheses of 6'-N-methyl-kanamycin and 3',4'-dideoxy-6'-N-methylkanamycin B active against resistant strains having 6'-N-acetylating enzymes, *J. Antibiot.* 25:743–745.

Umezawa, H., Ueda, M., Maeda, K., Yagishita, K., Kando, S., Okami, Y., Utahara, R., Osato, Y., Nitta, K. and Kakeuchi, T., 1957, Production and isolation of a new antibiotic kanamycin, *J. Antibiot.* 10:181–189.

Vakulenko, S.B. and Entina, E.G., 1990, Nucleotide sequence of *aacC2* gene from a clinical strain of *Escherichia coli*, *Antibiot. Khimioter.* 35:46–50.

Van Pelt, J.E., Iyengar, R. and Frey, P.A., 1986, Gentamicin nucleotidyltransferase. Stereochemical inversion at phosphorus in enzymatic 2'-deoxyadenylyl transfer to tobramycin, *J. Biol. Chem.* 261:15995–15999.

Van Pelt, J.E. and Northrop, D.B., 1984, Purification and properties of gentamicin nucleotidyltransferase from *Escherichia coli*: Nucleotide specificity, pH optimum, and the separation of two electrophoretic variants, *Arch. Biochem. Biophys.* 230:250–263.

Van Pelt, J.E., Mooberry, E.S. and Frey, P.A., 1990, ^{1}H, ^{13}C, and ^{31}P Nuclear magnetic resonance spectral assignments for tobramycin, 2"-(adenosine-5'-phosphoryl)-tobramycin and 2"-(adenosine-5'-thiophosphoryl)-tobramycin, *Arch. Biochem. Biophys.* 280:284–291.

Vliegenthart, J.S., Ketelaar-van Gaalen, P.A. and van de Klundert, J.A., 1989, Nucleotide sequence of the *aacC2* gene, a gentamicin resistance determinant involved in a hospital epidemic of multiply resistant members of the family Enterobacteriaceae, *Antimicrob. Agents Chemother.* 33:1153–1159.

Vliegenthart, J.S., Ketelaar-van Gaalen, P.A. and van de Klundert, J.A., 1991, Nucleotide sequence of the *aacC3* gene, a gentamicin resistance determinant encoding aminoglycoside-(3)-N-acetyltransferase III expressed in *Pseudomonas aeruginosa* but not in *Escherichia coli*, *Antimicrob. Agents Chemother.* 35:892–897.

Vögtli, M. and Hütter, R., 1987, Characterisation of the hydroxystreptomycin phosphotransferase gene (*sph*) of *Streptomyces glaucescens*: nucleotide sequence and promoter analysis, *Mol. Gen. Genet.* 208:195–203.

Waksman, S.A. and Lechevalier, H.A., 1949, Neomycin, a new antibiotic active against streptomycin-resistant bacteria, including tuberculosis organisms, *Science.* 109:305–307.

Wang, Y., Hamasaki, K. and Rando, R.R., 1997, Specificity of aminoglycoside binding to RNA constructs derived from the 16S rRNA deconding region an the HIV-RRE activator region, *Biochemistry.* 36:768–779.

Weinstein, M.J., Luedemann, G.M., Oden, E.M., Wagman, G.H., Rosselet, J.P., Marquez, J.A., Coniglio, C.T., Charney, W., Herzog, H.L. and Black, J., 1963, Gentamicin, a new antibiotic complex from *Micromonospora*, *J. Med. Chem.* 6:463–464.

Weinstein, M.J., Marquez, J.A., Testa, R.T., Wagman, G.H., Oden, E.M. and Waitz, J.A., 1970, Antibiotic 6640, a new *Micromonospora*-produced aminoglycoside antibiotic, *J. Antibiotic.* 23:551–554.

Werstuck, G., Zapp, M.L. and Green, M.R., 1996, A non-canonical base pair within the human immunodificiency virus Rev-responsive element is involved in both Rev and small molecule recognition, *Chem. Biol.* 3:129–137.

Williams, J.W. and Northrop, D.B., 1976, Purification and properties of gentamincin acetyltransferase I, *Biochemistry.* 15:125–131.

Williams, J.W. and Northrop, D.B., 1978a, Kinetic mechanism of gentamicin acetyltransferase I, *J. Biol. Chem.* 253:5902–5907.

Williams, J.W. and Northrop, D.B., 1978b, Substrate specificity and structure-activity relationships of gentamicin acetyltransferase I, *J. Biol. Chem.* 253:5908–5914.

Williams, J.W. and Northrup, D.B., 1979, Synthesis of a tight-binding, multisubstrate analog inhibitor of gentamicin acetyltransferase, *J. Antibiot.* 32:1147–1154.

Woo, P.W.K., Dion, H.W. and Bartz, Q.R., 1971, Butirosins A and B, aminoglycoside antibiotics. I. Structural units. *Tet. Lett.*:2617–2620.

Woodcock, J., Moazed, D., Cannon, M., Davies, J. and Noller, H.F., 1991, Interaction of antibiotics with A- and P-site-specific bases in 16S ribosomal RNA, *EMBO J.* 10:3099–3103.

Wright, G.D. and Ladak, P., 1997, Overexpression and characterization of the chromosomal aminoglycoside 6'-*N*-acetyltransferase from *Enterococcus faecium*, *Antimicrob. Agents Chemother.* 41:956–960.

Wu, H.Y., Miller, G.H., Guzman Blanco, M., Hare, R.S. and Shaw, K.J., 1997, Cloning and characterization of an aminoglycoside 6'-N-acetyltransferase gene from *Citrobacter freundii* which confers an altered resistance profile, *Antimicrob. Agents Chemother.* 41:2439–2447.

Xu, R.-M., Carmel, G., Kuret, J. and Cheng, X., 1996, Structural basis for selectivity of the isoquinoline sulfonamide family of protein kinase inhibitors, *Proc. Natl. Acad. Sci. USA.* 93:6308–6313.

Yenofsky, R.L., Fine, M. and Pellow, J.W., 1990, A mutant neomycin phosphotransferase II gene reduces the resistance of transformants to antibiotic selection pressure, *Proc. Natl. Acad. Sci. USA.* 87:3435–3439.

Young, M.L., Bains, M., Bell, A. and Hancock, R.E., 1992, Role of *Pseudomonas aeruginosa* outer membrane protein OprH in polymyxin and gentamicin resistance: isolation of an OprH-deficient mutant by gene replacement techniques, *Antimicrob. Agents Chemother.* 36:2566–2568.

Zalacain, M., Gonzalez, A., Guerrero, M.C., Mattaliano, R.J., Malpartida, F. and Jimenez, A., 1986, Nucleotide sequence of the hygromycin B phosphotransferase gene from *Streptomyces hygroscopicus*, *Nucleic Acids Res.* 14:1565–1581.

Zalacain, M., Malpartida, F., Pulido, D. and Jimenez, A., 1987a, Cloning and expression in *Escherichia coli* of a hygromycin B phosphotransferase gene from *Streptomyces hygroscopicus*, *Eur. J. Biochem.* 162:413–418.

Zalacain, M., Pardo, J.M. and Jimenez, A., 1987b, Purification and characterization of a hygromycin B phosphotransferase from *Streptomyces hygroscopicus*, *Eur. J. Biochem.* 162:419–422.

Zapp, M.L., Stern, S. and Green, M.R., 1993, Small molecules that selectively block RNA binding of HIV-1 Rev protein inhibit Rev function and viral production, *Cell.* 74:969–978.

Zhang, C.-C., 1996, Bacterial signalling involving eukaryotic-type protein kinases, *Mol. Microbiol.* 20:9–15.

Zhang, F., Strand, A., Robbins, D., Cobb, M.H. and Goldsmith, E.J., 1994, Atomic structure of the MAP kinase ERK2 at 2.3 Å resolution, *Nature.* 367:704–11.

Zhou, J. and Adams, J.A., 1997, Is there a catalytic base in the active site of cAMP-dependent protein kinase? *Biochemistry.* 36:2977–2984.

5

HOW β-LACTAMASES HAVE DRIVEN PHARMACEUTICAL DRUG DISCOVERY

From Mechanistic Knowledge to Clinical Circumvention

Karen Bush[1] and Shahriar Mobashery[2]

[1]Drug Discovery
R. W. Johnson Pharmaceutical Research Institute
Raritan, New Jersey 08869
[2]Department of Chemistry
Wayne State University
Detroit, Michigan 48202

1. INTRODUCTION

Although antibiotic resistance has only recently become a recognized topic for the popular press, resistance has been the major stimulus for the pharmaceutical development of novel β-lactam antibiotics. Benzylpenicillin (Penicillin G), the first member of this important class of antibacterial agents, was initially used to counteract Gram-positive infections, particularly those caused by *Streptococcus pneumoniae*, the scourge of hospitals in the 1940s. Before penicillins found widespread clinical utility, it was discovered that certain bacterial enzymes, the β-lactamases, had the ability to hydrolyze the lactam ring of these antibiotics and render them ineffective as antibacterial agents (Abraham and Chain, 1940; Kirby, 1944). When resistance to penicillin was soon selected rapidly by β-lactamase-producing bacteria, it became obvious that the hydrolytic β-lactamases could potentially destroy the utility of this potent class of antibiotics. The pharmaceutical industry has proceeded to identify novel β-lactams over the past 40 years in an attempt to keep ahead of the continuous evolution of new β-lactamases with altered hydrolytic properties. Two approaches were undertaken: development of agents stable to hydrolysis by the major β-lactamases, and identification of potent inhibitors for these enzymes. The topics germane to these strategies will be addressed in this manuscript.

Resolving the Antibiotic Paradox, edited by Rosen and Mobashery.
Kluwer Academic / Plenum Publishers, New York, 1998.

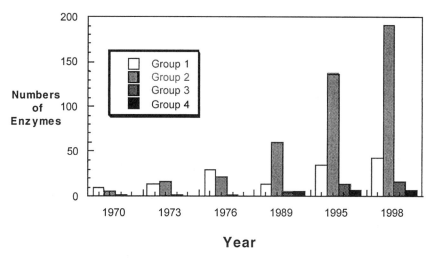

Figure 1. Increasing numbers of characterized β-lactamases in published literature are depicted according to the year the data were compiled.

2. CLASSIFICATION AND NUMBER OF β-LACTAMASES

2.1. Functional Classification Schemes

Jack and Richmond (1970), Richmond and Sykes (1973), Sykes and Matthew (1976), and Bush, Jacoby and Medeiros (1995) have all classified β-lactamases based upon substrate profiles, inhibition profiles, isoelectric points and molecular size. Early schemes were limited, in that methodology was not adequate to measure low rates of hydrolysis and molecular sizes were often inaccurate due to the methods used. For example, the class A β-lactamases SHV-1 and PSE-2 were reported in 1979 to have molecular sizes of 17,000 and 41,000, respectively, based on molecular sieving, and a size of 12,400 for PSE-2 based on ultracentrifugation; after amino-acid sequences were determined in the late 1980s these enzymes were found to have molecular sizes of 28,800 and 27,500, respectively. Also, many substrates and inhibitors, such as imipenem and clavulanic acid, now considered to be critical for defining functional β-lactamase subgroups, were not available prior to 1976 when the early studies were published.

The most current functional classification is that of Bush et al. (1995) in which 188 discrete β-lactamases were identified. That functional classification, based on one first proposed in 1989 (Bush, 1989) and expanded in 1995, was designed empirically to try to correlate function with known molecular structure as best as possible at the time. When the scheme was first introduced, only 19 of the 84 β-lactamases in the scheme had any sequence information, and substrate/inhibitor profiles were the most important attributes for a newly described β-lactamase. Today, sequencing has become so routine that most new β-lactamases will be classified according to molecular structure, and functional classifications will be useful to define the properties important for microbiologists and clinicians.

Molecular classes can be divided into two major subdivisions, those enzymes that utilize serine at the active site and those that require a divalent cation, generally Zn^{2+}, for hydrolysis. Functional classes were established such that serine-based enzymes in molecular classes C (Jaurin and Grundstrom, 1981), and A (Ambler, 1980) and D (Huovinen et al., 1988) correlated to functional groups 1 and 2, respectively (Bush, 1989; Bush et al., 1995). The zinc-based enzymes of molecular class B (Ambler, 1980) are members of functional class 3 (Bush, 1989). A final functional group 4 includes β-lactamases that will eventually be assigned to one of the other groups when the molecular characteristics are better defined.

At the present time the number of unique β-lactamases has risen to at least 255. As seen in Figure 1, the largest increase in β-lactamases is the serine-based group 2 enzymes. Many of the more recently described enzymes fall into the subgroup of extended-spectrum β-lactamases (ESBLs) derived from the common TEM and SHV β-lactamases. The fewest characterized enzymes in any molecular class include the class B metallo-β-lactamases in functional group 3. Some of these metalloenzymes have the broadest substrate specificity of any β-lactamase, a development that has affected a number of drug discovery programs. β-lactamases such as the CcrA enzymes from *Bacteroides fragilis* can hydrolyze virtually every β-lactam class with the exception of the monobactams [Yang et al., 1992]. In addition, these enzymes are not inhibited by the standard β-lactamase inactivators, so that their production in a clinically relevant isolate virtually negates the use of β-lactams for the treatment of infection.

2.2. Mechanisms of Action

β-Lactam antibiotics belong to a group of enzyme inactivators which are referred to as mechanism-based inactivators. This group of enzyme inactivators exploits the normal catalytic processes of the targeted enzymes in the onset of inhibition. The enzyme inactivation is usually covalent and functionally irreversible. It is known that β-lactam antibiotics inhibit the processes of cell-wall biosynthesis (Tipper and Strominger, 1965; Ghuysen, 1991; Ghuysen et al., 1996; Ghuysen, 1997), and specifically the transpeptidation reaction which results in cross-linking of the bacterial cell wall. This reaction is catalyzed by certain enzymes which are collectively known as penicillin-binding proteins (PBPs). They are referred to as such since they were identified to be covalently modified by penicillins. This covalent modification of PBPs is the critical step which deprives the bacterium of the biological function of these enzymes, namely cross-linking of the cell wall, which leads to bacterial cell death.

The transpeptidase reaction of these PBPs facilitates the trading of one amide bond for another in the course of the cross-linking reaction. This was an expedient development in evolution of bacteria since ATP, the reagent used in typical amide bond-forming reactions is lacking in the periplasmic space of these organisms where the cross-linking reaction takes place. These enzymes have utilized an active-site-serine strategy to make possible the transpeptidation reaction.

The peptidoglycan has features such as D-Ala, D-Glu, diaminopimelate, and amide linkages via the D-Glu side chain which are uniquely bacterial (Fig. 2). The active-site serine of these enzymes attacks the carbonyl of the penultimate D-Ala, with concomitant departure of the terminal D-Ala, to give rise to an acyl-enzyme intermediate. An amine from the side chain of another peptidoglycan, either that of a diaminopimelate or a modified lysine derivative, approaches the ester of the acyl-enzyme intermediate to give the cross-linked species.

It was suggested insightfully by Tipper and Strominger that the backbone of a β-lactam antibiotic, such as a typical penicillin, mimics the topology of the acyl-D-Ala-D-Ala portion of the bacterial peptidoglycan (Tipper and Strominger, 1965; Fig. 3). Hence, the β-

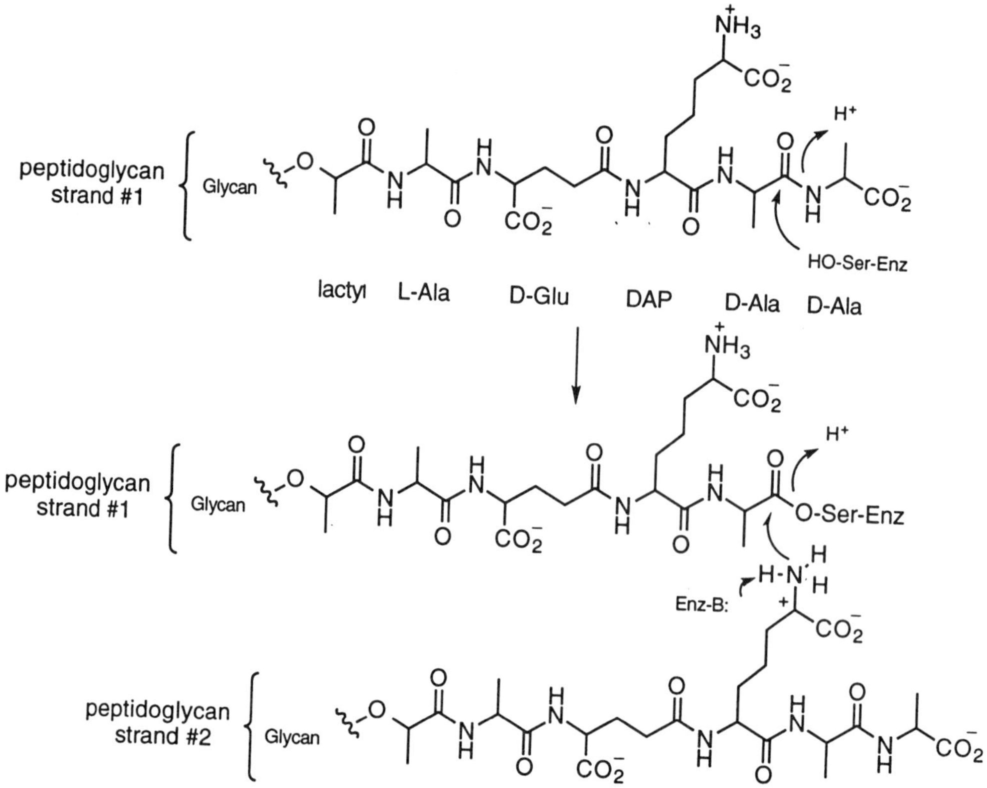

Figure 2. A representative transpeptidation reaction in Gram-negative bacteria catalyzed by some PBPs commences by acylation of the active-site serine of the enzyme by one strand of peptidoglycan. The approach of the second strand of the peptidoglycan to the ester of the acyl-enzyme intermediate results in the cross-linked cell wall.

lactam would modify the active-site serine of PBPs via its carbonyl group, which spatially corresponds to that of the penultimate D-Ala of the peptidoglycan strand. The penicillin structure in its entirety would obviously remain tethered to the enzyme as an integral part of the "acyl-enzyme intermediate", and it would present a steric barrier to the approach of the second strand of peptidoglycan at the ester carbonyl. Therefore, transpeptidation is prevented, and the enzyme is no longer available for its normal function, since it is covalently modified in the active site.

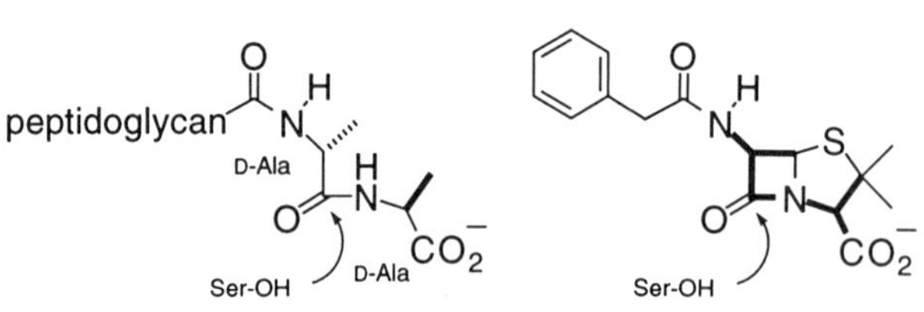

Figure 3. Penicillin G (right-hand structure) is depicted here as a mimic of the topology of the C-terminal portion of the peptidoglycan (left-hand structure). The carbonyl of the penultimate D-Ala corresponds spatially to that of the β-lactam carbonyl. Both acylate the active-site serine of the PBP.

2.3. Evolution

We know that the above-mentioned function of β-lactam antibiotics leads to bacterial death. It has been suggested that the organisms which produce these agents do so in order to ward off their competition for resources with other microorganisms (Medeiros, 1997). Production of these antibacterial agents by the producer organisms, which include non-β-lactam-susceptible fungi and actinomycetes, as well as susceptible bacteria (Wells et al., 1982), would have created a selection pressure for non-producing bacteria to acquire resistance to them. This resistance was most likely manifested initially by the ability of soil bacteria to develop enzymes which modify the structures of natural antibiotics, thus rendering them inactive. Specifically, bacterial β-lactamases hydrolyze the critical β-lactam moiety of these antibiotics to manifest resistance to the antibiotic.

Recent structural data clearly indicate that despite low amino-acid sequence homology between and among PBPs and β-lactamases, the general topology of these enzymes has been preserved, so they are all related (Lobkovsky et al., 1993; Knox et al., 1996; Massova and Mobashery, 1998). In addition, recent mechanistic evidence also underscores concepts in the details of the catalytic processes which support this kinship (Strynadka et al., 1992; Jelsch et al., 1993; Dubus et al., 1994; Dubus et al. 1996; Miyashita et al., 1995; Bulychev et al., 1997). With the exception of one PBP and a few β-lactamases which are dependent on zinc for their chemistries, most of the enzymes of both families utilize the active-site serine strategy for their respective reactions. Hence, the typical β-lactamase undergoes acylation of its active-site serine by the antibiotic, analogous to its reaction with PBPs. The difference lies in the rates of deacylation for the two groups of enzymes. The acyl-enzyme intermediates of PBPs do show some ability to undergo deacylation. This rate of deacylation could show a half-life of minutes to hours (Frère and Joris, 1985; Bush et al., 1987) and it may represent a basal level for this reaction which is unpromoted by the protein. β-Lactamases, on the other hand, have acquired the ability to promote a water molecule for the deacylation step. As such they are efficient enzymes which undergo acylation and deacylation in two separate steps, rapidly completing hydrolysis of β-lactam substrates with turnover numbers as high as 1500 s^{-1}.

If one considers that the ester moiety of the acyl-enzyme intermediate of this nascent β-lactamase is flat, the approach of the hydrolytic water can take place either from the top, or from the bottom of the ester group. The end result will be the same, namely hydrolysis of the β-lactam substrate regardless of which direction for the approach of the hydrolytic water is pursued by the primordial enzyme. Recent mechanistic studies indicate that indeed both routes for the approach of the hydrolytic water have been adapted by the better studied members of the classes A and C of β-lactamases (Bulychev et al., 1997; Massova and Mobashery, 1998). In β-lactam terminology, the water approaches the carbonyl of the ester from the α or β face of the ester group in classes A and C of β-lactamases, respectively (Bulychev et al., 1997; Massova and Mobashery, 1998). Furthermore, the two mechanisms for promotion of these water molecules are distinct. The water molecule is promoted by Glu-166 of class A enzymes and that in the case of class C enzymes is by the environment created by the side chain of Tyr-150 and the ring nitrogen of the acyl-enzyme intermediate itself. The implications of how the processes for the deacylation step may have developed were discussed in greater detail by Massova and Mobashery (1998).

Recently, an extensive sequence alignment of approximately 150 enzymes representing PBPs and β-lactamases has been performed (Massova and Mobashery, 1998; Fig. 4; The class B metallo-β-lactamases were not included, as their origins may be distinct from that of active-site-serine enzymes). This analysis showed that PBPs diversified early in evolutionary time-scale. Subsequently, in relatively more recent evolutionary periods, β-lactamases evolved from different classes of PBPs. This view is consistent with the observations for relatively recent evolution of the efficient deacylation step, perhaps driven by evolution of biosynthesis for β-lactam antibiotics (Aharonowitz and Cohen, 1992).

3. β-LACTAMS OF COMMERCIAL UTILITY BEFORE 1975

3.1. Penicillins

Availability of benzylpenicillin (1), the first β-lactam drug to be used clinically, was considered a major advance in the treatment of Gram-positive bacteria, especially for streptococcal infections that were a significant cause of mortality. Streptococci remained fully susceptible to penicillin until the late 1970s (Tarpay, 1978); although the incidence of penicillin-resistant streptococci is increasing, the majority of *S. pneumoniae* remain susceptible to penicillin and amoxicillin (Thornsberry et al., 1997). These organisms are one of a very few genera of bacteria that have never been reported to produce a β-lactamase, partially explaining the continued success of penicillin therapy. However, in the early 1940s, staphylococci, bacteria that co-existed with streptococci *in vivo*, were >90% susceptible to penicillin (Kirby, 1944); only a minority of isolates were capable of producing either plasmid-mediated or chromosomal β-lactamases. Unfortunately, these β-lactamase-producing isolates were quickly selected during penicillin therapy for streptococcal infections, and soon became a factor that appeared to doom the therapeutic use of penicillin.

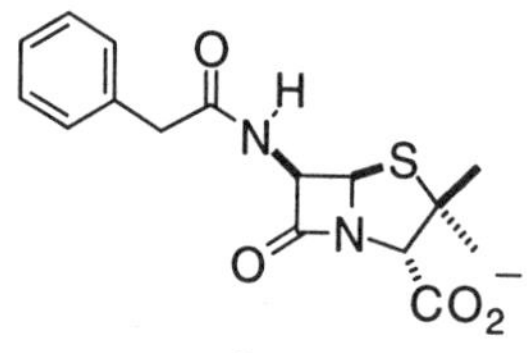

1

3.2. Semi-Synthetic Penicillins and Cephalosporins

Development of novel β-lactams has been closely associated with advances in natural products chemistry. The identification of 6-aminopenicillanic acid (2) and cephalosporin C (3) in the late 1950s provided medicinal chemists with appropriate β-lactam

Figure 4. Multiple-sequence alignment of β-lactamases and PBPs. The columns from left to right indicate whether the organism is Gram-positive (+) or Gram-negative (-), the nature of the protein [penicillin-binding protein (P); class A (A), class C (C), or class D (D) β-lactamases, or transglycosylase (T)]. The pound sign indicates a protein with available crystal coordinates, and the asterisk signifies a crystallized protein for which the coordinates are still not available to public. The column to the far right gives the source of the enzyme. A somewhat different version of this dendrogram was reported by Massova and Mobashery (1998) earlier.

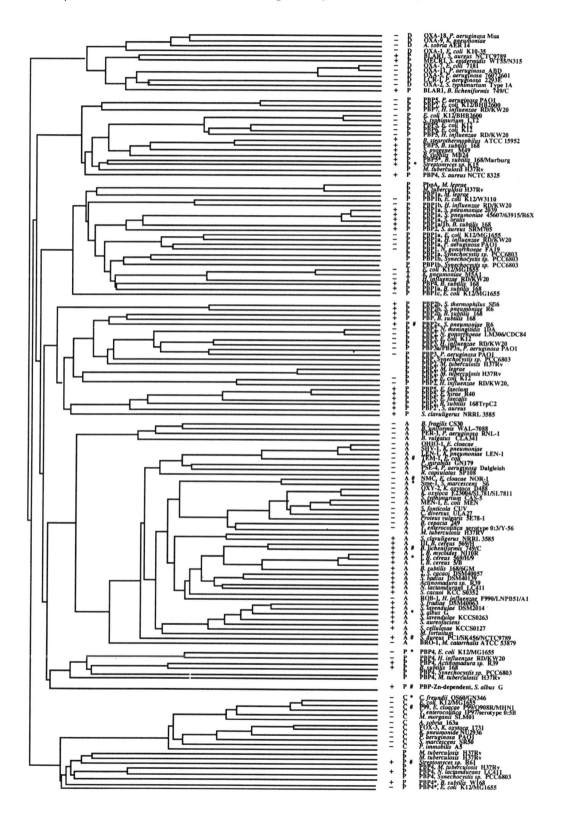

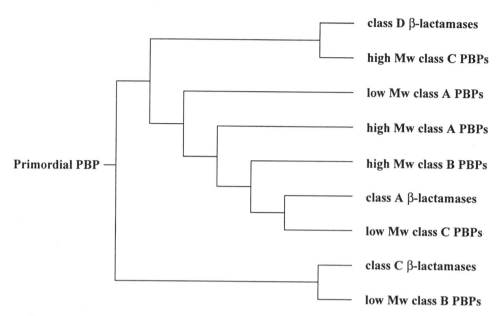

	class D β-lactamases
	high Mw class C PBPs
	low Mw class A PBPs
	high Mw class A PBPs
Primordial PBP	high Mw class B PBPs
	class A β-lactamases
	low Mw class C PBPs
	class C β-lactamases
	low Mw class B PBPs

scaffolds, allowing them to modify the basic β-lactam structure. Semi-synthetic isoxa-zolyly penicillins, such as methicillin (**4**) and oxacillin (**5**), and "first-generation" cepha-losporins, such as cephaloridine (**6**) and cephalothin (**7**), exhibited improved stability to the staphylococcal β-lactamases, enzymes that strongly preferred simple penicillins as substrates. The clinical importance of the Gram-positive β-lactamases diminished as a re-sult. The stage was now set for the emergence of potent, broad-spectrum, β-lactamases which were produced predominantly by Gram-negative enterobacteriaceae.

Figure 5. The schematic of the findings of Figure 4 are summarized here (Mw stands for molecular weight). The designation of PBPs into classes A, B, and C is according to Ghuysen (1991 and 1997).

4. β-LACTAMASE INHIBITORS

As stated earlier, the environmental evolution of β-lactams may have driven evolution of β-lactamases. The advent of β-lactamases could have resulted in the obsolescence of β-lactam antibiotics active against the antibiotic-susceptible strains. Organisms such as streptomycetes were able to produce both antibacterial and β-lactamase inhibitory β-lactams to retain the utility of their original antibiotics (Brown et al., 1976; Perez-Llarena et al., 1997). Or, the inhibitors, both protein (Doran et al., 1990; Strynadka et al., 1996) and β-lactams (such as clavulanic acid; Brown et al., 1976; Baggaley et al., 1997) inhibited the activity of the resistance enzymes, making possible the continued effectiveness of the otherwise β-lactamase-susceptible antibiotic. This strategy in microbial systems has an obvious corollary in the pharmaceutical approach, which has proven quite successful (*vide infra*).

4.1. Clinical Need

Plasmid-mediated β-lactamases in Gram-negative bacteria began to be identified in the early 1960s. The most infamous of these was the TEM β-lactamase, described almost simultaneously from *E. coli, Salmonella typhimurium* and *Salmonella paratyphi* B clinical isolates (Datta and Kontomichalou, 1965). This enzyme, initially known as the "RTEM" β-lactamase, quickly became a reference standard in the β-lactamase literature, and was widely used as the most important plasmid-mediated β-lactamase in both the academic world and in the pharmaceutical industry. The enzyme was found in virtually every species of enterobacteriaceae, and in most collections in the 1980s represented >50% of all plasmid-mediated β-lactamases in ampicillin-resistant Gram-negative pathogens (Bush and Sykes, 1987). The occurrence of a transposon-encoded TEM-1 in *Neisseria gonorrhea*, first reported in 1976 (Percival et al., 1976) in at least two multi-drug resistant plasmids (Perine et al., 1977), resulted in a panic world-wide when it became apparent that single dose penicillin therapy was no longer effective against many gonococcal strains (Percival et al., 1976). One plasmid in *N. gonorrhea* was specifically identified with an England-Far Eastern set of strains which also carried an additional conjugative plasmid (Perine et al., 1977). The second plasmid-mediated RTEM apparently originated in West Africa (Perine et al., 1977). To make the situation worse, the first plasmid also carried markers for tetracycline resistance, so that two staples in the drug armamentarium against gonococcal infections were now compromised.

By the mid 1970s several pharmaceutical companies had mobilized their efforts to identify novel β-lactamase inhibitors, specifically targeting the RTEM β-lactamase, but also evaluating the activity of their inhibitors against the earliest extended-spectrum β-lactamase, the K1 enzyme from *Klebsiella oxytoca* (also classified as *Klebsiella pneumoniae* or *Klebsiella aerogenes*) and against the class C cephalosporinase from *Enterobacter cloacae* P99. All of these enzymes had been purified and characterized so that basic biochemical information for these enzymes was available at that time (Datta and Richmond, 1966; Marshall et al., 1972).

The search for inhibitors focused upon natural products, as this had been the source for novel antimicrobial agents up to that point. Major contenders in the field were the British companies, Glaxo and Beecham, with Beecham emerging as the company that was the first to identify clavulanate from *Streptomyces clavuligerus* (**8**; Brown et al., 1976, also known as clavulanic acid in the acidic form). Many other natural product inhibitors were later identified, including olivanic acids (**9**) of the carbapenem class (Butterworth et al., 1979), and the sulfated macrolide izumenolide (**10**, Bush et al., 1980). However, there was a reluctance to continue these studies into the early 1980s when the commercial introduction of clavulanic acid and sulbactam (**11**, English et al., 1978) was proposed as combination products with β-lactamase-susceptible penicillins. In the United States, there was concern in the industry that β-lactam inhibitor combinations (e.g., amoxicillin/clavulanic acid and ampicillin/sulbactam) would not find favor with the regulatory agencies, and that antibiotic combinations would never be approved for clinical use. For this reason, and because of the potency of clavulanic acid, the interest in these areas waned, and only one other combination, piperacillin/tazobactam (**12**, Jacobs et al., 1986) was eventually approved. Clinically, these drugs afforded significant advantages over other antimicrobial agents, in that they could be used to treat Gram-negative bacteria that produced many of the plasmid-mediated β-lactamases. However, all three inhibitors had the same limitations: all inhibited the same class of β-lactamases, the class A enzymes, but not the chromosomal class C cephalosporinases.

4.2. Clavulanic Acid

Clavulanic acid, a β-lactam inhibitor of β-lactamases, biosynthesized by *S. clavuligerus* (Brown et al., 1976; Baggaley et al., 1997), has been in clinical use since the mid 1980s in two combinations: amoxicillin/clavulanate (Leigh et al., 1981) and ticarcillin/clavulanate (Roselle et al., 1985). The compound is an efficient and irreversible inactivator of class A β-lactamases (Fisher et al., 1978; Reading and Farmer, 1981). This clavam inhibits class C β-lactamases in *in vitro* experiments less effectively than class A enzymes (Reading and Cole, 1977; Reading and Farmer, 1981), resulting in the inability to observe synergistic activity for clavulanate combinations against most clinical isolates producing class C cephalosporinases (Dumon et al., 1979).

The inhibition chemistry for class A enzymes starts by acylation of the active-site serine (**8**→ **13**). At the acyl-enzyme intermediate stage the species **13** may undergo deacylation to give turnover, or it may expel its leaving group from C5 to give rise to the linear form of the acyl-enzyme intermediate (**14**). The linear species leads to irreversible inactivation of the enzyme (**14**→ **15**→ **16**). Turnover and inactivation processes take place with reasonably similar rate constants, so clavulanate is not turned over many times before the onset of irreversible inactivation of the enzyme. The number of molecules of inactivator which are turned over before inactivation of the enzyme is referred to as the partition ratio, and that for the TEM-1 and the closely related TEM-2 β-lactamases ranges between 160 and 115, respectively (Fisher et al., 1978; Imtiaz et al., 1993).

Two fates await the linear acyl-enzyme intermediate. Either the iminium double bond would be tautomerized to give the species **17**, or a nucleophile may be trapped at the iminium carbon, followed by deprotonation at C6 and the expulsion of the amine leaving group (**14** → **15** → **16**). The former would give rise to an α,β-conjugated ester, which because of its relative chemical stability resists the deacylation chemistry. Therefore, species **17** would deacylate given time, and it is referred to as the transiently inhibited species. The process of conversion of **15** to **17** gives irreversible inactivation of the enzyme. Molecular modeling with the crystal structure of the enzyme had suggested that Ser-130, an invariant residue in class A β-lactamases, was the likely residue to be trapped by **14** (Imtiaz et al., 1993), an assertion which was subsequently shown to be true for the TEM β-lactamase experimentally (Brown et al., 1996; Brown et al., 1997) In essence, both the processes which would lead to transient inhibition and irreversible inactivation involve deprotonation at C6, so the issue becomes whether the nucleophile interception takes place or not, to give one or the other. Inactivation by clavulanate proceeds rapidly for susceptible TEM β-lactamases, such that inhibition of β-lactamase in the presence of the favorable penicillin substrates can proceed, permitting the penicillin to survive to inhibit the bacterial PBP.

4.3. Penicillanate Sulfones

Clavulanic acid with its unique biological activity inspired many investigations of its mechanism of action (Charnas et al., 1978; Fisher et al., 1978; Reading and Farmer, 1981). As it was appreciated that clavulanate acylated the active-site serine of β-lactamases readily, followed by the expulsion of the departing group from C5 to give the linear species **14** which led to enzyme inactivation, it became obvious that such chemistry may be applicable to certain β-lactam derivatives which can easily be accessible synthetically. The first commercially successful derivative was sulbactam (**11**; English et al., 1978). A variant on the structure of sulbactam is tazobactam (**12**), which has superior kinetic properties in its inactivation of β-lactamases (Bush et al., 1993; Payne et al., 1994). Both sulbactam and tazobactam have found clinical use in the following combinations: sulbactam with either ampicillin or cefoperazone and tazobactam with piperacillin.

The mechanisms of action of these two compounds are essentially identical to that of clavulanic acid and will not be discussed here in any detail. Suffice it to say that these compounds also result in both transiently inhibited and irreversibly inhibited species

(Bush et al., 1993; Imtiaz et al., 1994; and the references cited therein). They do so with kinetic parameters which are somewhat different than those of clavulanic acid. An interesting feature of the interactions of sulbactam (and possibly tazobactam) with β-lactamases is the fact that in contrast to clavulanic acid (Imtiaz et al., 1993), the departure of the C5 sulfonate is not assisted by enzyme (Imtiaz et al., 1994).

4.4. Clinical Response Delayed (IRTs)

Resistance to the β-lactamase inhibitor combinations has been delayed compared to the rapid emergence of resistance to other β-lactams. The fact that the antimicrobial and biochemical features of two disparate agents must be overcome to give effective resistance has resulted in a slower response by bacteria. Inhibitor-resistant TEM-derived enzymes (IRTs) were first reported from France in 1992 (Vedel et al., 1992), but their appearance at this time has been confined to Western Europe. At present, there are at least 15 IRTs and one SHV-derived inhibitor-resistant β-lactamase.

Four natural mutations of consequence have been detected in the TEM β-lactamase which give resistance to clavulanic acid inhibition. The mutations have been detected at positions 69, 244, 275, and 276 of the TEM β-lactamase (Belaaouaj et al., 1994; Zhou et al., 1994; Henquell et al., 1995). The majority of these structure modifications appear to result in reduced affinity to clavulanic acid in the natural enzymes. The most common residue at position 244 for class A β-lactamases is an arginine. The side chain of this arginine is coordinated to a structurally conserved water molecule which would appear to serve as the source for an important proton in the process of formation of the inactivating species 14 of clavulanic acid (Imtiaz et al., 1993). Mutations at this position reduce the rate constant for inactivation of the enzyme more dramatically than they alter the affinity of the enzyme for clavulanic acid (Imtiaz et al., 1993).

Another mutation of consequence to resistance to inhibition by clavulanic acid is that of Ser-130-Gly seen in the SHV-10 β-lactamase from an *E. coli* clinical isolate (Prinarakis et al., 1997). Since this amino acid has been shown to be the site of covalent modification by clavulanic acid in the TEM β-lactamase (Brown et al., 1996; Brown et al., 1997), the mutant enzyme should resist inhibition by clavulanic acid, which appears to be the case. This mutant enzyme retains much of its activity against penicillins, but activity against cephalosporins was drastically reduced (Prinarakis et al., 1997).

One possible reason that this set of β-lactamase variants has not spread so rapidly is that the inhibitor-resistant TEM variants have become less efficient in hydrolyzing normally good substrates for TEM-1, so that the producing organisms retain susceptibility to cephalosporins such as cephalothin (Lemozy et al., 1995), as well as to normally poor substrates such as aztreonam and imipenem (Vedel et al., 1992). It is also important to note that the decreased inhibitor response is not the same for all three inhibitors; the combination of piperacillin/tazobactam seems to be more effective than other combinations against organisms producing these enzymes (Vedel et al., 1992; Lemozy et al., 1995). This may be related to the frequent use and availability of oral therapy with amoxicillin/clavulanic acid, thus sensitizing the bacterial flora to clavulanic acid rather than to the sulfones, sulbactam and tazobactam, which both appear in parenteral formulations.

5. EXPANDED-SPECTRUM β-LACTAMS

5.1. Penicillins, Cephalosporins, and Monobactams

At the same time, natural product investigators were searching for novel natural inhibitors of class A β-lactamases, medicinal chemists were looking carefully at additional synthetic modifications of the 6-aminopenicillanic acid and 7-aminocephalosporanic acid nuclei as scaffolds for future modifications. As a result, during the late 1970s and early 1980s expanded-spectrum penicillins with activity against both Gram-positive and Gram-negative bacteria, and cephalosporins with increased stability to hydrolysis by class A and class C β-lactamases were developed. Ureidopenicillins such as azlocillin (**20**), mezlocillin (**21**) and piperacillin (**22**) emerged, with piperacillin, the only one of the three to achieve modest success commercially (Durckheimer et al., 1985). These penicillins, especially azlocillin and piperacillin, had better activity against Gram-negative bacteria with notably good activity against *Pseudomonas aeruginosa,* but were readily hydrolyzed by the ubiquitous TEM and SHV β-lactamases (Neu, 1983).

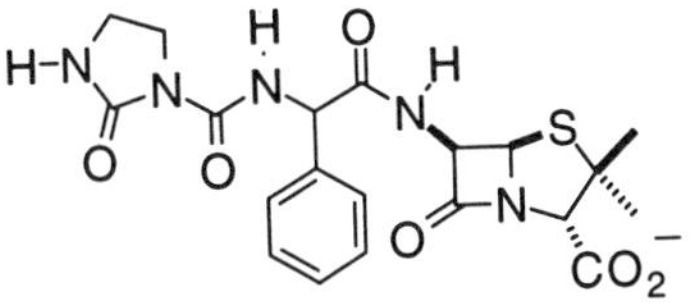

20

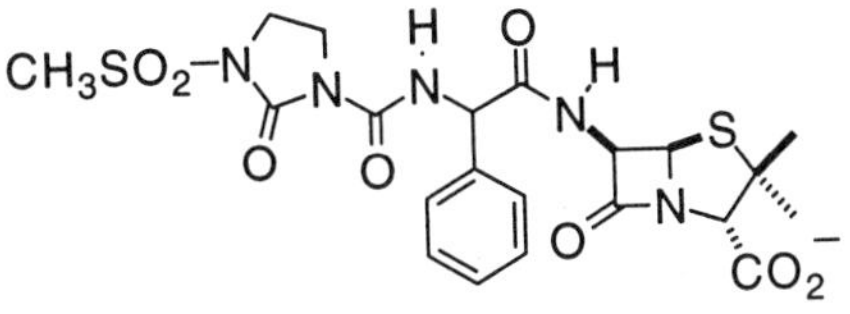

21

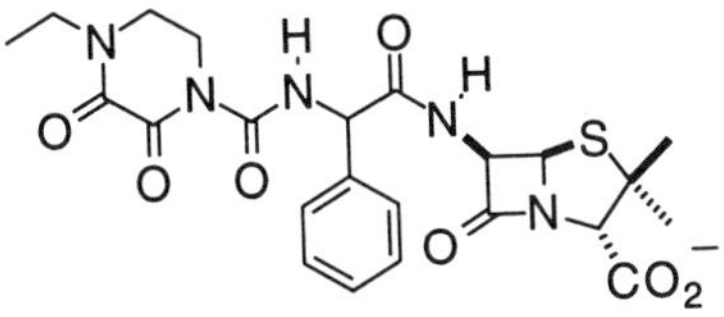

22

Development of the aminothiazolyl cephalosporins was a major breakthrough in the saga of β-lactam antibiotics. Agents such as cefotaxime (**23**), ceftriaxone (**24**), cefoperazone (**25**) and ceftazidime (**26**) had spectra of activity that included many difficult-to-treat enterobacteriaceae, with good anti-pseudomonal activity particularly noted for cefoperazone and ceftazidime (Durckheimer et al., 1985). Modest activity against Gram-positive bacteria was an advantage for agents such as ceftazidime, when empirical therapy could be instituted with these drugs. In addition to the expanded-spectrum cephalosporins, the monobactam aztreonam (**27**) was developed, based upon monocyclic naturally-occurring β-lactams (Sykes et al., 1982). Although this agent satisfied the definition of Paul Ehrlich's "magic bullet" with no useful Gram-positive activity, but excellent activity against Gram-negative aerobic bacteria, including *P. aeruginos*a, it achieved only modest success clinically.

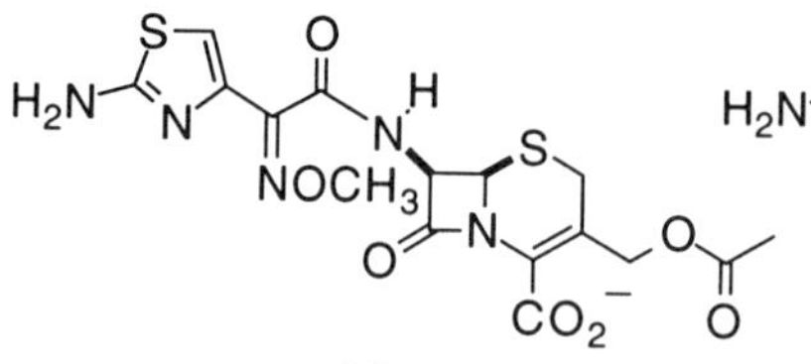

23 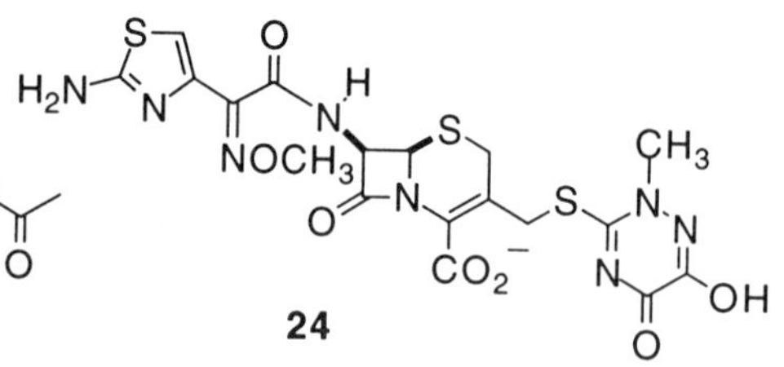　　　　　　　　　　　**24**

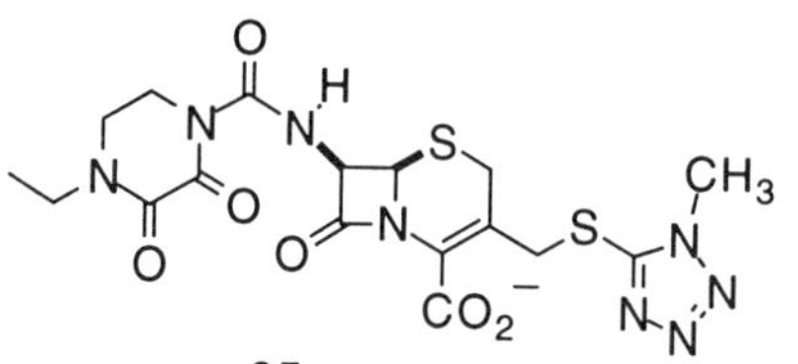

25 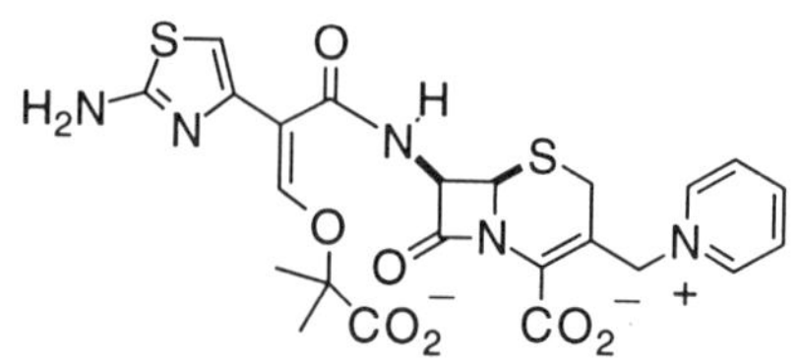　　　　　　　　　　**26**

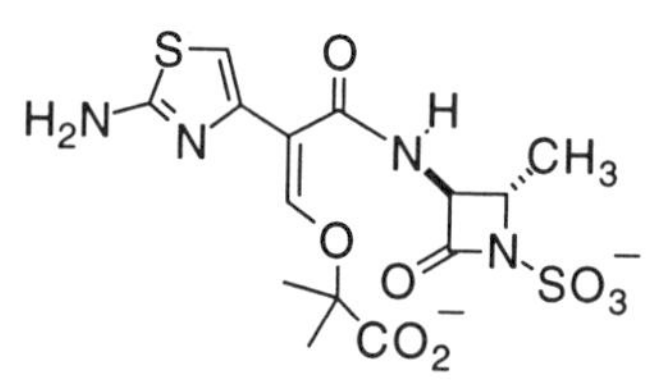

27

Most importantly, stability of these antibiotics to hydrolysis by most clinically relevant β-lactamases was excellent. During the development of aztreonam in the early 1980s, a major effort was made by Squibb scientists to identify any β-lactamases that were capable of hydrolyzing ceftazidime or aztreonam, both of which share the same aminothiazolyl side chain. The PSE-2 and K1 chromosomal β-lactamases from *Klebsiella oxytoca* were the only characterized enzymes with hydrolysis rates for aztreonam >1% that for benzylpenicilllin (**1**) or cephaloridine (**6**) (Sykes et al., 1982). When ceftazidime was used as a substrate, no β-lactamases in common culture collections were capable of hydrolyzing this cephalosporin at easily detectable rates (Bush, personal observation). Attempts to predict possible β-lactamase-mediated resistance to these new agents centered on the chromosomal class C cephalosporinases and the selection of enterobacteriaceae derepressed for high-level production of the class C enzymes (Gootz et al., 1982).

5.2. Rapid Clinical Response

After introduction of the expanded-spectrum penicillins, no enzymes were identified with altered hydrolytic properties for these penicillins, agents which were not found widely in the clinical setting. However, the hydrolysis that was observed with the TEM and SHV β-lactamases allowed the enzymes to confer resistance, especially when high-level production occurred in organisms harboring these β-lactamases. Therefore, these penicillins may have contributed to resistance development by the later cephalosporins by selecting for organisms retaining high copy plasmids encoding the TEM and SHV β-lactamases.

Resistance to the aminothiazole-containing cephalosporins emerged quite rapidly, however, in a fashion never anticipated by the "β-lactamase experts" of the early 1980s.

Variants of the common TEM and SHV β-lactamases began to appear shortly after the introduction of these cephalosporins into clinical usage, first in *Klebsiella pneumoniae* and later in almost all enterobacteriaceae (Knothe et al., 1983; Sirot et al., 1987; Petit et al., 1990). The most important characteristic of the producing organisms was their decreased susceptibility to either cefotaxime or ceftazidime, or both. Susceptibility to aztreonam decreased in parallel with that for ceftazidime. These first variant TEM and SHV enzymes differed from their parents by 1–3 amino acids, none of which was immediately associated with residues known to be involved with the active site (Knox, 1995). Coincidentally, outbreaks of ESBL-producing organisms were frequently associated with hospitals that were using large amounts of cefotaxime or ceftazidime (Petit et al., 1990; Meyer et al., 1993). In some cases, the progression of sequential nucleotide changes could be traced within a single patient who developed more resistant infections during the course of therapy with an expanded-spectrum cephalosporin (Rasheed et al., 1997).

Initially, ESBLs appeared to have well-defined substrate specificities, such that the early enzymes were often classified as being either "cefotaximases" or "ceftazidimases." The early dogma indicated that all ESBLs were susceptible to inhibition by the β-lactamase inhibitor combinations, so there was a feeling of confidence that therapy would always be available for ESBL-producing organisms. However, ESBLs based on the TEM enzyme have been identified with reduced affinities for clavulanic acid (Perilli et al., 1997; Sirot et al., 1997).

The structural reasons for the enhanced activity toward these poor substrates to these enzymes is of considerable interest. A well-studied example of these expanded-spectrum cephalosporins is cefepime (**34**). In a recent study, it was shown that the affinity of cefepime for the ubiquitous TEM-1 β-lactamase (as measured by the value for the dissociation constant, K_s) was evaluated at the exceedingly high value of 10.3 mM (Taibi et al., 1996). K_m values >2 mM have been previously reported for other expanded-spectrum cephalosporins and aztreonam with the closely related TEM-2 enzyme (Gutmann et al., 1988; Bush and Singer, 1989, Vakulenko et al., unpublished results). Such concentrations are practically unattainable within the periplasm; hence enzymes like TEM-1, cannot reach saturation with cephalosporins such as cefepime. This is one reason for the survivability of cefepime, and that of other expanded-spectrum cephalosporins, in the face of challenge by class A β-lactamases. However, when saturation was attained with cefepime in *vitro* experiments with purified enzyme, the enzyme was acylated, and given time, deacylation occurred (Taibi et al., 1996). The rate constants for acylation and deacylation were severely depressed compared to other penicillin or earlier cephalosporin substrates for the enzyme, and the deacylation step was rate-limiting (Taibi et al., 1996). These unfavorable parameters stem from the fact that expanded-spectrum cephalosporins have large substituents in their C7 positions. The poor steric interactions of these groups with the enzyme active sites reduce affinity for the formation of the preacylation complex ("Michaelis complex"), but also adversely affect the magnitude of the microscopic rate constants for acylation and deacylation.

It has been shown that mutations in an Ω-loop near the active site of class A enzymes impart enhanced activity toward expanded-spectrum cephalosporins (Sowek et al., 1991; Knox, 1995). Some of these mutant variants were characterized recently to show that substitutions at position 164 had the ability to increase the values for both the microscopic rate constants for acylation and deacylation significantly (Taibi et al., 1996). It is of considerable interest that this site is approximately 13 Å away from the active-site serine, and its effects on substrate binding are entirely indirect. It has been suggested that mutations at this site would restructure the conformation of the Ω-loop such that the active-site cavity where the bulky C7 side chain of the expanded-spectrum cephalosporin would fit has effectively been enlarged. For example, the manifestation of the R164N mutation in the TEM-1 β-lactamase is that the value for K_s for cefepime is lowered to 0.7 mM (from 10.3 mM for the parental enzyme), which places the affinity in the range for K_m for typical first-generation cephalosporin substrates for the wild-type enzyme (Taibi et al., 1996). Hence, saturation of the enzyme may become feasible (if agents are dosed parenterally).

Additional mutations in the parental TEM and SHV β-lactamases resulting in enhanced activity against expanded-spectrum cephalosporins are continually being identified. An ongoing summary of these changes is maintained by Jacoby and Bush at www.lahey.hitchcock.org/pages/lhc/studies/webt.htm. A recent review by Knox provides a structural context for the resistance phenotype for some of these enzyme variants (Knox, 1995). The structural reason for the enhanced activity has not been studied, or is not readily discerned, in all known cases. However, it has been suggested in a few examples that the manifestation of the mutation is in enlargement of the active-site cavity to accommodate the large C7 side chain of these cephalosporins. These examples include mutational replacement of amino acids at positions 238 (Huletsky et al., 1993) and 242 (Bonomo et al., 1995). Both these residues are on β-strand B3, near the active site of the class A β-lactamases.

The origins of the TEM variants remain somewhat controversial. It is likely that not all the point mutations giving ESBL or IRT activity, are selected for during therapy. For many years, the high frequency of TEM-1-producing isolates in clinical collections of isolates was based upon isoelectric points, especially in the days before sequencing became routine. Therefore, it is likely that many of the silent nucleotide changes, or the "modulating" mutations (Huang and Palzkill, 1997) that by themselves appear to confer no obvious phenotypic advantage to the enzyme, have been in the "noise" of the genetic background for many years. The use of the newer expanded-spectrum agents has then served to increase the frequency of mutation for the last, more deleterious, mutation that is readily identified in a clinical population.

6. CARBAPENEMS

The development of carbapenems for clinical use was a major accomplishment in the mid to late 1970s. During the process of identifying natural product-derived β-lactamase inhibitors, the search for novel β-lactam structures was emphasized. A number of β-lactamase inhibitors were found by Beecham to be simple β-lactam molecules that were members of the olivanic acid family (9, Butterworth et al., 1979), better recognized as carbapenems. Concurrently, Merck scientists identified a highly unstable, β-lactam with an extremely potent, broad-spectrum, antimicrobial activity (Kahan et al., 1979). The carbapenem thienamycin (28) was a chemist's nightmare and a microbiologist's fantasy. Subsequent to structure elucidation, it became obvious that the chemical instability of thienamycin was due to an intermolecular aminolysis reaction. The amine of the C2 substituent would attack the strained β-lactam ring in another molecule of the antibiotic, resulting in the opening of the ring and the attendant loss of activity. This observation also explained the concentration dependence for the instability of thienamycin; the higher the concentration, the more rapid was the loss of activity. Due to the perseverance of a group of Merck chemists, formimidoyl-thienamycin, or imipenem (29), was eventually developed as one of the most effective antimicrobial agents in the current armamentarium (Birnbaum et al., 1985; Buckley et al., 1992). Because of the higher pK_a for the formimidoly functionality, it remains protonated at physiological pH, and hence non-nucleophilic, avoiding the aminolysis reaction. Not only did the molecule have a superior antibacterial profile, including anti-pseudomonal activity, it also displayed high hydrolytic stability to most clinically important β-lactamases of the time.

28   29

6.1. Imipenem

The broad-spectrum and potent antibacterial activity of imipenem, combined with its stability to the hydrolytic action of most β-lactamases, heralded this agent as a nearly ideal antibiotic. These desirable traits of imipenem make it a valuable antibiotic to the present day. Indeed, it remains as an antibiotic of "last resort" in the face of the clinical challenge by bacteria harboring many different kinds of β-lactamases (Buckley et al., 1992).

However, the creative work of the Merck chemists in rendering the structure of thienamycin stable by their preparation of imipenem was not the last hurdle for this antibiotic before its introduction to clinic. Animal studies indicated that imipenem serves as an adventitious substrate for a kidney dipeptidase, a zinc-dependent enzyme also known as renal dehydropeptidase (Kropp et al., 1982; Kim et al., 1982). The outstanding properties of imipenem warranted the exploration of suitable inhibitors for this human "β-lactamase". Cilastatin was developed as a potent inhibitor of the kidney enzyme (Kahan et al., 1983; Graham et al., 1987; D'Amato et al., 1990) and is currently marketed in combination with imipenem as another example of a β-lactamase inhibitor combination that has achieved clinical success (Buckley et al., 1992).

Imipenem has a number of structural features which sets it apart from other β-lactam antibiotics. These features are important for both its interactions with PBPs and β-lactamases. It has a carbon atom at position 1, and a double bond at position 2. Whereas the carbon at position 1 is not likely to play a structurally important role in interactions with the target proteins, the nature of the double bond in the five-membered ring is important. This double bond makes the site of attachment of the ring carboxylate (C3) planar, hence the spatial orientation of the atoms of the carboxylate are different than the corresponding atoms in penicillins and cephalosporins. This carboxylate is known to make important interactions with specific residues in β-lactamases in anchoring of the molecule in the active site (Moews et al., 1990; Ellerby et al., 1990; Strynadka, 1992), and it is likely to make similar electrostatic contacts in the active sites of PBPs. Furthermore, the nature and orientation of the C6 substituent is unprecedented. The 1R-hydroxyethyl group is appended as a C6α group, and it is not a modified amine, as is typical in most β-lactam antibiotics. As will be elaborated below, this feature makes critical contribution to stability of imipenem to β-lactamases.

Although imipenem is well known for its tight binding to PBP 2 in Gram-negative bacteria, it binds well to multiple PBPs. The mechanism of killing in Gram-negative organisms is thought to be due to the initial binding to PBP 2, resulting in disruption of cell division and the formation of spherical forms (Spratt et al., 1977). Subsequently, other PBPs become saturated, notably the bifunctional PBPs 1a and 1b in *E. coli* and their counterparts in other Gram-negative bacteria. This results rapidly in lysis, causing a cidal event. In *S. aureus* imipenem binds well to all four major PBPs, accounting for its excellent activity against Gram-positive bacteria (Yang et al., 1995). Though early studies of carbapenems with β-lactamases involved several members of this family of antibiotics (Charnas and Knowles, 1981; Easton and Knowles, 1982), the best studied compound has been imipenem (Zafaralla and Mobashery, 1992; Matagne et al., 1993; Taibi and Mobashery, 1995), the focus of the following discussion.

Carbapenems such as imipenem are excellent substrates for class B metallo-β-lactamases and a small subgroup of serine β-lactamases (*vide infra*), but are very poor substrates for the most common serine-dependent β-lactamases. Many class A β-lactamases show high affinity for imipenem (lower micromolar range for the dissociation constants), which rapidly acylates the active-site serine, but deacylates slowly (Taibi and Mobashery, 1995). Knowles and colleagues were first to note that hydrolysis of carbapenems by the TEM β-lactamase shows biphasic kinetics (Charnas and Knowles, 1981; Easton and Knowles, 1982). A relatively rapid phase for turnover of carbapenems undergoes an attenuation in rate to give rise to a slower phase for turnover. The rate of turnover for this second phase with imipenem is measured in several hours. Hence, imipenem is not only a good antibiotic because of its favorable interactions with PBPs, it is also an effective inhibitor of class A β-lactamases. The structural basis for this inhibition, which is due to slow deacylation of the acyl-enzyme intermediate(s), is discussed below.

In recent work on rational design of inhibitors for β-lactamases, it was shown that introduction of the C6α-hydroxymethyl group on a penicillanate nucleus (compound **30**) was sufficient to give rapid acylation of the TEM-1 β-lactamase, but the acyl-enzyme intermediate resisted deacylation for several hours (Miyashita et al., 1995; Maveyraud et al., 1996). This compound showed biphasic kinetics for both enzyme acylation and deacylation, indicative of the existence of at least two distinct acyl-enzyme intermediates in turnover of **30**. The recent X-ray structure for one of these acyl-enzyme species revealed that the hydroxyl group of the hydroxymethyl moiety of **30** made a hydrogen bond to the hydrolytic water molecule in the active site of the TEM-1 enzyme (Maveyraud et al., 1996). This hydrogen bond would attenuate the nucleophilicity of the hydrolytic water, but more importantly, the hydroxymethyl group presented a steric barrier to the travel of the hydrolytic water toward the ester carbonyl of the acyl-enzyme intermediate, accounting for the longevity of the species. This hydrogen bond is of course dynamic in nature. From time to time it breaks and allows for the rotation of the moiety away from the hydrolytic water molecule, opening access to the ester carbonyl for the water molecule. This type of process does indeed take place to result in deacylation of the intermediate and recovery of activity in several hours. It is important to note that the carbonyl of the ester function remains ensconced within the oxyanion hole of the enzyme, an interaction which is believed to result directly from the fitting of the β-lactam carbonyl of the substrate in the preacylation ("Michaelis") complex. This fitting in the oxyanion hole of the ester group is also believed to be important for the activation of the carbonyl group for attack by the hydrolytic water molecule.

Similarly, the effect of the 1*R*-hydroxyethyl group on hydrolysis of the two penicillanate derivatives **31** and **32** has been measured (Miyashita et al., 1996). These studies have shown that hydroxyethyl group at position C6α of **31** attenuates the rate of turnover of the compound by 10000-fold over that of **32**, and deacylation is rate-limiting for **31** (Miyashita et al., 1996). Molecular modeling supports a role for the 6α-1*R*-hydroxymethyl group similar to that for the 6α-hydroxymethylpenicillanate.

30   **31**   **32**

The structure of the immediate acyl-enzyme intermediate for imipenem is believed to be similar. In essence, the presence of 1R-hydroxyethyl group at C6α of imipenem should slow down deacylation by interfering with the approach of the hydrolytic water at the ester carbonyl, as discerned from molecular modeling. However, it would appear that the addition of the methyl group to the hydroxymethyl moiety to give rise to the 1R-hydroxyethyl function, no matter what prochiral position were to be modified, generates relatively unfavorable steric interactions in the active site of the TEM-1 β-lactamase. Such unfavorable interactions would appear to facilitate a conformational change in the immediate ("canonical") acyl-enzyme intermediate, resulting in a different acyl-enzyme intermediate with apparent lower energy content. A crystal structure for this species has recently been solved at 1.8 Å (Maveyraud et al., 1998), giving a clear picture for the unprecedented conformational alteration in the enzyme, which ultimately retards deacylation even beyond that seen with the immediate acyl-enzyme intermediate. This structure also accounts for the biphasic kinetics seen with the class A β-lactamases, two phases for the turnover profile for two different acyl-enzyme intermediates.

6.2. Meropenem

Meropenem (**33**), recently approved for clinical use, has a spectrum of antimicrobial activity that parallels that for imipenem (Edwards et al., 1989). Both have potent broad-spectrum activity against both aerobic and anaerobic bacteria. Meropenem is 2–4-fold more active than imipenem against Gram-negative bacteria, whereas imipenem retains a slight edge in potency against Gram-positive bacteria. Meropenem, with a C1-β-methyl substituent, is more stable to the mammalian renal dehydropeptidase than imipenem and does not require an accompanying peptidase inhibitor to protect it *in vivo* from hydrolysis (Harrison et al., 1993). Meropenem is also more stable than imipenem to hydrolysis by a subgroup of the metallo-β-lactamases (Rasmussen and Bush, 1997), although this stability may not translate into clinical susceptibility.

33

6.3. Clinical Response

Imipenem has often been classified as a "reserve" drug, one that is held for only the most serious infections. However, with the proliferation of ESBLs, more hospitals have found it necessary to use larger quantities of imipenem. Although many have been awaiting an explosion of carbapenem-hydrolyzing enzymes, including the metallo-β-lactamases which hydrolyze imipenem effectively, this has not happened. Even though Japanese workers have identified at least two different plasmid-mediated metallo-β-lactamases in *Bacteroides fragilis* (Bandoh et al., 1992), *Pseudomonas aeruginosa, Serratia marcescens* and other enterobacteriaceae (Minami et al., 1996), the frequency of these enzymes has remained at a low level. Instead, class A carbapenem-hydrolyzing β-lactamases are becoming more visible. Surprisingly, none of the carbapenem-hydrolyzing enzymes has become a major threat to the use of these potent antibacterial agents even though imipenem has been in clinical use for over a decade.

6.3.1. Metallo-β-Lactamases. Metallo-β-lactamases are the "step-children" of the β-lactamase family. They bear virtually no sequence homology to the serine β-lactamases, and are not really closely related to each other. These enzymes are all assumed to contain at least one active-site zinc atom that is required for catalysis, but beyond this feature they vary considerably. Substrate profiles vary considerably and little molecular conservation is observed within this family of β-lactamases that has only nine fully conserved amino acids. These enzymes tend to have little in common with one another other than their ability to hydrolyze imipenem. To confound the problems, most of these enzymes appear as "secondary" β-lactamases, with two or three enzymes produced per strain, each with a different substrate specificity. Attempts to devise a single strategy to counteract their actions will be difficult.

Rasmussen and Bush have proposed three distinct functional subgroups of the metallo-β-lactamases (Rasmussen and Bush, 1997). The largest subgroup of enzymes, found in some strains of *B. fragilis*, most strains of *S. maltophilia*, and on plasmids in Japan, possesses a very broad spectrum of activity. Most β-lactams are hydrolyzed by these enzymes, with the notable exception of the monobactams. One subgroup of metallo-enzymes contains a single member, the broad spectrum enzyme from *Legionella gormanii* that hydrolyzes penicillins and cephalosporins much more effectively than imipenem. To date there has been no structural information about the third unique subgroup of metallo-β-lactamases from *Aeromonas* spp. These enzymes recognize only carbapenems as good β-lactam substrates and appear to be only distantly related to the other metallo-β-lactamases (Massida et al., 1991). Again, these enzymes co-exist with at least one or two other β-lactamases that confer resistance to penicillins and cephalosporins, so they are not required to hydrolyze these classes of antibiotics for protection.

The mechanism of action of the metalloenzymes from the first subgroup is of considerable interest, based upon recent crystallographic information (Carfi et al., 1995; Concha et al., 1996). They would appear to require two zinc ions in their active sites (Concha et al., 1996). Although the mechanism of active-site binding is subject to dispute, the open nature of the active site provides much space for binding of various β-lactams, hence the broad substrate specificity of most of these enzymes. There does not appear to be an acyl-enzyme intermediate in the course of substrate turnover by these enzymes. It has been proposed that a water molecule is promoted by the enzyme to give a one-step hydrolysis of the β-lactam in substrates (Bounaga et al., 1998).

6.3.2. Serine-Based Carbapenem-Hydrolyzing Enzymes. Serine-dependent carbapnem-hydrolyzing β-lactamases comprise the smallest functional group of β-lactamases (Bush et al., 1995). Initially only five strains producing these group 2f β-lactamases had been positively identified: two London isolates producing the Sme-1 β-lactamase (Yang et al., 1990), one strain from France producing the NMC-A enzyme (Nordmann et al., 1993) and two California isolates, both of which probably produced the IMI-1 enzyme (Rasmussen et al., 1996). Most notably, isolation of these strains occurred before the clinical introduction of imipenem. Recently a set of isolates of *S. marcescens* from Boston, Minneapolis, and Los Angeles have been found to produce enzymes very similar to the Sme-1 enzyme (Carmeli and Quinn, personal communication). This small group of carbapenem-hydrolyzing serine enzymes may, in fact, be much larger than originally suspected, perhaps due to recent widespread use of imipenem. The crystal structures for the Sme-1 and the NMC-A enzymes have recently been determined (correspondence with J. P. Samama). It is notable that the general topology of these enzymes is essentially identical to those of other class A β-lactamases. The structural information on these enzymes would undoubtedly shed further light on their unique properties in the immediate future.

7. FUTURE

As the result of the current use of β-lactams, the enzymes that are expected to proliferate will be: ESBLs, in response to the expanded-spectrum cephalosporins, including cefepime (**34**) and cefpirome (**35**); IRTs, as the β-lactamase inhibitor combinations continue to be used; metallo-β-lactamases, as a response to the increasing number of carbapenems that are under development, particularly if an orally active agent is approved; and staphylococci variants, as a response to the development of potent β-lactams to treat methicillin-resistant *S. aureus*. The number of possible TEM variants in clinical isolates is currently over 60, but Palzkill's group has shown that all but 43 amino acids in the TEM sequence can be modified to give active enzyme in laboratory selection procedures (Huang et al., 1996). The possibility for further mutation of the staphylococcal enzymes has also been demonstrated in the laboratory (Voladri et al., 1996), but interest in β-lactamases from Gram-positive bacteria has surprisingly diminished in the past ten years, at a time when cloning and sequencing β-lactamases has become somewhat routine for the Gram-negative enzymes.

Because we were unprepared for the multitude of possible variations in the TEM structure resulting in major changes in substrate specificity, one can continue to speculate about further modifications. Will we see more enzymes acquire the ability to hydrolyze carbapenems as the result of point mutations? Can staphylococcal β-lactamases become more adept at hydrolyzing cephalosporins? And, if so, what will be the compensating effect on the other enzymatic properties of the parent enzyme? It is possible that like the IRTs, the loss of one function will result in a more positive response to another known group of β-lactams. However, as we have seen previously, it is difficult to predict the next changes that may occur.

34   **35**

Regulation of the level of β-lactamase activity has been one of the measures used by bacteria to deal with undesirable β-lactams in the environment. Concomitantly, decreased uptake of β-lactams into Gram-negative bacteria has often been associated with overproduction of β-lactamase. In organisms with these characteristics, resistance to β-lactam-containing agents may be synergistic compared to the effects of either mechanism acting alone (Bush et al., 1985). In addition, the description of efflux mechanisms for selected β-lactams in bacteria suggests that efflux may play a role in the decreased susceptibility observed in organisms such as *Pseudomonas aeruginosa* (Li et al., 1994). Overuse of agents that can select for mutants in these areas will certainly lead to an increase in the observed resistance phenotypes. In the laboratory, selection of permeability mutants is simple and occurs with high frequency (Bush et al., 1985). Therefore, it is not surprising to see clinical isolates produce an ESBL, followed by subsequent resistant isolates with porin mutations (Rasheed et al., 1997).

The final known mechanism of β-lactam resistance is the production of altered penicillin-binding proteins. The only organisms in which this has driven pharmaceutical development has been for MRSA and penicillin-resistant *Streptococcus pneumoniae* (Berger-Bachi, 1995; Coffey et al., 1995). These organisms are major public health problems that may not be easily treated with new β-lactam molecules.

β-lactam antimicrobial agents have proven to be safe, efficacious, and cost-effective over the past 50 years. The reliance of clinicians upon this class of antibiotics will not abate in the near future, and indeed we should anticipate dependence on these agents for the foreseeable future. However, the numbers are on the side of the microorganisms. These organisms reproduce rapidly, presenting proving grounds for selections of new phenotypes in response to various challenges. When a new class of antimicrobial agent successfully enters clinical practice, it faces the prospect of rapid obsolescence due to development of resistance. The only new class of antibacterial agents approved by the FDA since 1980, the fluoroquinolones, appeared to be compromised by the alarming swiftness with which resistance to all members of the drug class appeared in *S. aureus* and *P. aeruginosa* (Blumberg, et al., 1991; Coronado et al., 1995). However, this resistance has not yet been translated to all bacterial populations, a situation similar to that seen with the β-lactams. One can hope that such broadly active agents will be able to retain some of their activity as we search for their eventual replacements. We remain dependent on the existing antibacterial agents for the immediate future and care must be taken to prolong their clinical usefulness as long as possible. Knowledge of the mechanisms of action and resistance at the molecular level, such as described in this chapter, is essential to develop strategies that may counteract this resistance, while preserving clinical utility of antibiotics.

ACKNOWLEDGMENTS

The work at Wayne State University was supported by a grant from the National Institutes of Health.

REFERENCES

Abraham, E.P., and Chain, E., 1940, An enzyme from bacteria able to destroy penicillin, *Nature*, 146:837.

Aharonowitz, Y., and Cohen, G., 1992, Penicillin and cephalosporin biosynthetic genes: structure, organization, regulation, and evolution, *Ann. Rev. Microbiol.*, 46:461.

Ambler, R.P., 1980, The structure of β-lactamases, *Philos. Trans. R. Soc. Lond. [Biol]*, 289:321.

Baggaley, K.H., Brown, A.G., and Schofield, C.J., 1997, Chemistry and biosynthesis of clavulanic acid and other clavams, *Nat. Prod. Rep.*, 14:309.

Bandoh, K., Watanabe, K., Muto, Y., Tanaka, Y., Kato, N., and Ueno, K., 1992, Conjugal transfer of imipenem resistance in *Bacteroides fragilis*, *J. Antibiot. (Tokyo)*, 45:542.

Belaaouaj, A., Lapoumeroulie, C., Canica, M.M., Vedel, G., Nevot, P., Krishnamoorthy, R., and Paul, G., 1994, Nucleotide sequences of the genes coding for the TEM-like beta-lactamases IRT-1 and IRT-2 (formerly called TRI-1 and TRI-2), *FEMS Microbiol. Lett.*, 120:75.

Berger-Baechi, B., 1995, Factors affecting methicillin resistance in *Staphylococcus aureus*, *Int. J. Antimicrob. Agents*, 6:13.

Birnbaum, J., Kahan, F.M., Kropp, H., and MacDonald, J.S., 1985, Carbapenems, a new class of beta-lactam antibiotics, *The Amer. J. Med.*, 78 (suppl. 6A):3.

Blumberg, H. M., Rimland, D., Carroll, D. J., Terry, P., and Wachsmuth, I. K., 1991, Rapid development of ciprofloxacin resistance in methicillin-susceptible and resistant *Staphylococcus aureus*, *J. Infect. Dis.*, 163:1279.

Bonomo, R. A., Dawes, C. G., Knox, J.R., and Shlaes, D. M., 1995, Complementary roles of mutations at positions 69 and 242 in class A β-lactamases, *Biochim. Biophys. Acta*, 1247:121.

Bounaga, S., Laws, A.P., Galleni, M., and Page, M.I., 1998, The mechanism of catalysis and the inhibition of the *Bacillus cereus* zinc-dependent β-lactamase, *Biochem. J.*, 331(Pt 3):703.

Brown, A.G., Butterworth, D., Cole, M., Hanscomb, G., Hood, J.D., Reading, C., and Rolinson, G.N., 1976, Naturally occuring β-lactamase inhibitors with antibacterial activity, *J. Antibiot.*, 29:668.

Brown, R.P., Alpin, R.T., and Schofield, C.J., 1996, Inhibition of TEM-2 β-lactamase from *Escherichia coli* by clavulanic acid: observation of intermediates by electrospray ionisation mass spectrometry, *Biochemistry*, 35:12421.

Brown, R.P., Alpin, R.T., and Schofield, C.J., 1997, Mass spectrometric studies on the inhibition of TEM-2 β-lactamase by clavulanic acid derivatives, *J. Antibiot.*, 50:184.

Buckley, M.M., Brogden, R.N., Barradel, L.B., and Goa, K.L., 1992, Imipenem/ cilastatin. A reappraisal of its antibacterial activity, pharmacokinetic properties and therapeutic efficacy, *Drugs*, 44:408.

Bulychev, A., Massova, I., Miyashita, K., and Mobashery, S., 1997, Evolution of the versatile β-lactam hydrolase activity: from biosynthetic enzymes to drug resistance factors, *J. Am. Chem. Soc.*, 119:7619.

Bush, K., 1989, Characterization of β-lactamases, *Antimicrob. Agents Chemother.*, 33:259.

Bush, K., Bonner, D.P., and Sykes, R.B., 1980, Izumenolide--a novel beta-lactamase inhibitor produced by *Micromonospora*, *J. Antibiotics*, 33:1262.

Bush, K., Jacoby, G.A., and Medeiros, A.A., 1995, A functional classification scheme for β-lactamases and its correlation with molecular structure, *Antimicrob. Agents Chemother.*, 39:1211.

Bush, K., Macalintal, C., Rasmussen, B.A., Lee, V.J., and Yang, Y., 1993, Kinetic interactions of tazobactam with β-lactamases from all major structural classes, *Antimicrob. Agents Chemother.*, 37:851.

Bush, K., and Singer, S.B., 1989, Biochemical characteristics of extended broad spectrum β-lactamases, *Infection*, 17:429.

Bush, K., Smith, S.A., Ohringer, S., Tanaka, S.K., and Bonner, D.P., 1987, Improved sensitivity in assays for binding of novel beta-lactam antibiotics to penicillin-binding proteins of *Escherichia coli*, *Antimicrob. Agents Chemother.*, 31:1271.

Bush, K., and Sykes, R.B. 1987. Characterization and epidemiology of beta-lactamases, in: *The Antimicrobial Agents Annual*, Peterson P.K. and Verhoef J., eds., Elsevier, Amsterdam, p 371–382.

Bush, K., Tanaka, S.K., Bonner, D.P., and Sykes, R.B., 1985, Resistance caused by decreased penetration of β-lactam antibiotics into *Enterobacter cloacae*, *Antimicrob. Agents Chemother.*, 27:555.

Butterworth, D., Cole, M., Hanscomb, G., and Rolinson, G.N. 1979, Olivanic acids, a family of beta-lactam antibiotics with beta-lactamase inhibitory properties produced by *Streptomyces* species. I. Detection, properties and fermentation studies., *J. Antibiotics*, 32:287.

Carfi, A., Pares, S., Duee, E., Galleni, M., Duez, C., Frere, J.-M., and Dideberg, O., 1995, The 3-D structure of a zinc metallo-β-lactamase from *Bacillus cereus* reveals a new type of protein fold, *EMBO*, 14:4914.

Charnas, R.L., and Knowles, J.R., 1981, Inhibition of the RTEM β-lactamase *from Escherichia coli*. Interaction of enzyme with derivatives of olivanic acid, *Biochemistry*, 20:2732.

Charnas, R.L., Fisher, J., and Knowles, J.R., 1978, Chemical studies on the inactivation of *Escherichia coli* RTEM β-lactamase by clavulanic acid, *Biochemistry*, 17:2185.

Coffey, T.J., Dowson, C.G., Daniels, M., and Spratt, B.G., 1995, Genetics and molecular biology of β-lactam-resistant pneumococci, *Microb. Drug Resist.*, 1:29.

Concha, N.O., Rasmussen, B.A., Bush, K., and Herzberg, O., 1996, Crystal structure of the wide-spectrum binuclear zinc β-lactamase from *Bacteroides fragilis*, *Structure*, 4:823.

Condra, J. H., Schleif, W. A., Blahy, O. M., Gabryelski, L. J., Graham, D. J., Quintero, J. C., Rhodes, A., Robbins, H. L., Roth, E., Shivaprakash, M., Titus, D., Yang, T., Teppler, H., Squires, K. E., Deutsch, P. J., and Emini, E. A., 1995, In vivo emergence of HIV-1 variants resistant to multiple protease inhibitors, *Nature*, 374:569.

Coronado, V. G., Edwards, J. R., Culver, D. H., and Gaynes, R. P., 1995, National nosocomial infections surveillance system. ciprofloxacin resistance among nosocomial *Pseudomonas aeruginosa* and *Staphylococcus aureus* in the United States. *Infect. Control Hosp. Epidemiol.* 16:71.

D'Amato, C., Armignacco, O., Antonucci, G., Bordi, E., Bove, G., Decarli, G., De Mori, P., Rosci, M.A., and Visco, G., 1990, The efficacy and safety of imipenem/cilastatin in the treatment of severe bacterial infection, *J. Chemother.*, 2:100.

Datta, N., and Kontomichalou, P., 1965, Penicillinase synthesis controlled by infectious R factors in enterobacteriaceae, *Nature*, 208:239.

Datta, N., and Richmond, M.H., 1966, The purification and properties of a penicillinase whose synthesis is mediated by an R-factor in *Escherichia coli*, *Biochem. J.*, 98:204.

Doran, J.L., Leskiw, B.K., Aippersbach, S., and Jensen, S.E., 1990, Isolation and characterization of a β-lactamase-inhibitory protein from streptomyces clavuligerus and cloning and analysis of the corresponding gene, *J. Bacteriol.*, 172:4909.

Dubus, A., Ledent, P., Lamotte-Brasseur, J., and Frère, J.M., 1996, The roles of residues Tyr150, Glu272, and His314 in class C β-lactamases, *Proteins Struc. Func. Gen.*, 25:473.

Dubus, A., Normark, S., Kania, M., and Page, M.G.P., 1994, The role of tyrosine 150 in catalysis of β-lactam hydrolysis by AmpC beta-lactamase from *Escherichia coli* investigated by site-directed mutagenesis, *Biochemistry*, 33:8577.

Dumon, L., Adriaens, P., Anne, J., and Eyssen, H., 1979, Effect of clavulanic acid on the minimum inhibitory concentration of benzylpenicillin, ampicillin, carbenicillin, or cephalothin against clinical isolates resistant to beta-lactam antibiotics, *Antimicrob. Agents Chemother.*, 15:315.

Durckheimer, W., Blumbach, J., Lattrell, R., and Scheunemann, K.H., 1985, Recent developments in the field of beta-lactam antibiotics, *Angew. Chem. Int. Ed. Engl.*, 24:180.

Easton, C.J., and Knowles, J.R., 1982, Inhibition of the RTEM β-lactamase from *Escherichia coli*. Interaction of the enzyme with derivatives of olivanic acid, *Biochemistry*, 21:2857.

Edwards, J.R., Turner, P.J., Wannop, C., Withnell, E.S., Grindey, A.J., and Nairn, K., 1989, In vitro antibacterial activity of SM-7338, a carbapenem antibiotic with stability to dehydropeptidase I., *Antimicrob. Agents Chemother.*, 33:215.

Ellerby, L.M., Escobar, W.A., Fink, A.L., Mitchinson, C., and Wells, J., 1990, The role of lysine-234 in β-lactamase catalysis probed by site-directed mutagenesis, *Biochemistry*, 29:5797.

English, A.R., Retsema, J.A., Girard, A.E., Lynch, J.E., and Barth, W.E., 1978, CP-45.899, a beta-lactamase inhibitor that extends the antibacterial spectrum of beta-lactams: initial bacteriological characterization., *Antimicrob. Agents Chemother.*, 14:414.

Fisher, J., Charnas, R.L., and Knowles, J.R., 1978, Kinetic studies on the inactivation of *Escherichia coli* RTEM beta-lactamase by clavulanic acid, *Biochemistry*, 17:2180.

Frère, J.-M., and Joris, B., 1985, Penicillin-sensitive enzymes in peptidoglycan biosynthesis, *CRC Crit. Rev. Microbiol.*, 11:299.

Ghuysen, J.-M., Charlier, P., Coyette, J., Duez, C., Fonzé, E., Fraipont, C., Goffin, C., Joris, B., and Nguyen-Distèche, M., 1996, Penicillin and beyond: evolution, protein fold, multimodular polypeptides, and multiprotein complexes, *Microb. Drug Resist.*, 2:163.

Ghuysen, J.M., 1991, Serine β-lactamases and penicillin-binding proteins, *Annu. Rev. Microbiol.*, 45:37.

Ghuysen, J.M., 1997, Penicillin-binding proteins. Wall peptidoglycan assembly and resistance to penicillin: facts, doubts and hopes, *J. Int. Antimicrobial Agents*, 8:45.

Gootz, T.D., Sanders, C.C., and Goering, R.V., 1982, Resistance to cefamandole: derepression of beta-lactamases by cefoxitin and mutation in *Enterobacter cloacae*, *J. Infect. Dis.*, 146:34.

Graham, D.W., Ashton, W.T., Barash, L., Brown, J.E., Brown, R.D., Canning, L.F., Chen, A., Springer, J.P., and Rogers, E.F., 1987, Inhibition of the mammalian β-lactamase renal dipeptidase (dehydropeptidase-I) by (Z)-2-(acylamino)-3-substituted-propenoic acids, *J. Med. Chem.*, 30:1074.

Gutmann, L., Kitzis, M.D., Billot-Klein, D., Goldstein, F., Tran Van Nhieu, G., Lu, T., Carlet, J., Collatz, E., and Williamson, R., 1988, Plasmid-mediated β-lactamase (TEM-7) involved in resistance to ceftazidime and aztreonam, *Rev. Infect. Dis.*, 10:860.

Harrison, M.P., Haworth, S.J., Moss, S.R., Wilkinson, D.M., and Featherstone, A., 1993, The disposition and metabolic fate of 14C-meropenem in man, *Xenobiotica*, 23:1311.-1323.

Henquell, C., Chanal, C., Sirot, D., Labia, R., and Sirot, J., 1995, Molecular characterization of nine different types of mutants among 107 inhibitor-resistant TEM β-lactamases from clinical isolates of *Escherichia coli*, *Antimicrob. Agents Chemother.*, 39:427.

Huang, W., and Palzkill, T., 1997, A natural polymorphism in β-lactamase is a global suppressor, *Proc. Natl. Acad. Sci. USA*, 94:8801.

Huang, W., Petrosino, J., Hirsch, M., Shenkin, P.S., and Palzkill, T., 1996, Amino acid sequence determinants of β-lactamase structure and activity, *J. Mol. Biol.*, 258:688.

Huletsky, A.; Knox, J. R., and Levesque, R. C., 1993, The role of Ser238 and Lys240 in the hydrolysis of third-generation cephalosporins by SHV-type β-lactamases probed by site-directed mutagenesis and three-dimensional modeling, *J. Biol. Chem.*, 268:3690.

Huovinen, P., Huovinen, S., and Jacoby, G.A., 1988, Sequence of PSE-2 beta-lactamase, *Antimicrob. Agents Chemother.*, 32:134.

Imtiaz, U., Billings, E., Knox, J.R., Manavathu, E.K., Lerner, S.A., and Mobashery, S., 1993, Inactivation of class A β-lactamases by clavulanic acid: the role of arginine-244 in a proposed nonconcerted sequence of events, *J. Am. Chem. Soc*, 115:4435.

Imtiaz, U., Billings, E.M., Knox, J.R., and Mobashery, S., 1994, A structure-based analysis of the inhibition of class A β-lactamases by sulbactam, *Biochemistry*, 33:5728.

Jack, G.W., and Richmond, M.H., 1970, Comparative amino acid contents of purified β-lactamases from enteric bacteria, *FEBS Lett.*, 12:30.

Jacobs, M.R., Aronoff, S.C., Johenning, S., and Yamabe, S., 1986, Comparative activities of the β-lactamase inhibitors YTR 830 and sulbactam combined with extended-spectrum penicillins against ticarcillin-resistant Enterobacteriaceae and pseudomonads, *J. Antimicrob. Chemother.*, 18:177.

Jaurin, B., and Grundstrom, T., 1981, *amp C* cephalosporinase of *Escherichia coli* K-12 has a different evolutionary origin from that of β-lactamases of the penicillinase type, *Proc. Natl. Acad. Sci. USA*, 78:4897.

Jelsch, C., Mourey, L., Masson, J.M., and Samama, J.P., 1993, Crystal structure of *Escherichia coli* TEM1 β-lactamase at 1.8 Å resolution, *Proteins*, 16:364.

Kahan, F.M., Kropp, H., Sundelof, J.G., and Birnbaum, J.J., 1983, Thienamycin: development of imipenem-cilastatin, *Antimicrob. Chemother.*, 12(Suppl. D):1–35.

Kahan, J.S., Kahan, F.M., Goegelman, R., Currie, S.A., Jackson, M., Stapley, E.O., Miller, T.W., Miller, A.K., Hendlin, D., Mochales, S., Hernandez, S., Woodruff, H.B., and Birnbaum, J., 1979, Thienamycin, a new β-lactam antibiotic. I. Discovery, taxonomy, isolation, and physical properties, *J. Antibiot.*, 32:1.

Kim, H.S., and Campbell, B.J., 1982, β-lactamase activity of renal dipeptidase against N-formimidoyl-thienamycin, *Biochem. Biophys. Res. Commun.*, 108:1638.

Kirby, W.M.M., 1944, Extraction of a highly potent penicillin inactivator from penicillin resistant staphylococci, *Science*, 99:452.

Knothe, H., Shah, P., Krcmery, V., Antal, M., and Mitsuhashi, S., 1983, Transferable resistance to cefotaxime, cefoxitin, cefamandole and cefuroxime in clinical isolates of *Klebsiella pneumoniae* and *Serratia marcescens*, *Infection*, 11:315.

Knox, J. R., 1995, Extended-spectrum and inhibitors-resistant TEM-type β-lactamases: mutations, specificity, and three-dimensional structure, *Antimicrob. Agents Chemother.*, 39:2593.

Knox, J.R., Moews, P.C., and Frère, J.M., 1996, Molecular evolution of bacterial β-lactam resistance, *Chem. Biol.*, 3:937.

Kropp, H., Sundelof, J.G., Hajdu, R., and Kahan, F. M., 1982, Metabolism of thienamycin and related carbapenem antibiotics by the renal dipeptidase, dehydropeptidase, *Antimicrob. Agents Chemother.*, 22:62.

Leigh, D.A., Bradnock, K., and Merriner, J.M., 1981, Augmentin (amoxicillin and clavulanic acid) therapy in complicated infections due to beta-lactamase producing bacteria, *J. Antimicrob. Chemother.*, 7:229.

Lemozy, J., Sirot, D., Chanal, C., Huc, C., Labia, R., Dabernat, H., and Sirot, J., 1995, First characterization of inhibitor-resistant TEM (IRT) beta-lactamase in *Klebsiella pneumoniae* strains, *Antimicrob. Agents Chemother.*, 33:2580.

Li, X.-Z., Ma, D., Livermore, D.M., and Nikaido, H., 1994, Role of efflux pump(s) in intrinsic resistance of *Pseudomonas aeruginosa*: Active efflux as a contributing factor to β-lactam resistance, *Antimicrob. Agents Chemother.*, 38:1742.

Lobkovsky, E, Moews, P.C., Liu,H., Zhao,H., Frère, J.M., and J. R. Knox, 1993, Evolution of an enzyme activity: crystallographic structure at 2-Å resolution of cephalosporinase from the ampC gene of *Enterobacter cloacae* P99 and comparison with a class A penicillinase, *Proc. Natl. Acad. Sci. USA*, 90:11257.

Marshall, M.J., Ross, G.W., Chanter, K.V., and Harris, A.M., 1972, Comparison of the substrate specificities of the β-lactamases from *Klebsiella aerogenes* 1082E and *Enterobacter cloacae* P99, *Appl. Microbiol.*, 23:765.

Massova, I., and Mobashery, S., 1998, Kinship and diversification of bacterial penicillin-binding proteins and β-lactamases, *Antimicrob. Agents Chemother.* 42:1.

Massida, O., Rossolini, G.M., and Satta, G., 1991, The *Aeromonas hydrophila cphA* gene: Molecular heterogeneity among Class B metallo-β-lactamases, *J. Bacteriol.*, 173:4611.

Matagne, A., Lamotte-Brasseur, J., and Frère, J.M., 1993, Interactions between active-site serine β-lactamases and so-called β-lactamase-stable antibiotics. Kinetic and molecular modelling studies, *Eur. J. Biochem.*, 217:61.

Maveyraud, L., Massova, I., Brick, C., Miyashita, K., Samama, J.P., and Mobashery, S., 1996, Crystal-structure of 6α-(hydroxymethyl) penicillanate complexed to the TEM-1 β-lactamase from *Escherichia coli*: evidence on the mechanism of action of a novel inhibitor designed by a computer-aided process, *J. Am. Chem. Soc.*, 118:7435.

Maveyraud, L., Mourey, L., Kotra, L.P., Pedelacq, J.D., Guille, V., Mobashery, S., and Samama, J.P., 1998, Structural basis for clinical longevity of carbapenem antibiotics in the face of challenge by the common class A β-lactamases from the antibiotic-resistant bacteria, *J. Am. Chem. Soc.*, 120:9748.

Medeiros, A.A., 1997, Evolution and dissemination of β-lactamases accelerated by generation of β-lactam antibiotics, *Clin. Inf. Diseases*, 24:S19.

Meyer, K.S., Urban, C., Eagan, J.A., Berger, B.J., and Rahal, J.J., 1993, Nosocomial outbreak of *Klebsiella* infection resistant to late-generation cephalosporins, *Ann. Int. Med.*, 119:353.

Minami, S., Akama, M., Araki, H., Watanabe, Y., Narita, H., Iyobe, S., and Mitsuhashi, S., 1996, Imipenem and cephem resistant *Pseudomonas aeruginosa* carrying plasmids coding for class B β-lactamase, *J. Antimicrob. Chemother.*, 37:433.

Miyashita, K., Massova, I., and Mobashery, S., 1996, Quantification of the extent of attenuation of the rate of turnover chemistry of the TEM-1 β-lactamase by the α-1*R*-hydroxyethyl group in substrates, *Bioorg. Med. Chem. Lett.*, 6:319.

Miyashita, K., Massova, I., Taibi, P., and Mobashery, S., 1995, Design, synthesis and evaluation of a potent mechanism-based inhibitor for the TEM β-lactamase with implications for the enzyme mechanism, *J. Am. Chem. Soc.*, 117:11055.

Moews, P.C., Knox, J.R., Dideberg, O., Charlier, P., and Frère, J.M., 1990, β-lactamase of *Bacillus licheniformis* 749/C at 2 Å resolution, *Proteins Struct., Funct.* 7:156.

Neu, H.C., 1983, β-Lactamase stability of cefoxitin in comparison with other β-lactam compounds, *Diagn. Microbiol. Infect. Dis.*, 1:313.

Nordmann, P., Mariotte, S., Naas, T., Labia, R., and Nicolas, M.-H., 1993, Biochemical properties of a carbapenem-hydrolyzing β-lactamase from *Enterobacter cloacae* and cloning of the gene into *Escherichia coli*, *Antimicrob. Agents Chemother.*, 37:939.

Payne, D.J., Cramp, R., Winstanley, D.J., and Knowles, D.J.C., 1994, Comparative activities of clavulanic acid, sulbactam, and tazobactam against clinically important β-lactamases, *Antimicrob. Agents Chemother.*, 38:767.

Percival, A., Corkill, J.E., Arya, O.P., Rowlands, J., Alergany, C.D., Rees, E., and Annels, E.H., 1976, Penicillinase-producing gonococci in Liverpool, *The Lancet*, 2:1379.

Perez-Llarena, F.J., Liras, P., Rodriguez-Garcia, A., and Martin, J.F., 1997, A regulatory gene (ccaR) required for cephamycin and clavulanic acid production in *Streptomyces clavuligerus*: amplification results in overproduction of both β-lactam compounds., *J. Bacteriol.*, 179:2053.

Perilli, M., Felici, A., Franceschini, N., DeSantis, A., Pagani, L., Luzzaro, F., Oratore, A., Rossolini, G.M., Knox, J.R., and Amicosante, G., 1997, Characterization of a new TEM-derived beta-lactamase produced in a *Serratia marcescens* strain, *Antimicrob. Agents Chemother.*, 41:2374.

Perine, P.L., Schalla, W., Siegel, M.S., Thornsberry, C., Biddle, J., Wong, K.-H., and Thompson, S.E., 1977, Evidence for two distinct types of penicillinase-producing *Neisseria gonorrhoeae*, *The Lancet*, 2:993.

Petit, A., Gergaud, G., Sirot, D., Courvalin, P., and Sirot, J., 1990, Molecular epidemiology of TEM-3 (CTX-1) beta-lactamase, *Antimicrob. Agents Chemother.*, 34:219.

Prinarakis, E.E., Miriagou, V., Tzelepi, E., Gazouli, M., and Tzouvelekis, L.S., 1997, Emergence of an inhibitor-resistant beta-lactamase (SHV-10) derived from an SHV-5 variant, *Antimicrob. Agents Chemother.*, 41:838.

Rasheed, J.K., Jay, C., Metchock, B., Berkowitz, F., Weigel, L., Crellin, J., Steward, C., Hill, B., Medeiros, A.A., and Tenover, F.C., 1997, Evolution of extended-spectrum beta-lactam resistance (SHV-8) in a strain of *Escherichia coli* during multiple episodes of bacteremia, *Antimicrob. Agents Chemother.*, 41:647.

Rasmussen, B.A., and Bush, K., 1997, Carbapenem-hydrolyzing β-lactamases, *Antimicrob. Agents Chemother.*, 41:223.

Rasmussen, B.A., Bush, K., Keeney, D., Yang, Y., Hare, R., O'Gara, C., and Medeiros, A.A., 1996, Characterization of IMI-1 β-lactamase, a class A carbapenem-hydrolyzing enzyme from *Enterobacter cloacae*, *Antimicrob. Agents Chemother.*, 40:2080.

Reading, C., and Cole, M., 1977, Clavulanic acid: a beta-lactamase inhibitor from *Streptomyces clavuligerus*, *Antimicrob. Agents Chemother.*, 11:852.

Reading, C., and Farmer, T., 1981, The inhibition of beta-lactamases from Gram-negative bacteria by clavulanic acid, *Biochem. J.*, 199:779.

Richman, D. D., 1995, Protease uninhibited. *Nature*, 374:494.

Richmond, M.H., and Sykes, R.B., 1973, The β-lactamases of gram-negative bacteria and their possible physiological role, *Adv. Microb. Physiol.*, 9:31.

Roselle, G.A., Bode, R., Hamilton, B., Bibler, M., Sullivan, R., Douce, R., Staneck, J.L., and Bullock, W.E., 1985, Clinical trial of the efficacy and safety of ticarcillin and clavulanic acid, *Antimicrob. Agents Chemother.*, 27:291.

Sirot, D., Recule, C., Chaibi, E.B., Bret, L., Croize, J., Chanal-Claris, C., Labia, R., and Sirot, J., 1997, A complex mutant of TEM-1 beta-lactamase with mutations encountered in both IRT-4 and extended-spectrum TEM-15, produced by an *Escherichia coli* clinical isolate, *Antimicrob. Agents Chemother.*, 41:1322.

Sirot, D., Sirot, J., Labia, R., Morand, A., Courvalin, P., Darfeuille-Michaud, A., Perroux, R., and Cluzel, R., 1987, Transferable resistance to third-generation cephalosporins in clinical isolates of *Klebsiella pneumoniae*: identification of CTX-1, a novel β-lactamase, *J. Antimicrob. Chemother.*, 20:323.

Sowek, J. A., Singer, S. B., Ohringer, S., Mally, M. F., Dougherty, T. J., Gougoutas, J. Z., and Bush, K., 1991, Substitution of lysine at position 104 or 240 of TEM β-lactamase enhances the effect of serine-164 substitution of hydrolysis or affinity for cephalosporins and the monobactam aztreonam, *Biochemistry*, 30:3179.

Spratt, B.G., Jobanputra, V., and Zimmermann, W., 1977, Binding of thienamycin and clavulanic acid to the penicillin-binding proteins of *Escherichia coli* K-12, *Antimicrob. Agents Chemother.*, 12:406.

Strynadka, N.C., Adachi, H., Jensen, S.E., Johns, K., Sielecki, A., Betzel, C., Sutoh, K., and James, M.N., 1992, Molecular structure of the acyl-enzyme intermediate in β-lactam hydrolysis at 1.7 Å resolution, *Nature*, 359:700.

Strynadka, N.C.J., Jensen, S.E., Alzari, P.M., and James, M.N.G., 1996, A potent new mode of β-lactamase inhibition revealed by the 1.7 Å X-ray crystallographic structure of the TEM-1-BLIP complex, *Nature Struct. Biol.*, 3:290.

Sykes, R.B., Bonner, D.P., and Bush, K., Georgopapadakou, N.H., 1982, Azthreonam (SQ 26,776), a synthetic monobactam specifically active against aerobic gram-negative bacteria, *Antimicrob. Agents Chemother.*, 21:85.

Sykes, R.B., and Matthew, M., 1976, The β-lactamases of gram-negative bacteria and their role in resistance to β-lactam antibiotics, *J. Antimicrob. Chemother.*, 2:115.

Taibi, P., and Mobashery, S., Mechanism of turnover of imipenem by the TEM β-lactamase revisited, *J. Am. Chem. Soc.*, 1995, 117:7600.

Taibi, P., Massova, I., Vakulenko, S.B., Lerner, S.A., and Mobashery, S., 1996, Evidence for structural elasticity of β-lactamases in the course of catalytic turnover of the novel cephalosporin cefepime, *J. Am. Chem. Soc.*, 118:7441.

Tarpay, M., 1978, Importance of antimicrobial susceptibility testing of *Streptococcus pneumoniae*, *Antimicrob. Agents Chemother.*, 14:628.

Thornsberry, C., Ogilvie, P., Kahn, J., and Mauriz, Y., 1997, Surveillance of antimicrobial resistance in *Streptococcus pneumoniae, Haemophilus influenzae*, and *Moraxella catarrhalis* in the United States in 1996–1997 respiratory season Thornsberry, Clyde; Ogilvie, P., Kahn, J., and Mauriz, Y., *Diagn. Microbiol. Infect. Dis.*, 29:249.

Tipper, D.J., and Strominger, J.L., 1965, Mechanism of action of penicillins: a proposal based on their structural similarity to acyl-D-alanyl-D-alanine, *Proc. Natl. Acad. Sci. U.S.A.*, 54:1133.

Vakulenko, S., Taibi-Tronche, P., Toth, M., Massova, I., Mobashery, S., and Lerner, S.S., Unpublished results.

Vedel, G., Belaaouaj, A., Gilly, L., Labia, R., Philippon, A., Névot, P., and Paul, G., 1992, Clinical isolates of *Escherichia coli* producing TRI β-lactamases: novel TEM-enzymes conferring resistance to β-lactamase inhibitors, *J. Antimicrob. Chemother.*, 30:449.

Voladri, R.K.R., Tummuru, M.K.R., and Kernodle, D.S., 1996, Structure-function relationships among wild-type variants of *Staphylococcus aureus* β-lactamase: importance of amino acids 128 and 216, *J. Bacteriol.*, 178:7248.

Wells, J.S., Hunter, J.C., Astle, G.L., Sherwood, J.C., Ricca, C.M., Trejo, W.H., Bonner, D.P., and Sykes, R.B., 1982, Distribution of β-lactam and β-lactone producing bacteria in nature, *J. Antibiotics*, 35:814.

Yang, Y., Bhachech, N., and Bush, K., 1995, Biochemical comparison of imipenem, meropenem and biapenem: permeability, binding to penicillin-binding proteins, and stability to hydrolysis by β-lactamases, *J. Antimicrob. Chemother.*, 35:75.

Yang, Y., Rasmussen, B.A., and Bush, K., 1992, Biochemical characterization of the metallo-β-lactamase Ccr A from *Bacteroides fragilis* TAL3636, *Antimicrob. Agents Chemother.*, 36:1155.

Yang, Y., Wu, P., and Livermore, D.M., 1990, Biochemical characterization of a β-lactamase that hydrolyzes penems and carbapenems for two *Serratia marcescens* isolates, *Antimicrob. Agents Chemother.*, 34:755.

Zafaralla, G., and Mobashery, S., 1992, Facilitation of the $\Delta^2 \rightarrow \Delta^1$ pyrroline tautomerization of carbapenem antibiotics by the highly conserved arginine-244 of class A β-lactamases during the course of turnover, *J. Am.
Chem. Soc.*, 114:1505.

Zhou, X.Y., Bordon, F., Sirot, D., Kitzis, M.-D., and Gutmann, L., 1994, Emergence of clinical isolates of *Escherichia coli* producing TEM-1 derivatives or an OXA-1 β-lactamase conferring resistance to β-lactamase
inhibitors, *Antimicrob. Agents Chemother.*, 38:1085.

6

ANTIFOLATE RESISTANCE MECHANISMS FROM BACTERIA TO CANCER CELLS WITH EMPHASIS ON PARASITES

Marc Ouellette, Éric Leblanc, Christoph Kündig, and
Barbara Papadopoulou

Centre de Recherche en Infectiologie du CHUL
Département de Microbiologie
Université Laval
Québec, Canada G1V 4G2

INTRODUCTION

Reduced folates serve as co-factors in a variety of one-carbon transfer reactions including the biosynthesis of thymidylate, of purine nucleotides, and of the amino acids serine and methionine. Dihydrofolate reductase (DHFR) and thymidylate synthase (TS) catalyze consecutive reactions in the *de novo* synthesis of dTMP. In protozoa and plants, these two enzymes are fused resulting in a DHFR-TS protein (Ferone and Roland, 1980). The enzyme DHFR is the target for the action of antifolates, which are widely used during chemotherapeutic interventions. Commonly used antifolates are shown in Figure 1. The folate antagonist trimethoprim (TMP) is used to treat bacterial infections caused by urinary tract or enteric pathogens (Huovinen et al., 1995). The antifolate pyrimethamine (PYR) is used against the protozoan parasites *Plasmodium* and *Toxoplasma* (Borst and Ouellette, 1995) whereas trimetrexate with leucovirin is used in fungal infections caused by *Pneumocystis carinii* (Hitchings, 1989). The antifolate methotrexate (MTX) is widely used for the treatment of various forms of cancer as well as for the treatment of rheumatoid arthritis, psoriasis and some autoimmune diseases (Gorlick et al., 1996). The primary structures of DHFR from a variety of organisms share very little homology, hence explaining, in part, the specificity and activity of different antifolates against targeted organisms. The basis for this selectivity was studied further by using comparative enzymology and structural analyses. Differences in the kinetic properties of the various DHFRs are likely to contribute to the selectivity of antifolates (Schweitzer et al., 1990).

Resolving the Antibiotic Paradox, edited by Rosen and Mobashery.
Kluwer Academic / Plenum Publishers, New York, 1998.

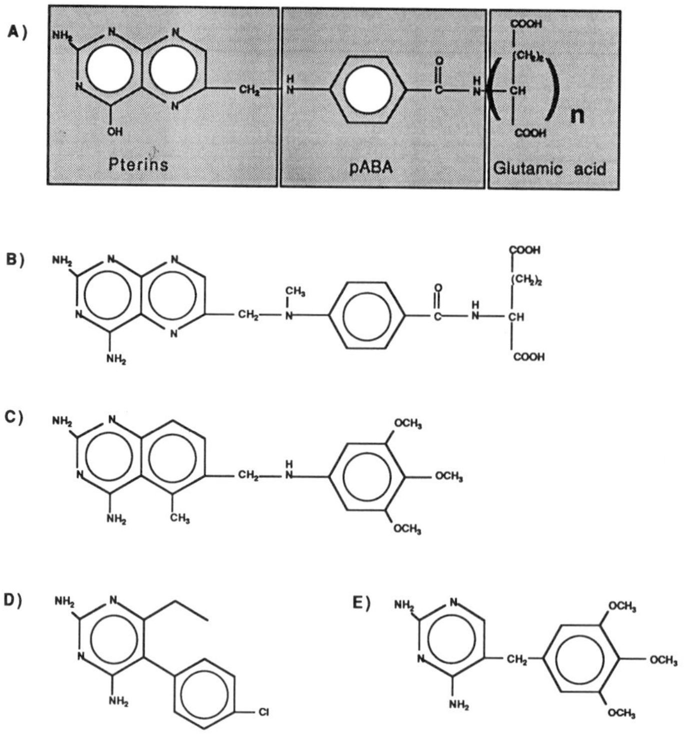

Figure 1. Structure of folic acid and of antifolates. A) Folic acid; B) methotrexate; C) trimetrexate; D) trimethoprim; E) pyrimethamine.

Synthesis of Reduced Folates

Folates are made of three building blocks; a pteridine, p-aminobenzoic acid (PABA) and glutamic acid (Fig. 1A). Some organisms are capable to synthesize folates *de novo*, others, such as mammals, rely on folates from the environment and require specific transport systems and receptors for their folate requirements. Bacteria and several eukaryotic cells can synthesize the pteridine backbone from GTP (Fig. 2). The first and rate limiting step is catalyzed by GTP cyclohydrolase I. Organisms that can synthesize folates *de novo* need to conjugate the pteridine to PABA. This is catalyzed by the enzyme dihydropteroate synthase (DHPS) (Fig. 2), a target of sulfonamides, the first class of antimicrobial agents developed to treat bacterial infections in humans with a satisfactory margin of selectivity. The enzyme dihydrofolate synthase (DHFS) catalyzes the addition of glutamic acid to dihydropteroate leading to the synthesis of 7,8-dihydrofolate. Nearly all the intracellular folates in microorganisms and animal cells occur as polyglutamates with four- to six-glutamate residues attached to the PABA moiety (Fig. 1A). Polyglutamated folates are often more efficient substrates for many folate-dependent enzymes. The enzyme DHFR reduces dihydrofolate into tetrahydrofolate. This reduced folate will be modified to serve as a carbon donor for the synthesis of thymidylate catalyzed by TS (Fig. 2).

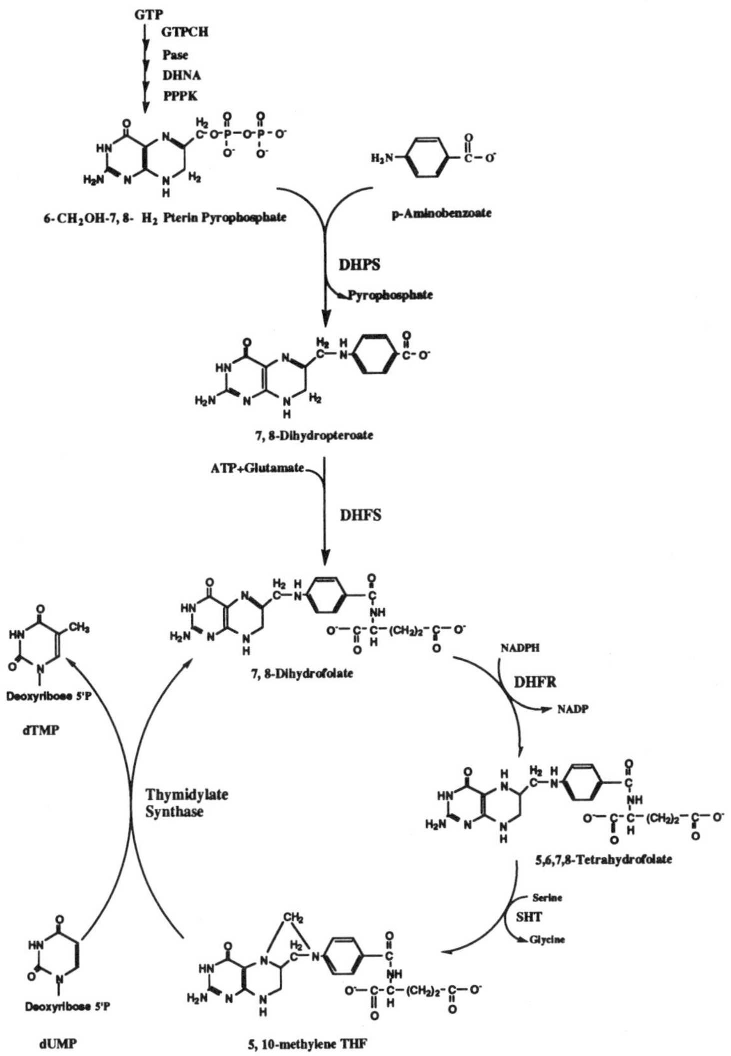

Figure 2. Folate metabolism. In some organisms pterins can be synthesized de novo from GTP. Dihydropteroate is made by the conjugation of a pterin to p-aminobenzoic acid which is catalyzed by dihydropteroate synthase (DHPS). The addition of glutamic acid by dihydrofolate synthase (DHFS) lead to dihydrofolate which is reduced to tetrahydrofolate by dihydrofolate reductase (DHFR). The latter reduced folate is modified by a serine hydroxymethyl transferase (SHT) which serve as a carbon donor for the synthesis of thymidine by thymidilate synthase (TS).

ANTIFOLATE RESISTANCE IN BACTERIA

Sulfonamides and Trimethoprim

The discovery of the antibacterial activity of the dye prontosil by the German chemist Domagk in 1935 led to the discovery of sulfonamides. The mechanism of action of sulfonamides was elucidated by Woods in 1940 where he showed that sulfonamide prevented the incorporation of PABA into pteroic acid (reviewed in Jukes, 1987). Several microorganisms require PABA to synthesize their folates whereas their hosts obtain their folates from dietary sources, hence explaining the selectivity of sulfonamides. Trimethoprim (TMP) (Fig. 1D) is a synthetic antibacterial agent that was developed in the 1950s during the synthesis of several 2,-4 diaminopyrimidines as antagonist of the enzyme DHFR. TMP has a wide spectrum of antibacterial activity and exhibits high specificity for the bacterial DHFRs compared to the mammalian ones.

As sulfonamides and TMP inhibit important steps of the same pathway, both drugs have been used in combination (e.g. co-trimoxazole, Fansidar) since the late 60s. This is supported by synergistic interactions between the two classes of drugs *in vitro*. However, the synergism of the combination TMP-sulfonamides *in vivo* is, at best, of marginal importance in the treatment of bacterial infections. Scientific and clinical considerations would suggest that for most bacterial infections, TMP alone is superior to co-trimoxazole (Brumfitt and Hamilton-Miller, 1995). The combination of both drugs seems more effective in the treatment of parasitic infections, however. Although both classes of drugs were introduced more than 30 years ago, they still find wide applications. As both drugs are relatively inexpensive they can also be used in the treatment of infections in developing countries. However, a marked and steady increase in the rate of resistance to TMP and sulfonamides is decreasing the usefulness of these drugs.

Resistance to Sulfonamides

Resistance to sulfonamides in Gram negative enteric bacteria is due to plasmid encoded DHPS, encoded by the *sul* genes, that have diverged considerably from the chromosomal bacterial DHPS (Huovinen et al., 1995). The *sul1* gene is part of integrons; these specialized mobile genetic elements are facilitating the genesis of multiresistance operons (Ouellette and Kündig, 1997). Sulfonamide resistance in *Neisseria meningitidis* is mediated by mutation in the chromosomal *dhps* gene (Fermer et al., 1995). Sequencing of the chromosomal *dhps* of sulfonamide resistant clinical isolates of *Staphylococcus aureus* indicated that as many as 14 residues may be involved in resistance (Hampele et al., 1997). None of these residues have been formally proven to be involved in resistance, however.

Resistance to Trimethoprim

The most common way by which bacteria resist the antifolate TMP is by a by-pass mechanism. This is achieved by virtue of the synthesis of a plasmid encoded DHFR that is TMP insensitive. More than 15 different plasmid DHFRs, that can be divided in two large families as defined by amino acid sequence analysis, have been described in gram negative bacteria (Huovinen et al., 1995). Resistance to TMP has spread most importantly in urinary tract and enteric pathogens while respiratory tract pathogens (such as *Haemophilus influenzae*, *Streptococcus pneumoniae* and *Moraxella catarrhalis*) have been spared by the emergence of resistance. This may be due to the inability of plasmids encoding the *dhfr* genes to replicate into the latter group of bacteria. Mutations in the *dhfr* chromosomal gene of *H. influenzae* can cause resistance. These mutations are either in the promoter region or in the structural DHFR gene (de Groot et al, 1996). Chromosomal mediated resistance will spread less efficiently than plasmid mediated resistance.

Two plasmid TMP-resistant DHFRs named S1 and S2 have been characterized in *Staphylococcus* species (Rouch et al., 1989; Dale et al., 1995). The S2 gene was recently found in *Listeria monocytogenes* (Charpentier and Courvalin, 1997). A single amino acid substitution in the active site of the chromosomal *S. aureus dhfr*, resulting in the loss of a hydrogen bond between TMP and the protein, can also lead to resistance (Dale et al., 1997).

Transport Related Mechanisms

Transport systems involved in either uptake or efflux are not critical in determining clinical antifolate resistance in bacteria. Nevertheless, decreased uptake of MTX has been described in strains of *Enterococcus faecium* selected stepwise *in vitro* for MTX resistance (Tamura et al., 1997). Bacterial multidrug efflux pumps have been shown to extrude several unrelated drugs outside the cell and may account for intrinsic resistance to a number of drugs (Lewis et al., 1997). Interestingly, TMP and sulfonamides were shown to be substrates of the MexAB/OprM multidrug efflux pump of *Pseudomonas aeruginosa* (Kohler et al., 1996) suggesting that efflux may be a further resistance mechanism against antifolates in some bacterial species.

ANTIFOLATE RESISTANCE IN CANCER CELLS

The folic acid analog MTX (amethopterin) (Fig. 1B) was first synthesized in 1948 and its biological activity was determined soon after where it was found to prolong the survival of mice transplanted with leukemia cells (reviewed in Jukes, 1987). Considerable work has been done on the mechanism of action and mechanisms of resistance to MTX (Bertino, 1993, Huennekens, 1996). While the activity of MTX against malignancies was being established in the 50s, its cellular target was found to correspond to DHFR. The main mechanisms of resistance to MTX are reduced uptake of the drug; increased or mutated DHFR; and finally decreased polyglutamate formation.

Transport Mutations

MTX is transported into cells by the carrier system used for the active transport of reduced folates. MTX transport deficiency due to decreased activity of the reduced folate carrier (RFC1) leads to resistance to MTX in several cell lines. The human RCF1 has been cloned by virtue of its ability to complement a mutant cell defective in the uptake of MTX (Williams and Flintoff, 1995). The importance of RCF1 in MTX resistance was recently established in various cell lines and in clinical specimens. Decreased RCF1 expression at the RNA level was associated with impaired MTX transport and clinical resistance (Gorlick et al., 1997; Moscow et al., 1997).

As cells without a RCF1 can still grow, cells must fulfill their folates requirement by other routes. Indeed, several glycosyl-phosphatidylinositol-anchored folate receptors (FR) are important for the uptake of folates and antifolates (Anthony, 1996). In at least one study, decreased expression of one of these FR was correlated with transport defective MTX resistance in human cells (Saikawa et al., 1993).

The RCF1 transporter mediates bi-directional transport of MTX and the steady state accumulation of the drug is dependent on the rate of influx and efflux (Zhao et al., 1997). Other routes of MTX (and folates) efflux have been described in cancer cells (Schlemmer and Sirotnak, 1992; Henderson et al., 1994). Interestingly, a Chinese hamster ovary line selected for resistance to the lipophilic antifolate PYR exhibited a marked decreased in the efflux of folic acid (Assaraf and Goldman, 1997) suggesting that down regulation of this export system may lead to resistance. Although the mammalian multidrug resistance efflux pump MDR1 does not confer resistance to MTX it can be amplified following selection with the lipophilic analog trimetrexate (Assaraf et al., 1989) and MDR1 can confer resistance to MTX in a folate transporter deficient background (de Graaf et al., 1996).

DHFR Amplification and Mutation

It has been known for a long time that acquired resistance to MTX in tumor cells was often caused by an increase in the level of DHFR (Bertino, 1993). The basis for this increased level was shown to correspond to amplification of the DHFR gene (Alt et al., 1978). Several investigators have used the *dhfr* locus and MTX selection to study the mechanisms of gene amplification and DNA replication in mammalian cells (Hamlin and Ma 1990). Amplification of DHFR is also observed in lines selected for resistance to the lipophilic analog trimetrexate (Assaraf et al., 1989). DHFR amplification is not a simple curiosity found in tumor cell lines generated in the laboratory. Indeed, DHFR gene amplification is responsible for resistance in acute lymphoblastic leukemia, which have relapsed after a first course of MTX treatment. Interestingly, *dhfr* amplification was correlated with mutation in p53 (Goker et al., 1995), a protein important in the cell cycle control. Suppression of other tumor suppressor genes, or their regulators such as the retinoblastoma gene and the cyclin D1, can also influence the level of MTX resistance by modulating the level of DHFR transcripts (Gorlick et al., 1996).

Resistance to MTX can also be achieved by point mutation in DHFR that lower the inhibition of MTX. Mutations at three positions (G15W; L22R; L22F; F31W; F31S) have been characterized in tumor cell lines (Schweitzer et al., 1990; Melera, 1991). Mutations at the hydrophobic residues at position 22 and 31 alter the folate-binding region of DHFR. Point mutations in DHFR do not seem to account frequently for clinical resistance in cancer, however (Gorlick et al., 1996; Spencer et al., 1996).

Decreased Polyglutamylation

MTX is a prodrug and requires polyglutamylation for cellular retention (Chabner et al., 1985). Decreased polyglutamylation will lead to decreased retention and efflux of MTX out of the cell. MTX is polyglutamated by the enzyme folylpolyglutamate synthase (FPGS). The human FPGS has been cloned (Garrow et al., 1992) and its altered transcriptional or post-transcriptional regulation is correlated with acquired antifolate resistance (Gorlick et al., 1996; Roy et al., 1997). MTX-polyglutamates, are transported into lysosomes where they are hydrolyzed to the monoglutamate form by a γ-glutamyl hydrolase (GGH). The human GGH gene was cloned (Yao et al., 1996) and an increase in GGH activity leading to MTX-monoglutamate and increased extrusion of the drug corresponds to a further mechanism of resistance to MTX (Rhee et al., 1993). In addition of being potent inhibitors of DHFR, MTX-polyglutamates are potent inhibitors of enzymes involved in purine biosynthesis. Decreased polyglutamylation may lead to decreased inhibition of the latter enzymes. The extent of MTX polyglutamylation formation in tumor cells is an important determinant of the efficacy of MTX treatment. The ratio between GGH and FPGS was found to be a good indicator of the levels of MTX-polyglutamate and may serve as a diagnostic predictor of the clinical response to MTX therapy and outcome (Longo et al., 1997).

ANTIFOLATE RESISTANCE IN PARASITES

In protozoa DHFR and TS are fused resulting in a DHFR-TS bifunctional protein. The DHFR antagonists pyrimethamine (PYR) (Fig. 1) and proguanil have played a major role in prophylaxis and treatment of *Plasmodium falciparum* infection and they are often used in conjunction with sulfadoxine, a combination known as Fansidar. Many protozoa, however, are incapable of synthesizing their own folates and they must obtain them from the environment via specific transporters. Other protozoa supplement the folates they make themselves with imported folates. Resistance against antifolates has been studied intensively in protozoa and in addition to already known mechanisms of resistance, novel ones have been discovered.

Mutations in DHFR and DHPS

The most commonly found resistance mechanism to PYR in *P. falciparum* is a single point mutation, S108N, in the DHFR domain (Cowman et al., 1988; Peterson et al., 1988). The DHFR of cycloguanil-resistant *P. falciparum* field strains contains a S108T mutation along with another mutation (Foote et al, 1990; Peterson et al., 1990). These latter isolates are not cross-resistant to PYR. To become resistant to both antifolates, a S108N mutation along with few other key point mutations are required (Foote et al, 1990; Peterson et al., 1990). The role of some of these mutations have now been tested by gene transfection (vanDijk et al., 1995; Wu et al., 1996). In cell lines selected *in vitro*, other DHFR amino acid residues, in addition to position 108, were altered and these may confer higher levels of resistance (Borst and Ouellette, 1995). A recent study of 141 field samples has indicated that 11 DHFR variants over wild-type are associated with PYR resistance (Wang et al., 1997a). By far the most predominant mutated residue is located at position 108 but the exact role of several of the other mutations pinpointed is still requiring functional testing. Nevertheless, several mutated DHFRs were purified and characterized. Results indicated that the accumulation of mutations at specific residues was selected in nature to optimize resistance to PYR (Sirawaraporn et al., 1997).

Although mutations in the DHFR have not been found in PYR resistant *Toxoplasma gondii*, introduction of mutations into the *T. gondii* DHFR-TS at positions corresponding to mutations found in *P. falciparum* and reintroduction of the mutated gene into *T. gondii*, led to PYR resistant parasites (Donald and Roos, 1993). The DHFR-TS of *Cryptosporidium parvum* was shown to contain several non conserved residues at positions for which point mutations have been shown to correlate with antifolate resistance in other DHFRs (Vasquez et al, 1996). This may explain the inefficacy of conventional microbial antifolate treatments against *C. parvum*.

Overproduction of DHFR by gene duplication (Inselburg et al., 1987; Cowman and Lew, 1989) will confer PYR resistance in *Plasmodium* lines selected under laboratory conditions. Although none of the currently available antifolates is suitable for treatment of leishmaniasis, considerable work has been done in laboratory induced MTX resistance. Amplification of the *dhfr-ts* gene is frequently observed in *Leishmania major* cells selected for MTX (Coderre et al., 1983; Beverley, 1991). Amplification of *dhfr-ts* has not been observed in other *Leishmania* species but when a preferred MTX resistance mechanism was unavailable in *Leishmania tarentolae*, *dhfr-ts* was amplified upon MTX selection (Kündig et al., 1996). In at least one case the DHFR overproduced in *L. major* had a point mutation (Arrebola et al., 1994) in a position known to correlate with MTX resistance in mammalian DHFRs. Transfection of this mutated allele confirmed that the mutation increased the level of MTX resistance (Arrebola et al., 1994). Nevertheless, the mutation occurred in the amplified gene and not in the chromosomal single copy gene.

The DHPS of *Plasmodium* (Brooks et al., 1994; Triglia and Cowman, 1994) and of *T. gondii* (Pashley et al., 1997) were characterized. In contrast to the bacterial DHPS, which are monofunctional, the parasitic DHPS are part of bifunctional proteins, hydroxymethyl-dihydropterin pyrophosphokinase (PPPK)-DHPS. PPPK catalyze the step immediately before DHPS in the *de novo* folate pathway (Fig. 2). In *Pneumocystis carinii*, the protein is trifunctional with dihydroneopterin aldolase-PPPK and-DHPS domains (Volpe et al., 1993). The DHPS of sulfadoxine resistant and sensitive malaria parasites were found to differ in sequence (Brooks et al., 1994; Triglia and Cowman, 1994). Analysis of a genetic cross indicated tight linkage between DHPS mutations and resistance to sulfonamides (Wang et al., 1997b). In the same study, the IC50 of sulfonamides was influenced markedly by exogenous folates. This phenotype did not segregate with DHPS but possibly with a gene close to DHFR (Wang et al., 1997b). Analysis of 141 *P. falciparum* clinical strains from diverse origins revealed that point mutation in DHPS of resistant isolates were detected at 13 different positions (Wang et al., 1997a). A good correlation was also found between the number and frequency of DHPS mutations and the history of Fansidar usage in the different geographical areas.

Transport Mutations

Leishmania is capable to synthesize folate de novo although the exact mechanism is unknown (Borst and Ouellette, 1995; Nare et al., 1997a). Radioactive biopterin is converted into folates (Beck and Ullman, 1991) but, at least in *L. major*, radioactive PABA is not incorporated into folates (Ellenberger and Beverley, 1987a). None of the sulfonamides tested has shown activity against *Leishmania* (Petrillo-Peixoto and Beverley, 1987; Kaur et al., 1988) suggesting that if *Leishmania* has a DHPS it must have diverged considerably from other DHPS. Whatever the non-conventional route *Leishmania* use for their *de novo* folate synthesis, it still rely heavily on import under standard conditions. *Leishmania* have a common folate/MTX transporter, and mutations in the gene for this transporter lead to MTX resistance (Dewes et al., 1986; Ellenberger and Beverley, 1987b; Kaur et al., 1988; Papadopoulou et al., 1993; Gamarro et al., 1994). Two mutant transport phenotypes have been observed in *Leishmania*; one that decreases uptake by 2–5 fold and one that decreases uptake by more than 50-fold (Ouellette et al., 1995). Genes involved in folate transport are starting to be isolated (Nare et al., 1997a) which will permit to study their role in resistance.

Leishmania cells without measurable folate transport grow perfectly well under standard laboratory conditions. Their folates are therefore obtained by either other routes of entry or by increased *de novo* synthesis. An interesting link between folate and pterin metabolism has been made in *L. donovani*. In contrast to wild type *L. donovani* cells, mutants with a defective folate transporter are unable to thrive in folate-deficient medium supplemented with pterins (Beck and Ullman, 1990). It is not obvious how a defect in a folate transporter could prevent biosynthesis of folates from biopterin. Recent work in our laboratory has indicated however, one strategy by which *L. tarentolae* can grow without a folate transporter (see below).

Novel Mechanisms of Resistance

One locus that is frequently amplified in MTX resistant *Leishmania* species is the H locus (Beverley, 1991; Ouellette and Papadopoulou 1993). In addition to MTX, several other drugs can induce the amplification of the H locus. At least two drug resistance genes have been isolated on the H locus. One is the ABC transporter PgpA (Ouellette et al., 1990). Transfection of the *pgpA* gene indicated that it is involved in arsenite and antimonite resistance (Callahan and Beverley, 1991; Papadopoulou et al., 1994a) and may recognize metals conjugated to glutathione and/or trypanothione (Grondin et al., 1997; Légaré et al., 1997). The second gene is *ptr1* (also known as LTDH or HMTXR) whose transfection confers high level antifolate resistance in *Leishmania* (Papadopoulou et al., 1992; Callahan and Beverley, 1992). PTR1 is part of the short chain dehydrogenases /reductases (SDR), a large family of proteins involved in various oxido-reduction reactions in different organisms (Jörnvall et al., 1995). This family of proteins has a universally conserved YXXXK motif and disruption of any of the two conserved residues in PTR1 will render the enzyme inactive (Leblanc et al., 1998). Amplification of a gene encoding for a SDR corresponds to a novel resistance mechanism and to understand the mechanism by which PTR1 confers resistance, genetic and biochemical analysis were performed (Borst and Ouellette, 1995; Nare et al., 1997a).

Either *L. tarentolae* or *L. major ptr1* null mutants generated by gene targeting were shown to be hypersensitive to MTX and to lose the ability of growing on biopterin-supplemented folate deficient medium (Bello et al., 1994; Papadopoulou et al., 1994b). The biochemical characterization of PTR1 has indicated that it exhibits an NADPH-dependent reductase activity; it reduces pterins and folates, with the most oxidized form of pterins being the preferred substrate (Bello et al., 1994; Wang et al., 1997c; Nare et al., 1997b). The main function of PTR1 is to salvage oxidized pterins (Bello et al., 1994); a secondary function is reduction of folates. Wild-type levels of PTR1 contribute to around 10% of reduced folates (Nare et al., 1997b) but amplification of its gene under MTX selection will furnish the cells with sufficient reduced folates to grow. PTR1 therefore serves as an alternative route for the synthesis of reduced folates and its amplification will lead to MTX resistance (Borst and Ouellette, 1995; Nare et al., 1997a). The role of PTR1 and DHFR-TS in folate metabolism and resistance to antifolates is illustrated in Fig. 3. A PTR1 homologue was recently characterized in *Trypanosoma cruzi* and its transfection also leads to MTX resistance (Robello et al., 1998).

The group of S. Beverley has set up transfection techniques that permit the cloning of *Leishmania* genes by functional complementation (Ryan et al, 1993). We used this ap-

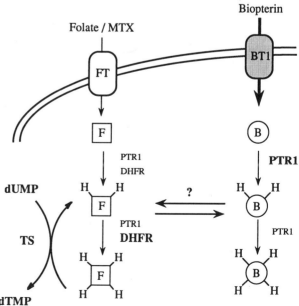

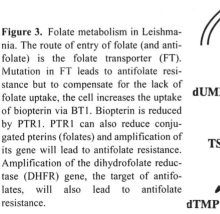

Figure 3. Folate metabolism in Leishmania. The route of entry of folate (and antifolate) is the folate transporter (FT). Mutation in FT leads to antifolate resistance but to compensate for the lack of folate uptake, the cell increases the uptake of biopterin via BT1. Biopterin is reduced by PTR1. PTR1 can also reduce conjugated pterins (folates) and amplification of its gene will lead to antifolate resistance. Amplification of the dihydrofolate reductase (DHFR) gene, the target of antifolates, will also lead to antifolate resistance.

proach to isolate novel antifolate resistance genes in *Leishmania*. Cosmid libraries of *Leishmania* species cloned into expression vectors were transfected into *Leishmania* which were then selected on MTX containing plates. One gene isolated in this manner was characterized, and its product corresponds to a membrane protein that is identical to the gene product of *orfG* (Myler et al., 1994). OrfG is part of a region known as CD1/LD1 that is frequently amplified in *Leishmania* strains from the lab and from the field (Segovia and Ortiz, 1997) The LD1 region was in search of a function and MTX resistance (and folate metabolism) may be one of these. The probable membrane location of OrfG incited us to look whether resistance could be mediated by efflux of MTX. In *Candida albicans*, the major facilitator efflux pump BENR may be involved in MTX resistance (Ben Yacov et al., 1994). Accumulation of MTX (or folate) was identical in orfG transfectants and wild-type cells. However, the uptake of biopterin was markedly increased suggesting that OrfG is a biopterin transporter (Kündig et al., 1997). Using a different selection scheme Moore and Beverley also found that orfG (named BT1) was a biopterin transporter (Moore and Beverley, 1996). An increased uptake of pterins, the main building block of folates, mediated by increased BT1 activity, is likely to contribute in increasing folate synthesis which in turns will lead to MTX resistance (Fig. 3). We have also analyzed *L. tarentolae* MTX resistant mutants to see whether BT1 plays a role in resistance. Remarkably, in every mutant for which resistance was mediated by a marked reduced uptake of MTX (and folate) biopterin uptake mediated by BT1 was increased. Since *Leishmania* cells depend mainly on folates from the environment for their growth, they seem to compensate for the lack of folate uptake (necessary for survival in the presence of MTX) by increasing the uptake of a precursor (Kündig et al., 1997).

COMMON THEMES OF ANTIFOLATE RESISTANCE MECHANISMS IN LIVING ORGANISMS

This chapter illustrates that organisms are not lacking of imagination and means to counteract antifolates. The various mechanisms are summarized in Table 1. Nevertheless, there are common themes between mammalian cells and microorganisms that are worth mentioning. The target of antifolates is DHFR and several resistance mechanisms are revolving around DHFR. Amplification of the *dhfr* gene, or its increased transcription, will often lead to MTX resistance in cancer cells and in *Leishmania*. Mutations in DHFR will also confer resistance provided that these mutations decrease the affinity of the enzyme for the inhibitor. Mutations may decrease the catalytic activity of the enzyme however, and this may require gene amplification. Nevertheless, some bacteria or *P. falciparum* with mutations in their single copy *dhfr* gene are growing normally suggesting that some DHFRs are more tolerant to mutations. When bacteria don't amplify and/or mutate their chromosomal *dhfr* gene they acquire novel genes whose gene products have DHFR activity but are insensitive to TMP. A similar by-pass mechanism is also observed in *Leishmania* where PTR1, with no sequence homology to DHFR, can nevertheless reduce folates. PTR1 is much less sensitive to MTX than DHFR-TS (Nare et al., 1997b). In organisms that depend on folates from the environment, mutation in the folate transporter will lead to decreased antifolate transport and hence to increased resistance. Although cells can now resist to antifolates they need to compensate for the lack of folate uptake. Cancer cells are likely to use other routes of entry while *Leishmania* cells may increased the uptake of the precursor biopterin. Increased efflux of MTX or decreased efflux of folates, are also other transport mutations that can contribute to antifolate resistance. MTX is a prodrug and it is

Table 1. Antifolate resistance mechanisms

Mechanisms	Bacteria	Cancer cells	Parasites
Gene amplification	+	+++	++
Target mutation	++	++	+++
By-pass mechanism	+++		++
Reduced uptake	+	+++	++
Modification		++	
Uptake of precursors			+

polyglutamylated. Although folates are polyglutamylated in most organisms, the drugs PYR and TMP are not. In contrast, MTX can be modified, and decreased activity of FPGS or increased hydrolysis of the glutamate tail by GGH will lead to decreased cellular retention of MTX and hence to MTX resistance. Interestingly, although folates are polyglutamated in *Leishmania* (Santi et al., 1987) MTX is not (Ellenberger et al., 1989). At this stage, it is not know whether FPGS of *Leishmania* can discriminate between folate and methotrexate and whether modification of the drug can lead to MTX resistance. *Leishmania* has an MTX-hydrolyzing enzymatic activity (Kaur et al., 1988; Ellenberger et al., 1989) which could potentially confer MTX resistance by modifying the drug. This has not yet been observed, however.

Our understanding of antifolate resistance is providing the tools, with PCR primers, to diagnose rapidly the resistance genotype and this could be useful to determine the appropriate therapy to combat microbial or neoplasic diseases. These tools may even serve to reach prognosis while using MTX for chemotherapy. Work on the mechanisms of resistance is also providing novel insights in folate metabolism and in pinpointing novel intracellular targets for which drugs could be developed. Our understanding of resistance mechanisms has indeed guided the design of new folate antagonists (Gorlick et al., 1996). Our continuing effort in understanding drug resistance mechanisms in general should lead to the generation of drugs that will be closer to the 'magic bullet' concept established almost a century ago by Paul Ehrlich.

ACKNOWLEDGMENTS

This work was supported by NSERC to M.O. EL is the recipient of a FCAR studentship; C.K. is a post-doctoral fellow of the Schweizerischer Nationalfonds, B.P. is a MRC scholar and M.O. is a chercheur boursier of the Fonds de Recherche en Santé du Québec. MO is a recipient of a Burroughs Wellcome Fund New Investigator Award in Molecular Parasitology.

REFERENCES

Alt, F.W., Kellems, R.E., Bertino, J.R., and Schimke, R.T. 1978. Selective multiplication of dihydrofolate reductase genes in methotrexate-resistant variant of cultured murine cells. *J. Biol. Chem.* 253:1357.

Antony AC. 1996. Folate receptors. *Annu. Rev. Nutr.* 16:501–521.

Arrebola, R., Olmo, A., Reche, P., Garvey, E.P., Santi, D.V., Ruiz-Perez, L.M., and Gonzales-Pacanowska, D. 1994. Isolation and characterization of a mutant dihydrofolate reductase-thymidylate synthase from methotrexate-resistant *Leishmania* cells. *J. Biol. Chem.* 269:10590.

Assaraf Y.G., and Goldman I.D. 1997. Loss of folic acid exporter function with markedly augmented folate accumulation in lipophilic antifolate-resistant mammalian cells. *J. Biol. Chem.* 272:17460.

Assaraf Y.G., Molina A., and Schimke R.T. 1989. Sequential amplification of dihydrofolate reductase and multidrug resistance genes in Chinese hamster ovary cells selected for stepwise resistance to the lipid-soluble antifolate trimetrexate. *J. Biol. Chem.* 264:18326.

Beck, J.T., and Ullman, B. 1990. Nutritional requirements of wild-type and folate transport-deficient *Leishmania donovani* for pterins and folates. *Mol. Biochem. Parasitol.* 43:221.

Beck, J.T., and Ullman, B. 1991. Biopterin conversion to reduced folates by *Leishmania donovani* promastigotes. *Mol. Biochem. Parasitol.* 49:21.

Bello, A.R., Nare, B., Freedman, D., Hardy, L., and Beverley, S.M. 1994. PTR1: a reductase mediating salvage of oxidized pteridines and methotrexate resistance in the protozoan parasite Leishmania major. *Proc. Natl. Acad. Sci. USA* 91:11442

Ben-Yaacov, R., Knoller, S., Caldwell, G.A., Becher, J.M., and Koltin, Y. 1994. Candida albicans gene encoding resistance to benomyl and methotrexate is a multidrug resistance gene. *Antimicrob. Agents Chemother.* 38:648–652.

Bertino J.R. 1993. Ode to methotrexate. *J. Clin. Oncol.* 11:5.

Beverley, S.M. 1991. Gene amplification in *Leishmania. Annu. Rev. Microbiol.* 45:417.

Borst, P., and Ouellette, M. 1995. New mechanisms of drug resistance in parasitic protozoa. *Annu. Rev. Microbiol.* 49:427.

Brooks, D., Wang, P., Read, M., Watkins, W., Sims, P., and Hyde, J. 1994. Correlation of sulfadoxine resistance with point mutations located within the bifunctional hydroxymethyldihydrobiopterin pyrophosphokinase-dihydropteroate synthase gene of the human malaria parasite Plasmodium falciparum. *Eur. J. Biochem.* 224:397.

Brumfitt W, and Hamilton-Miller J.M. 1995. Combinations of sulphonamides with diaminopyrimidines: how, when and why? *J. Chemother.* 7:136.

Callahan, H.L. and Beverley, S.M. 1991. Heavy metal resistance : a new role for P-glycoproteins in *Leishmania. J. Biol. Chem.* 266:18427.

Callahan, H.L. and Beverley, S.M. 1992. A member of the aldoketo reductase family confers methotrexate resistance in *Leishmania. J. Biol. Chem.* 267:24165.

Chabner B.A., Allegra C.J., Curt G.A., Clendeninn N.J., Baram J., Koizumi S., Drake J.C., Jolivet J. 1985. Polyglutamation of methotrexate. Is methotrexate a prodrug ? *J. Clin. Invest.* 76:907.

Charpentier E., Courvalin P. 1997. Emergence of the trimethoprim resistance gene dfrD in Listeria monocytogenes BM4293. *Antimicrob. Agents Chemother.* 41:1134.

Coderre, J.A., Beverley, S.M., Schimke, R.T., and Santi, D.V. 1983. Overproduction of a bifunctional thymidylate synthetase-dihydrofolate reductase and DNA amplification in methotrexate-resistant *Leishmania tropica. Proc. Natl. Acad. Sci. USA* 80:2132.

Cowman, A.F. and Lew, A.M. 1989. Antifolate drug selection results in duplication and rearrangement of chromosome 7 in *Plasmodium chabaudi. Mol. Cell Biol.* 9: 5182.

Cowman, A.F., Morry, M.J., Biggs, B.A., Cross, G.A.M. and Foote, S.J. 1988. Amino acid changes linked to pyrimethamine resistance in the dihydrofolate reductase-thymidylate synthase gene of *Plasmodium falciparum. Proc. Natl. Acad. Sci. USA* 25: 9109.

Dale G.E., Broger C., D'Arcy A., Hartman P.G., DeHoogt R., Jolidon S., Kompis I., Labhardt A.M., Langen H., Locher H., Page M.G., Stuber D., Then R.L., Wipf B., Oefner C. 1997. A single amino acid substitution in *Staphylococcus aureus* dihydrofolate reductase determines trimethoprim resistance. *J. Mol. Biol.* 266:23.

Dale G.E., Langen H., Page M.G., Then R.L., Stuber D. 1995. Cloning and characterization of a novel, plasmid-encoded trimethoprim-resistant dihydrofolate reductase from *Staphylococcus haemolyticus* MUR313. *Antimicrob. Agents Chemother.* 39:1920.

De Graaf, D., Sharma, R.C., Mechetner, E.B., Schimke, R.T., and Roninson, I.B. 1996. P-glycoprotein confers methotrexate resistance in 3T6 cells with deficient carrier-mediated methotrexate uptake. *Proc. Natl. Acad. Sci. USA* 93:1238.

De Groot R., Sluijter M., de Bruyn A., Campos J., Goessens W.H., Smith A.L., and Hermans P.W. 1996. Genetic characterization of trimethoprim resistance in *Haemophilus influenzae. Antimicrob. Agents Chemother.* 40:2131.

Dewes, H., Ostergaard, H.L., and Simpson, L. 1986. Impaired drug uptake in methotrexate resistant *Crithidia fasciculata* without changes in dihydrofolate reductase activity or gene amplification. *Mol. Biochem. Parasitol.* 19:149.

Donald, R.G.K., and Roos, D.S. 1993. Stable molecular transformation of *Toxoplasma gondii*: a selectable dihydrofolate reductase-thymidylate synthase marker based on drug-resistance mutations in malaria. *Proc. Natl. Acad. Sci. USA* 90:11703.

Ellenberger, T.E., and Beverley, S.M. 1987a. Biochemistry and regulation of folate and methotrexate transport in *Leishmania major*. *J. Biol. Chem.* 262:10053.

Ellenberger, T.E., and Beverley, S.M. 1987b. Reductions in methotrexate and folate influx in methotrexate-resistant lines of *Leishmania major* are independent of R and H region amplification. *J. Biol. Chem.* 262:13501.

Ellenberger, T.E., Wright J.E., Rosowsky, A. and Beverley, S.M. 1989. Wild type and drug-resistant *Leishmania major* hydrolyze methotrexate to N-10-methyl-4-deoxy-4-aminopteroate without accumulation of methotrexate polyglutamates. *J. Biol. Chem.* 264:15960.

Fermer C., Kristiansen B.E., Skold O., and Swedberg G. 1995. Sulfonamide resistance in *Neisseria meningitidis* as defined by site-directed mutagenesis could have its origin in other species. *J. Bacteriol.* 177:4669–4675.

Ferone, R., and Roland, S. 1980. Dihydrofolate reductase-thymidylate synthetase a bifunctionnal polypeptide from *Crithidia fasciculata*. *Proc. Natl. Acad. Sci. USA* 77:5802.

Foote, S.J., Galatis, D. and Cowman, A.F. 1990. Amino acids in the dihydrofolate reductase-thymidylate synthase gene of *Plasmodium falciparum* involved in cycloguanil resistance differ from those involved in pyrimethamine resistance. *Proc. Natl. Acad. Sci. USA* 87: 3014.

Gamarro, F., Amador, M.V., Chiquero, M.J. , Légaré, D. , Ouellette, M. and Castanys, S. 1994. Multidrug resistance phenotype and P-glycoprotein overexpression in a methotrexate-resistant *Leishmania infantum*. *Biochem. Pharmacol.* 47: 1939.

Garrow T.A., Admon A., and Shane B. 1992. Expression cloning of a human cDNA encoding folylpoly(gamma-glutamate) synthetase and determination of its primary structure. *Proc. Natl. Acad. Sci. USA* 89:9151.

Goker E., Waltham M., Kheradpour A., Trippett T., Mazumdar M., Elisseyeff Y., Schnieders B., Steinherz P., Tan C., Berman E., et al. 1995. Amplification of the dihydrofolate reductase gene is a mechanism of acquired resistance to methotrexate in patients with acute lymphoblastic leukemia and is correlated with p53 gene mutations. *Blood* 86:677.

Gorlick R., Goker E., Trippett T., Steinherz P., Elisseyeff Y., Mazumdar M., Flintoff W.F., and Bertino J.R. 1997. Defective transport is a common mechanism of acquired methotrexate resistance in acute lymphocytic leukemia and is associated with decreased reduced folate carrier expression. *Blood*, 89:1013.

Gorlick R., Goker E., Trippett T., Waltham M., Banerjee D., and Bertino J.R. 1996. Intrinsic and acquired resistance to methotrexate in acute leukemia. *New Engl. J. Med.* 315:1041.

Grondin, K., Haimeur, A., Mukhopadhyay, R., Rosen, B.P., and Ouellette, M. 1997. Co-amplification of the γ-glutamylcysteine synthetase gene gsh1 and of the ABC transporter gene *pgpA* in arsenite-resistant Leishmania tarentolae. *EMBO J.* 16: 3057

Hamlin J.L., and Ma C. 1990. The mammalian dihydrofolate reductase locus. *Biochim. Biophys. Acta.* 1087:107.

Hampele I.C. D'Arcy A., Dale G.E., Kostreva D., Nielson J., Oefner C., Page M.G., Schonfeld H.J., Stuber D., Then R.L. 1997. Structure and function of the dihydropteroate synthase from *Staphylococcus aureus*. *J. Mol. Biol.* 268:21.

Henderson G.B., Hughes T.R., and Saxena M. 1994. Functional implications from the effects of 1-cholro-2,4-dinitrobenzene and ethacrynic acid on efflux routes for methotrexate and cholate in L1210 cells. *J. Biol. Chem.* 269:13382.

Hitchings H.G. 1989. Selective inhibitors of dihydrofolate reductase. *In Vitro Cell. Dev. Biol.* 25:303.

Huennekens FM. 1996. In search of dihydrofolate reductase. *Protein Sci.* 5:1201.

Huovinen P., Sundström L, Swedberg, G, and Sköld O. 1995. Trimethoprim and sulfanamide resistance. *Antimicrob. Agents Chemother.* 39:279.

Inselburg, J., Bzik, D.J. and Horii, T. 1987. Pyrimethamine resistant *Plasmodium falciparum*: overproduction of dihydrofolate reductase by a gene duplication. *Mol. Biochem. Parasitol.* 26: 121.

Jörnvall, H., Persson, B., Krook, M., Atrian, S., Gonzàles-Duarte, R., Jeffery, J., and Ghosh, D. 1995. Short-chain dehydrogenases/reductases (SDR). *Biochemistry* 34:6004.

Jukes, TH. 1987. Searching for magic bullets: early approaches to chemotherapy-antifolates, methotrexate. *Cancer Res.* 47:5528.

Kaur K., Coons, T., Emmet, K., and Ullman, B. 1988. Methotrexate-resistant *Leishmania donovani* genetically deficient in the folate-methotrexate transporter. *J. Biol. Chem.* 263:7020.

Kohler T., Kok M., Michea-Hamzehpour M., Plesiat P., Gotoh N., Nishino T., Curty L.K., Pechere J.C. 1996. Multidrug efflux in intrinsic resistance to trimethoprim and sulfamethoxazole in *Pseudomonas aeruginosa*. *Antimicrob. Agents Chemother.* 40:2288.

Kündig C, Grondin K, Leblanc É, Haimeur A, Papadopoulou B, and Ouellette M. 1996. Amplification of *ptr1* and *dhfr-ts* in *L. tarentolae* selected for methotrexate resistance. Molecular Parasitology meeting VII. Marine Biologicals Laboratories, Woods Hole, U.S.A Abstract 95

Kündig C, Haimeur A, Leblanc É, Grondin K, Papadopoulou B, and Ouellette M. 1997. Overexpression of bt1, a novel mechanisms of methotrexate resistance in *Leishmania*. Molecular Parasitology meeting VIII. Marine Biologicals Laboratories, Woods Hole, U.S.A. Abstract

Leblanc É., Papadopoulou B., Bernatchez C., Ouellette M. 1998. Residues involved in co-factor and substrate binding of the short chain dehydrogenase/reductase PTR1 producing methotrexate resistance in *Leishmania*. *Eur. J. Biochem.* in press

Légaré D., Papadopoulou B., Roy G., Mukhopadhyay R., Haimeur A., Dey S., Grondin K., Brochu C., Rosen B.P., and Ouellette M. 1997. Efflux systems and increased trypanothione levels in arsenite resistant *Leishmania* species. *Exp. Parasitol.* In press

Lewis, K., Hooper, D. and Ouellette, M. 1997. Multidrug resistance pumps provide broad defense. *ASM News*, 63:605.

Longo G.S., Gorlick R., Tong W.P., Lin S., Steinherz P., and Bertino J.R. 1997. Gamma-glutamyl hydrolase and folylpolyglutamate synthetase activities predict polyglutamylation of methotrexate in acute leukemias. *Oncol. Res.* 9:259.

Melera P.W. 1991. Acquired versus intrinsic resistance to methotrexate: diversity of the drug-resistant phenotype in mammalian cells. *Semin. Cancer Biol.* 2:245.

Moore J.B., Beverley S.M. 1996. Pteridine transport and recurrent amplification of extrachromosomal DNAs in Leishmania. Molecular Parasitology meeting VIII. Marine Biologicals Laboratories, Woods Hole, U.S.A Abstract 107.

Moscow J.A., Connolly T., Myers T.G., Cheng C.C., Paull K., and Cowan K.H. 1997. Reduced folate carrier gene (RFC1) expression and anti-folate resistance in transfected and non-selected cell lines. *Int. J. Cancer* 72:184.

Myler P.J., Lodes M.J., Merlin G. de Vos T., and Stuart K.D. 1994. An amplified DNA element in Leishmania encodes potential integral membrane and nucleotide-binding proteins. *Mol. Biochem. Parasitol.* 66:11.

Nare B., Luba J., Hardy L.W., and Beverley S.. 1997a. New approaches to *Leishmania* chemotherapy: pteridine reductase 1 (PTR1) as a target and modulator of antifolate sensitivity. *Parasitology*. 114:S101.

Nare, B., Hardy, L.W., and Beverley, S.M. 1997b. The roles of pterine reductase 1 and dihydrofolate reductase-thymidylate synthase in pteridine metabolism in the protozoan parasite Leishmania major. *J. Biol. Chem.* 272: 13883.

Ouellette, M. and Kündig C. 1997. Microbial multidrug resistance. *Int. J. Antimicrob. Agents.* 8: 179.

Ouellette, M. and Papadopoulou, B. 1993. Mechanisms of drug resistance in *Leishmania*. *Parasitol. Today.* 9:150.

Ouellette, M., Fase-Fowler, F., and Borst, P. 1990. The amplified H circle of methotrexate-resistant *Leishmania tarentolae* contains a novel P-glycoprotein gene. *EMBO J.* 9:1027.

Ouellette, M., Papadopoulou, B., Haimeur, A, Grondin, K. Leblanc, E., Légaré, D., and Roy, G. 1995. Transport of antimonials and antifolates in drug resistant Leishmania. In "Drug transport in antimicrobial and anticancer chemotherapy" in Georgopapadakou, N.H.ed. pp. 377–402 Marcel Dekker, NewYork, NY.

Papadopoulou, B., Roy, G., and Ouellette M., 1992. A novel antifolate resistance gene on the amplified H circle of *Leishmania* . *EMBO J.,* 11:3601.

Papadopoulou, B., Roy, G., and Ouellette M., 1993. Frequent amplification of a short chain dehydrogenase gene as part of circular and linear amplicons in methotrexate resistant *Leishmania*. *Nucleic Acids Res.* 21:4305.

Papadopoulou, B., Roy, G., Dey, S., Rosen, B.P. and Ouellette, M. 1994a. Contribution of the *Leishmania* P-glycoprotein related gene *ltpgpA* to oxyanion resistance. *J. Biol. Chem.* 269:11980.

Papadopoulou, B., Roy, G., Mourad, W., Leblanc, E. and Ouellette, M. 1994b. Changes in folate and pterin metabolism after disruption of the *Leishmania* H locus short-chain dehydrogenase gene. *J. Biol. Chem.* 269:7310.

Pashley T.V., Volpe F., Pudney M., Hyde J.E., Sims P.F., and Delves C.J. 1997. Isolation and molecular characterization of the bifunctional hydroxymethyldihydropterin pyrophosphokinase-dihydropteroate synthase gene from *Toxoplasma gondii*. *Mol. Biochem. Parasitol.* 86:37.

Peterson, D.S. Milhous, W.K. and Wellems, T.E. 1990. Molecular basis of differential resistance to cycloguanil and pyrimethamine in *Plasmodium falciparum*. *Proc. Natl. Acad. Sci. USA* 87: 3018.

Peterson, D.S., Walliker, D. and Wellems, T.E. 1988. Evidence that a point mutation in dihydrofolate reductase-thymidylate synthase confers resistance to pyrimethamine in *falciparum malaria*. *Proc. Natl. Acad. Sci. USA* 85, 9114.

Petrillo-Peixoto, M.L., and Beverley, S.M. 1987. In vito activity of sulfonamides and sulfones against Leishmania major promastigotes. *Antimicrob. Agents Chemother.* 31:1575.

Rhee, M.S., Wang, Y., Nair, M.G., and Galivan, J. 1993. Acquisition of resistance to antifolates caused by enhanced g-glutamyl hydrolase activity. *Cancer Res.* 53:2227.

Robello C., Navarro P., Castanys S., and Gamarro F. 1998. A pteridine reductase gene ptr1 contiguous to a P-glycoprotein confers resistance to antifolates in Trypanosoma cruzi. *Mol. Biochem Parasitol.* in press

Rouch D.A., Messerotti L.J., Loo L.S.L., Jackson C.A., and Skurray R.A. 1989. Trimethoprim resistance transposon Tn4003 from *Staphylococcus aureus* encodes genes for a dihydrofolate reductase and thymidylate synthetase flnaked by three copies of IS257. *Mol. Microbiol.* 3:161.

Roy K., Egan M.G., Sirlin S., and Sirotnak, F.M. 1997. Posttranscriptionally mediated decreases in folylpolygluta-mate synthetase gene expression in some folate analogue-resistant variants of the L210 cell. Evidence for an altered cognate mRNA in the variants affecting the rate of de novo synthesis of the enzyme. *J. Biol. Chem.* 272:6903.

Ryan, K.A., Garraway, L.A., Descoteaux, A., Turco, S.J., and Beverley, S.M. 1993. Isolation of virulence genes directing surface glycosyl-phosphatidylinositol synthesis by functional complementation of *Leishmania*. *Proc. Natl. Acad. Sci. USA* 90:8609.

Saikawa Y., Knight C.B., Saikawa T., Page S.T., Chabner B.A., and Elwood P.C. 1993. Decreased expression of the human folate receptor mediates transport-defective methotrexate resistance in KB cells. *J. Biol. Chem.* 268:5293.

Santi, D.V., Nolan, P., and Shane, B. 1987. Folylpolyglutamates in *Leishmania major*. *Biochem. Biophys. Res. Comm.* 146:1089.

Schlemmer S.R., and Sirotnak F.M. 1992. Energy-dependent efflux of methotrexate in L1210 leukemia cells. Evidence for the role of an ATPase obtained with inside-out plasma membrane vesicles. *J. Biol. Chem.* 267:14746.

Schweitzer, B.I., Dicker, A.P., and Bertino, J.R. 1990. Dihydrofolate reductase as a therapeutic target. *FASEB J.* 4:2441

Segovia M., and Ortiz G. 1997. LD1 amplification in *Leishmania*. *Parasitol Today* 13:342.

Sirawaraporn W., Sathitkul T., Sirawaraporn R., Yuthavong Y., Santi D.V. 1997. Antifolate-resistant mutants of Plasmodium falciparum dihydrofolate reductase. *Proc. Natl. Acad. Sci. USA.* 94:1124.

Spencer H.T., Sorrentino B.P., Pui C.H., Chunduru S.K., Sleep S.E., Blakley R.L. 1996. Mutations in the gene for human dihydrofolate reductase: an unlikely cause of clinical relapse in pediatric leukemia after therapy with methotrexate. *Leukemia* 10:439.

Tamura T., Baggott J.E., Johnston K.E., Li Q.J., and Antony AC. 1997. The form of folate affects the mechanisms of methotrexate resistance in *Enterococcus faecium*. Microbiology 143:2639.

Triglia, T., and Cowman, A.F. 1994. Primary structure and expression of the dihydropteroate synthetase gene of *Plasmodium falciparum*. *Proc. Natl. Acad. Sci. USA* 91:7149.

Van Dijk M.R., Waters A.P., Janse C.J. 1995. Stable transfection of malaria parasite blood stages. *Science* 268:1358.

Vasquez J.R., Gooze L., Kim K., Gut J., Peterson C., Nelson R.G. 1996. Potential antifolate resistance determinants and genotypic variation in the bifunctional dihydrofolate reductase-thymidylate synthase gene from human and bovine isolates of *Cryptosporidium parvum*. *Mol. Biochem. Parasitol.* 79:153.

Volpe F., Ballantine S.P., Delves C.J. 1993. The multifunctional folic acid synthesis fas gene of *Pneumocystis carinii* encodes dihydroneopterin aldolase, hydroxymethyldihydropterin pyrophosphokinase and dihydropteroate synthase. *Eur. J. Biochem.* 216:449

Wang P., Lee C.-S., Bayoumi R., Djimde A., Doumbo O., Swedberg G., Dao L., Mshinda H., Tanner M., Watkins W.M., Sims P.F.G., and Hyde J.E. 1997a. Resistance to antifolates in plasmodium falciparum monitored by sequence analysis of dihydropteroate synthetase and dihydrofolate reductase alleles in a large number of field samples of diverse origins. *Mol. Biochem. Parasitol.* 89:161.

Wang P., Read M., Sims P.F., and Hyde J.E. 1997b. Sulfadoxine resistance in the human malaria parasite *Plasmodium falciparum* is determined by mutations in dihydropteroate synthetase and an additional factor associated with folate utilization. *Mol. Microbiol.* 23:979

Wang, J., Leblanc, E. Chang C.-F., Papadopoulou, B., Bray, T. Whiteley, J. S.X. Lin and Ouellette, M. 1997c. Folate and pterin reduction by the *Leishmania tarentolae* H locus short-chain dehydrogenase/ reductase PTR1. *Arch. Biochem. Biophys.* 342:197.

Williams F.M., and Flintoff W.F. 1995. Isolation of a human cDNA that complements a mutant hamster cell defective in methotrexate uptake. *J. Biol. Chem.* 270:2987.

Wu Y., Kirkman L.A., and Wellems T.E. 1996. Transformation of *Plasmodium falciparum* malaria parasites by homologous integration of plasmids that confer resistance to pyrimethamine. *Proc. Natl. Acad. Sci. USA* 93:1130.

Yao R., Schneider E., Ryan T.J., Galivan J. 1996. Human gamma-glutamylhydrolase:cloning and characterization of the enzyme expressed in vitro. *Proc. Natl. Acad. Sci. USA.* 93:10134.

Zhao R, Seither R, Brigle KE, Sharina IG, Wang PJ, Goldman ID. 1997. Impact of overexpression of the reduced folate carrier (RFC1), an anion exchanger, on concentrative transport in murine L1210 leukemia cells. *J. Biol. Chem.* 272:21207.

7

RESISTANCE TO ANTITUBERCULAR DRUGS

Luiz A. Basso and John S. Blanchard

Department of Biochemistry
Albert Einstein College of Medicine
Bronx, New York 10461

INTRODUCTION

Historians established the existence of endemic tuberculosis from Egyptian mummies dating from 2000 to 4000 B.C. (reviewed by Bloom and Murray, 1992). Tuberculosis was prevalent in Europe throughout the middle ages. Newly crowned kings of England and France were believed to have special healing powers and the most desired treatment of tuberculosis was being touched by these kings. Tuberculosis was responsible for 20% of all deaths in London in 1651, and the disease may have accounted for a third of all deaths in Paris in the 19th century. As Europeans colonized the Americas and sub-Saharan Africa, the disease was passed to susceptible populations and spread worldwide (Young *et al.*, 1996). In 1882, Robert Koch identified an acid-fast bacterium, *Mycobacterium tuberculosis*, as the causative agent of tuberculosis (Koch, 1932). His criteria for proof that the organism he discovered caused tuberculosis have been widely adopted and have become known as Koch's postulates: isolation of the bacilli from the body, growth in pure culture, and reproduction of the same "morbid" condition by administering the isolated bacilli to animals. In 1908, the BCG (bacille Calmette-Guerin) vaccine was first used to immunize a patient, and is currently the most widely used vaccine in the world. Discovery of the antibacterial activity of prontosil in 1935 by Gerhard Domagk marked a fundamental change from pathogen-specific therapy to non-pathogen-specific therapy that allowed prompt and effective treatment of bacterial infections without the necessity of identifying the pathogens involved (Casadevall, 1996). The discovery of the antibacterial and antitubercular properties of streptomycin in 1944 (Schatz and Waksman), and both isoniazid and pyrazinamide in 1952 (Kushner *et al.*; Middlebrook), led to effective chemotherapies that decreased tuberculosis mortality rates in the United States and worldwide. The later introduction of ethionamide, rifampicin, ethambutol and ciprofloxacin to the arsenal used to treat tuberculosis seemed to provide an adequate number of effective antimicrobial agents.

The development of modern multi-drug antibiotic therapy permitted a continuous decrease in tuberculosis mortality rates. This trend continued from 1953, when U.S. surveillance programs were instituted, to the mid-1980s, when the number of new reported cases

Resolving the Antibiotic Paradox, edited by Rosen and Mobashery.
Kluwer Academic / Plenum Publishers, New York, 1998.

began to increase in the United States. Possible factors underlying the resurgence of tuberculosis have been proposed (Bloom and Murray, 1992): the HIV epidemic, increase in the homeless population, decline in health care structures and national surveillance. The resurgence of tuberculosis caused by the emergence of drug-resistant strains throughout the world (Heym et al., 1994; Kritski et al., 1996; Ristow et al., 1995; Frieden et al., 1993; Cohn et al., 1997) has led to an increased need for understanding the molecular mechanisms of drug action and drug resistance. A multi-drug resistant (MDR) strain is defined as one that has resistance to rifampicin and isoniazid (and occasionally other drugs). The emergence of MDR-TB in different parts of the world is particularly worrisome, given the poor therapeutic outcomes when isolates are resistant to both isoniazid and rifampicin (Goble et al., 1993; Fischl et al., 1992). In the United States, approximately 13% of new cases were found to be resistant to at least one of the five frontline antitubercular drugs: isoniazid, rifampicin, pyrazinamide, streptomycin and ethambutol (Bloch et al., 1994).

The response of the pharmaceutical industry to the progression of antibiotic resistance has involved three primary approaches to the development of chemotherapeutic agents: modification of existing agent classes, interference with resistance mechanisms to increase target access, and search for agents with novel mechanisms of action (Kessler, 1997). All antibiotics introduced clinically since 1960 are chemical modifications of existing basic structures (Bax, 1997). Future approaches may include exploitation of potential antibacterial targets, such as DNA or RNA methylation, RNA processing, protein processing, lipid synthesis, membrane assembly, cell division, and cytoplasmic and membrane transfer steps of peptidoglycan synthesis (Silver and Bostian, 1990; Coleman et al., 1994; Ghuysen, 1994).

BASICS OF CHEMOTHERPAY

Physiology of Tubercle Bacilli

Tuberculosis is caused by infection by *Mycobacterium tuberculosis*, which is a rod-shaped obligate aerobe, that survives best in an environment with a pO_2 of 100 to 140 mm Hg, 5% CO_2 and a physiologic pH of 7.4 (Grosset, 1980). Thus the bacilli colonize the walls of pulmonary cavities where oxygen tension is high and the medium is lightly alkaline. *M. tuberculosis* is a facultative, intracellular bacterial pathogen that survives and multiplies within phagosomes whose maturation has been arrested by the bacilli and that resist acidification (Clemens, 1996). The disease is spread from person to person almost exclusively by small-particle aerosols of sufficiently small size (1–5 μM) so that they are inhaled into the alveolar space, where they are deposited and the organism begins to replicate. Tubercle bacilli divide slowly with a doubling time of approximately 24 hours (Hiriyanna and Ramakrishnan, 1986). This slow doubling time increases the length of time required for chemotherapy and makes drug susceptibility determinations time-consuming. This slow growth is also the reason for an initially intensive drug therapy, useful in eliminating larger bacterial populations, followed by fewer drugs and less frequent doses for an extended period (total six months) in order to completely eradicate the bacilli. Mitchison (1985) has suggested that pathogenic mycobacterial populations be divided into four components: actively metabolizing and rapidly growing, semidormant in an acidic intracellular environment, semidormant in a nonacidic intracellular environment, and dormant. The latter categories appear to be unique properties of mycobacterial infections, with the organisms able to remain quiescent for years, or decades.

Chemotherapy

Effective tuberculosis chemotherapy must include early bactericidal action against rapidly growing organisms and subsequent sterilization of the semidormant and dormant populations of bacilli (Mitchison, 1985). The first-line drugs isoniazid, rifampicin, streptomycin, and ethambutol exhibit early bactericidal activity against actively metabolizing bacilli (Heifets, 1994). Pyrazinamide is active against the semidormant bacilli in acidic intracellular environments. The bacteriostatic second-line drugs ethionamide, cycloserine and para-aminosalicylic acid (PAS) are reserved to strengthen the treatment of drug-resistant disease or when certain bactericidal drugs are prohibited because of allergic response or toxicity (Dutt and Stead, 1997). The newer fluoroquinolones (sparfloxacin, ciprofloxacin and ofloxacin) are bactericidal against *M. tuberculosis.* Although usually not indicated as first-line therapeutic agent for the treatment of tuberculosis, the fluoroquinolones have an important role in the treatment of resistant organisms. The modern, standard "short-course" therapy (Mitchison, 1985; Stratton and Reed, 1986) for tuberculosis is based on a four-drug regimen of isoniazid, rifampicin, pyrazinamide, and ethambutol or streptomycin for two months, followed by treatment with a combination of isoniazid and rifampicin for an additional four months. This combination therapy must be strictly followed to prevent drug resistance and relapse, and direct observation of patient compliance is the most reliable way to ensure effective treatment and prevent the acquisition of resistance (Weis *et al.*, 1994).

Mycobacteria show a high degree of intrinsic resistance to most antibiotics and chemotherapeutic agents due to the low permeability of the cell wall (Jarlier and Nikaido, 1994). Hydrophilic agents traverse the cell wall slowly because of the low concentration of mycobacterial porins and their relatively inefficient solute transport. Lipophilic agents are retarded by the lipid bilayer which is of unusually low fluidity. Nevertheless, the cell wall barrier alone cannot produce significant levels of drug resistance.

Resistant mutants of *M. tuberculosis* occur naturally, irrespective of exposure to drugs (Canetti, 1965). *M. tuberculosis* resistant mutants to any single effective drug are present in any large bacterial population at a frequency of 1 x 10^{-6} (David, 1980). The frequency of mutants resistant to rifampicin is 1 x 10^{-8}, and 1 x 10^{-6} for isoniazid and streptomycin. Therefore the large extracellular population (10^7–10^9) of actively metabolizing and rapidly growing tubercle bacilli in cavitary lesions will contain 1000 to 10,000 organisms which are resistant to a single effective drug. Consequently, monotherapy or improperly administered two-drug therapy will select for drug-resistant mutants which ultimately may lead to drug resistance in the entire population of bacilli.

The most important factors in the emergence of drug-resistance include inappropriate treatment regimens and patient noncompliance in completing the prescribed courses of therapy (Huebner and Castro, 1995). Scrutiny of treatment strategies has resulted in recommendations for inclusion of as many as three or four additional drugs to the standard three-drug regimen of isoniazid, rifampicin, ethambutol, and pyrazinamide (Weltman and Rose, 1994).

RESISTANCE TO FIRST-LINE ANTITUBERCULAR DRUGS

Isoniazid

Isoniazid (INH, isonicotinic acid hydrazide, Figure 1) was first reported to be effective in the treatment of tuberculosis in 1952 (Berstein *et al.*, 1952). Both *M. tuberculosis*

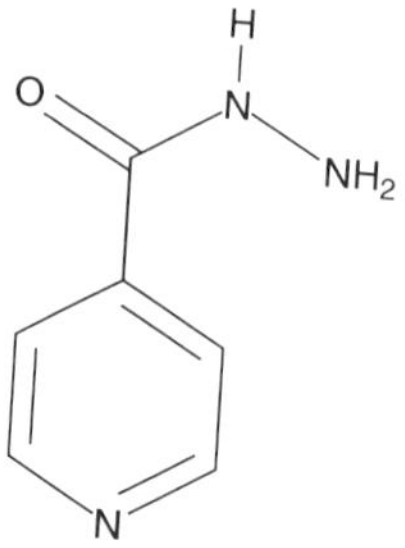

Figure 1. The structure of isoniazid.

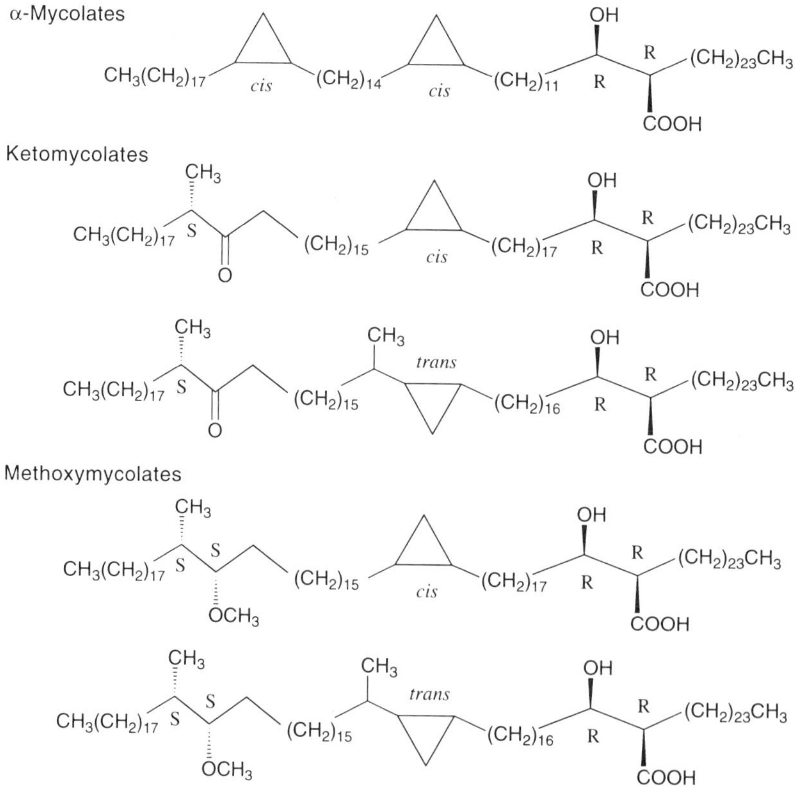

Figure 2. The structures of mycolic acids identified in *M. tuberculosis.*

and *M. bovis* BCG are susceptible to isoniazid in the range of 0.02–0.2 μg/ml (Heifets, 1994). Isoniazid is the oldest synthetic antitubercular, and the most prescribed drug for active infection and prophylaxis. Strains of *M. tuberculosis* resistant to isoniazid were reported shortly after the introduction of this drug (Middlebrook, 1952). A major target for isoniazid has recently been shown to be the product of the *inhA* gene (Banerjee et al., 1994), subsequently identified as an NADH-dependent enoyl-ACP (acyl carrier protein) reductase (Quémard et al., 1995). This enzyme exhibits specificity for long-chain (C_{16} > C_{18}) enoyl thioester substrates which is consistent with its suggested involvement in mycolic acid biosynthesis (Quémard et al., 1995).

Mycolic acids (Figure 2) are α-branched lipids, with a species-dependent saturated "short" arm of 20–24 carbon atoms and a "long" meromycolic acid arm of 50–60 carbon atoms, functionalized at regular intervals by cyclopropyl (α-mycolates), α-methyl ketone (ketomycolates), or α-methyl methylethers (methoxymycolates) groups. Mycolic acids form ester bonds to a unique polysaccharide, arabinogalactan. The arabinan chains, which consist of linked α-D-arabinosylfuranose-(1→5) residues, are attached to the galactan core through the C-5 of some of the 6-linked galactosylfuranose units. The galactan is attached to the peptidoglycan structure through a phosphodiester linkage to the C6 of a muramic acid residue via the diglycosylphosphoryl bridge, D-rhamnosepyranosyl-(1→3)-D-*N*-acetylglucosamine-(1→P)(Figure 3). The peptidoglycan component of mycobacterial cell walls is a polysaccharide chain composed of repeating *N*-acetyl-β-D-glucosaminyl-(1→4)-*N*-glycolyl-muramic acid units crosslinked by short peptide chains linked to the lactoyl groups of muramic acid residues (Figure 4). The muramic acid is *N*-glycolylated in *Mycobacterium* and *Nocardia*, in contrast to the *N*-acetylation found in all other bacteria, which may provide additional hydrogen bonding resulting in enhanced rigidity of the peptidoglycan structure (Brennan and Nikaido, 1995).

Mutations in the *inhA* structural gene (Banerjee et al., 1994; Kapur et al., 1995) and in the *inhA* locus promoter region (Morris et al., 1995; Musser et al., 1996) have been associated with isoniazid resistance. The *in vitro* generated S94A mutant of the enoyl reductase (Banerjee et al., 1994) displayed a higher K_m value for NADH (Quémard et al., 1995). Comparison of the crystal structure of binary complex of wild-type and the mutant enoyl reductases with NADH showed that disruption of a hydrogen bond network could account for the observed higher K_m value (Dessen et al., 1995). The mutations in the *inhA* gene locus accounts for approximately 25–30% of isoniazid resistance.

Some of the earliest studies of isoniazid-resistant clinical isolates of *M. tuberculosis* noted a correlation between resistance and attenuated catalase-peroxidase activity (Middlebrook, 1954; Middlebrook et al., 1954; Winder, 1960). The *katG* gene, which encodes the mycobacterial catalase-peroxidase enzyme, was cloned from *M. tuberculosis* (Zhang et al., 1992). Introduction of the wild-type *katG* gene into either *M. smegmatis* or *E. coli*, which are naturally less susceptible to isoniazid, or isoniazid-resistant strains of *M. tuberculosis* enhanced the sensitivity of these organisms to the drug (Zhang et al., 1993). Deletions of, or missense mutations in, the *katG* gene have been associated with decreased susceptibility to isoniazid in approximately 50% of clinical isolates of *M. tuberculosis* (Cockerill et al., 1995; Heym and Cole, 1992; Heym et al., 1995; Musser et al., 1996). Peroxidases have been shown to react with isoniazid to generate a number of oxidized products similar to those observed *in vivo* (Shoeb et al., 1985). A mechanism for the action of isoniazid has been proposed that involves the conversion of isoniazid, by the mycobacterial *katG*-encoded catalase-peroxidase, into a number of electrophilic intermediates capable of either oxidizing or acylating amino acid residues in proteins (Johnsson and Schultz, 1994). The amino acid residue of the enoyl reductase modified by the electro-

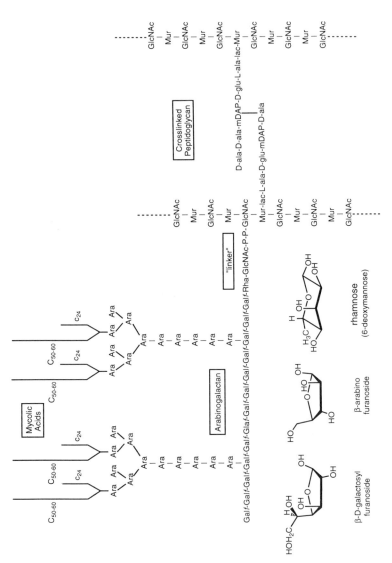

Figure 3. A representation of a portion of the mycobacterial cell wall.

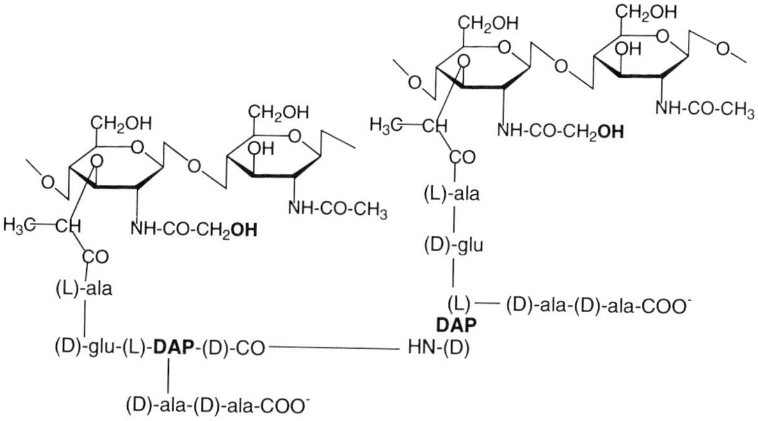

CH_2OH CH_2OH
OH
$NH-CO-CH_3$

H_3C-CH $NH-CO-CH_2OH$
CO
(L)-ala

(D)-glu

(L) — (D)-ala-(D)-ala-COO⁻
DAP

CH_2OH CH_2OH
OH
$NH-CO-CH_3$

H_3C-CH $NH-CO-CH_2OH$
CO
(L)-ala

(D)-glu-(L)-**DAP**-(D)-CO —————— HN-(D)

(D)-ala-(D)-ala-COO⁻

Figure 4. The structure of mycobacterial peptidoglycan.

philic drug metabolite was proposed to be cysteine-243 (Johnsson *et al.*, 1995), although subsequent studies suggested this not to be likely (Basso *et al.*, 1996). Although isoniazid does not bind to the *inhA*-encoded enoyl reductase (Quémard *et al.*, 1995), the catalase-peroxidase-activated drug intermediate binds to, and inhibits, the reductase in the presence of NADH (Johnsson *et al.*, 1995). Catalase-peroxidase-activated isoniazid was shown to bind exclusively to the enoyl reductase-NADH binary complex (Quémard *et al.*, 1996).

The three-dimensional structure determination of the ternary complex of *E. coli* enoyl reductase, NAD⁺ and diazoborine, an antibacterial agent that blocks production of lipolysaccharide, revealed a covalent bond between the 2' hydroxyl of nicotinamide ribose and the boron atom of the diazoborine (Baldock *et al.*, 1996). Inhibition is caused by the tight, but noncovalent binding, of this bisubstrate analog to the enzyme, which is the target for diazoborines (Bergler *et al.*, 1994). Replacement of glycine for serine at position 93 of the *E. coli* enoyl reductase causes diazoborine resistance (Bergler *et al.*, 1992).

The mycobacterial *inhA*-encoded enoyl reductase shares 40% amino acid sequence identity with the *E. coli* envM-encoded enoyl reductase (Banerjee *et al.*, 1994). The serine residue at position 94 of the enoyl reductase mutated to alanine in isoniazid-resistant mutants of *M. tuberculosis* (Banerjee *et al.*, 1994) and the glycine 93 residue of the enoyl reductase mutated to a serine residue in diazoborine-resistant mutants of *E. coli* (Bergler *et al.*, 1992) are both located in the nucleotide binding site. More recently, the three dimensional structure has been determined for the ternary complex of the wild-type enoyl reductase of *M. tuberculosis*, NADH and activated isoniazid (Rozwarski *et al.*, 1998). In this complex, generated by the *in vitro* reaction of manganese, isoniazid and oxygen (Zabinski and Blanchard, 1997) with the enzyme-NADH complex, the acylpyridine fragment of isoniazid is covalently attached to the C4 position of NADH (Figure 5). It is likely that the *in vivo* formation of a similar adduct between the electrophilic intermediate of isoniazid produced by oxidation of the drug by the catalase-peroxidase and the NADH-enoyl reductase complex would be similarly formed. Isoniazid is, therefore, a pro-drug, which is oxidized by the catalase-peroxidase to generate an intermediate that forms a bisubstrate analog with NADH, inhibiting the *M. tuberculosis* enoyl reductase, resulting in reduction of mycolic acid synthesis.

The molecular mechanism responsible for isoniazid resistance in approximately 20% of isoniazid-resistant clinical isolates is unknown. It has been suggested that increased expres-

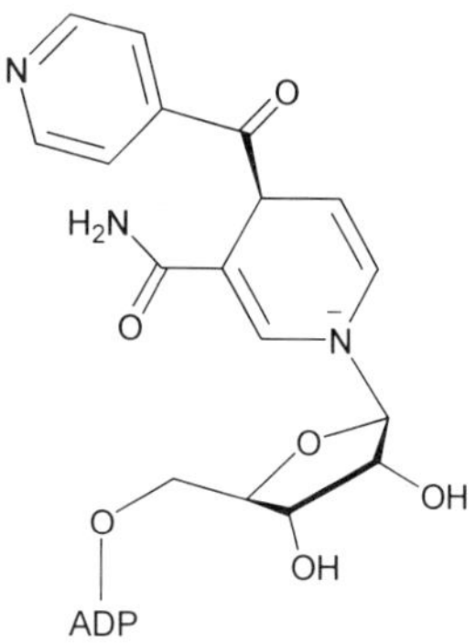

Figure 5. Structure of the activated-isoniazid-NADH covalent adduct (adapted from Rozwarski et al., 1998).

sion of an *ahpC*-like component of the alkyl hydroperoxidase complex can confer isoniazid resistance to some *M. tuberculosis* strains lacking mutations in *katG* and *inhA* genes (Dhandayuthapani *et al.*, 1996; Wilson and Collins, 1996). However, overexpression of this gene in *M. tuberculosis* results in no significant isoniazid resistance in the absence of additional *katG* mutations (Sherman *et al.*, 1996). Moreover, the virtual absence of mutations in the *ahpC* coding region or mutations in the *ahpC* promoter region in isoniazid-resistant clinical isolates with lesions at the *katG* or *inhA* loci (Sreevatsan *et al.*, 1997; Kelley *et al.*, 1997) suggest a secondary role of the *ahpC* gene in clinical isoniazid resistance. These observations leave open the issue of the molecular mechanism responsible for isoniazid resistance in approximately 20% of organisms lacking mutations in either the *katG* or *inhA* locus.

Rifampicin

Rifampicin (Figure 6), a semi-synthetic derivative of the natural product rifamycin, obtained from culture filtrates of *Streptomyces mediterranei*, was introduced in 1972 as an antitubercular drug (Woodley *et al.*, 1972). Rifampicin is bactericidal against *M. tuberculosis* with MIC values of 0.1–0.2 µg/ml (Heifets, 1994). Rifampicin has powerful sterilizing action because of its effectiveness in killing bacilli exhibiting even modest metabolic activity (Dickinson and Mitchison, 1981). Thus the introduction of rifampicin helped to shorten the course of treatment against drug-susceptible infections, and is now a key com-

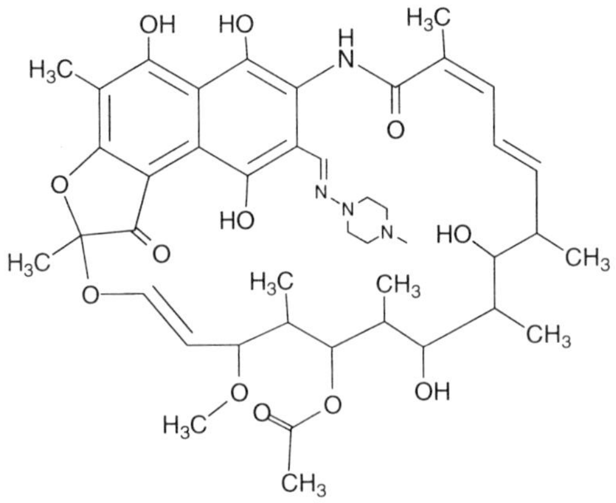

Figure 6. The structure of rifampicin.

ponent of all short-course multi-drug-treatment regimens of tuberculosis and leprosy (Mitchison, 1985).

Resistance to rifampicin is increasing rapidly as a result of its widespread use. Rifampicin-resistant tuberculosis, often observed in conjunction with isoniazid resistance, leads to a longer treatment period and significantly poorer chemotherapeutic outcomes. Resistance has been observed in 3.9% of all cases nationally, but in 9% of patients previously treated for tuberculosis (Bloch *et al.*, 1994). In a more recent survey of worldwide antitubercular drug resistance (Cohn *et al.*, 1997), primary resistance to rifampicin ranged from 0% to 3% (median, 0.2%) and acquired resistance ranged from 0% to 14.5% (median, 2.4%).

The rifampicin drug target in *Mycobacterium smegmatis* has been shown to be RNA polymerase (Levin and Hatfull, 1993). Rifampicin specifically inhibits the elongation of full-length transcripts, but has little or no effect on transcription initiation. The genes encoding the β subunit of the mycobacterial RNA polymerase, *rpoB*, have been sequenced from both *M. tuberculosis* (Donnabella *et al.*, 1994; Miller *et al.*, 1994) and *M. leprae* (Honore and Cole, 1993). The mutations in the *rpoB* gene that result in rifampicin resistance have been identified (Telenti *et al.*, 1993; Donnabella *et al.*, 1994; Honore and Cole, 1994; Williams *et al.*, 1994; Ohno *et al.*, 1996). These findings now allow for the rapid determination of the drug-susceptibility characterization of clinical isolates of *M. tuberculosis* using PCR-SSCP or automated DNA sequencing methods (Telenti *et al.*, 1993; Kapur *et al.*, 1994). More recently, an RNA/RNA mismatch assay has been proposed as a cost-effective, rapid, simple and specific method for detection of rifampicin resistance in *M. tuberculosis* (Nash *et al.*, 1997). However, since the quantitative relationship between specific alterations in the *rpoB* gene and susceptibility to rifampicin has not been unequivocally demonstrated, the identification of additional drug-resistant genes or further analysis of the relationship between MICs and gene alteration has been proposed (Ohno *et al.*, 1996; Taniguchi *et al.*, 1996).

The increasing occurrence of rifampicin-resistant *M. tuberculosis*, especially in individuals not previously treated for tuberculosis (Bloch *et al.*, 1994), is cause for significant concern. Few other antitubercular compounds are as rapidly effective as rifampicin, and although newer synthetic derivatives (rifabutin and rifapentin MIC's = 0.03–0.06 and 0.01–0.06) appear to be more effective than rifampicin (Heifets *et al.*, 1990), these compounds exhibit cross-resistance with rifampicin. Although the target and mechanisms of action and resistance of rifampicin in *M. tuberculosis* have been well documented in the past several years, more potent new analogs to replace rifampicin have not been developed.

The vast majority of rifampicin resistance-conferring mutations in the mycobacterial *rpoB*-encoded RNA polymerase are single nucleotide changes that result in single amino acid substitutions (>80%; Cole, 1994; Kapur *et al.*, 1994; Ohno *et al.*, 1996). The remaining mutations are insertions and deletions, but most mutations map to the presumed rifampicin binding site (Figure 7) between amino acid positions 511 and 533 (*E. coli* numbering system). The two most commonly encountered amino acid substitutions have so far been

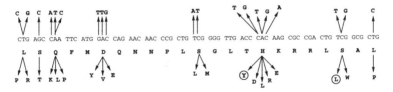

Figure 7. Mutations in the *rpoB* gene encoding the mycobacterial RNA polymerase that result in rifampicin resistance.

shown to occur at His526 and Ser531 (Williams *et al.*, 1994; Kapur *et al.*, 1994; Ohno *et al.*, 1996). Additional mutations have been mapped to positions 511, 512, 513, 516, 522 and 533 as seen in Figure 7. Mutations resulting in rifampicin resistance have also been identified outside of this region, including Ala381Val, Thr481Asn, and Ser509Arg mutations (Tanigushi *et al.*, 1996; Nash *et al.*, 1997). Point mutations have also been found in rifampicin-sensitive strains of *M. tuberculosis* in the *rpoB* gene (codon 521, 533, 679 or 687; Taniguchi *et al.*, 1996). These results suggest that mutations in the *rpoB* gene are largely, but not uniquely, associated with rifampicin resistance in *M. tuberculosis*.

Streptomycin

Streptomycin (Figure 8) was first shown to be an effective antitubercular drug in 1944 (Schatz and Waksman, 1944). The MIC of streptomycin against *M. tuberculosis* has been reported to be in the range 0.4–1.5 µg/ml (Heifets, 1994), making it one of the most effective early antitubercular drugs. The antibacterial activities of streptomycin, and related aminoglycosides, are due to their ability to cause misreading of the genetic code, inhibition of the initiation of mRNA translation and aberrant proofreading (Moazed and Noller, 1987). A common mechanism of resistance to aminoglycoside antibiotics in other bacteria is drug inactivation via acetylation, phosphorylation or adenylation (Benveniste and Davies, 1973). However, this mechanism of resistance via drug modification has not been reported in *Mycobacterium tuberculosis*. Instead two classes of mutations account for a large proportion of the high- and intermediate-level streptomycin resistance in *M. tuberculosis*. The first consists of point mutations in the ribosomal S12 protein, encoded by the *rpsL* gene, resulting in single-amino acid replacements (Finken *et al.*, 1993; Nair *et al.*, 1993; Meier *et al.*, 1994, 1996; Cooksey *et al.*, 1996; Sreevatsan *et al.*, 1996). These mutants account for approximately two thirds of the resistant mutations. Sequencing of the *rpsL* gene revealed that all mutations occurred in two highly conserved regions of the gene encoding one of two critical lysine residues (K43 and K88). In all cases, either K88 was converted to an arginine residue or K43 was converted to either an arginine or threonine residue. Ribosomal protein S12 stabilizes the pseudoknot structure formed by 16S rRNA (Noller, 1984), and thus amino acid substitutions in the *rpsL* gene product affect the higher-order structure of 16S rRNA (Allen and Noller, 1989).

The second class of mutations occur in the *rrs* gene that encodes the 16S rRNA (Douglass and Steyn, 1993; Finken *et al.*, 1993; Honore and Cole, 1993; Cooksey *et al.*,

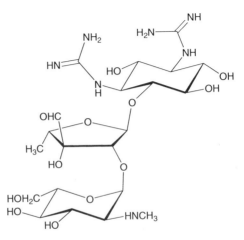

Figure 8. The structure of streptomycin.

1996; Sreevatsan *et al.*, 1996). Mutations in streptomycin-resistant *M. tuberculosis* have been mapped to two regions; the 530 loop and the 915 region of *rrs* gene (*E. coli* numbering). In the 530 loop, C→T transitions at positions 491, 512, and 516, and 513 are observed as well as A→C transversion at position 523 (*M. tuberculosis* numbering). Mutations in the 915 region were observed at positions 798 (C→T), 866 (A→G), 877 (G→A), 903 (C→G/A), 904 (A→G), and 906 (A→C) (*M. tuberculosis* numbering). The 530 loop region of 16S ribosomal RNA interacts with the 510 region bulge loop, and the resulting pseudoknot is thought to be stabilized by ribosomal protein S12 (Woese and Gutell, 1989). The highly conserved C912-A915 nucleotides (*E. coli* numbering) in the 915 region have been suggested to be a streptomycin binding site from protection studies with alkylating agents and nucleases (Montandon et al., 1986; Moazed and Noller, 1987).

Approximately one third of drug-resistant clinical isolates lack changes in *rpsL* or *rrs* genes, indicating that alternate mechanisms of streptomycin resistance exist in *M. tuberculosis* (Heym *et al.*, 1994; Kapur *et al.*, 1995, Cooksey *et al.*, 1996). It has been suggested that low-level streptomycin resistance in strains with wild-type *rpsL* and *rrs* genes is due to changes in the permeability for the drug (Meier *et al*, 1996), while high- and medium-level resistance are caused by alterations in *rpsL* and *rrs* genes, respectively.

Resistance to streptomycin appears in 5.7% of new cases and 7.7% of recurrent tuberculosis cases reported in the United States (Bloch *et al.*, 1994). In a recent worldwide survey of strains of *M. tuberculosis* resistant to antimycobacterial agents, primary resistance to streptomycin occurs in 3.5%, and acquired resistance in 4.9%, of the cases (Cohn *et al.*, 1997). In general, resistance to isoniazid and streptomycin was more common than was resistance to rifampicin or ethambutol.

Cross-resistance in *M. tuberculosis* to other related aminoglycosides (gentamicin, kanamycin, paromomycin and amikacin) has never been observed (Heifets and Lindholm-Levy, 1989; Meier *et al.*, 1996). Of the aminoglycosides, kanamycin and amikacin are important secondary agents for the treatment of tuberculosis. Amikacin, in particular, has emerged as a potentially important agent for treating infections of non-tuberculous mycobacteria (Böttger, 1994). Acquired resistance to amikacin in rapidly growing non-tuberculous mycobacteria has been described, but the mechanism of resistance is unknown (Wallace *et al.*, 1985). The lack of cross-resistance suggests that these compounds may be substituted for streptomycin in those cases where resistance has been determined (Blanchard, 1996). Since all of these compounds must be administered intravenously, whether streptomycin and related inhibitors of bacterial protein synthesis will continue to be considered as first-line antituberculars in short-course chemotherapies is not clear.

Ethambutol

Ethambutol (Figure 9) is a specific antitubercular bactericidal agent used in most modern combination antitubercular therapies. Its powerful antimycobacterial effects were first described in 1961 (Thomas *et al.*, 1961), and the *S,S* stereochemistry was shown to be

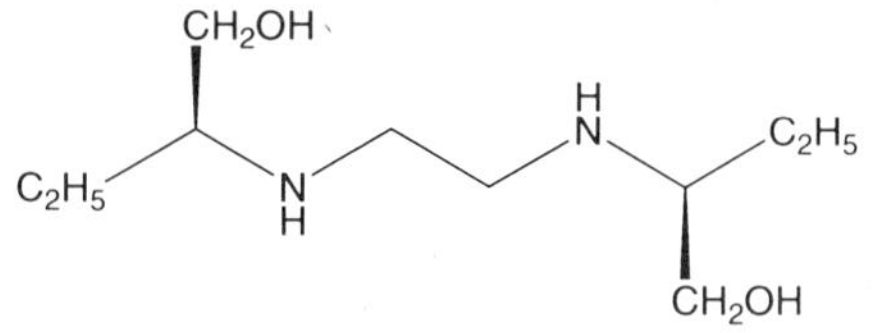

Figure 9. The structure of ethambutol.

essential for activity. Ethambutol is active only against actively multiplying bacteria and the MIC's in various types of liquid and solid media range from 0.5 to 2.0 µg/ml, in 7H12 BACTEC broth they range from 0.95 µg/ml to 3.8 µg/ml, and in 7H10 agar from 1.9 µg/ml to 7.5 µg/ml (Heifets, 1994).

Early studies on the effect of ethambutol showed that transfer of mycolic acids into the cell wall was inhibited as early as fifteen minutes after drug administration (Takayama *et al.*, 1979), and even more rapid effects were seen in the accumulation of trehalose mono- and dimycolates (Kilburn and Takayama, 1981). These experimental observations suggested that the biochemical target was involved in the construction of the outer envelope of the mycobacterial cell wall (Sareen and Khuller, 1990). The structure and composition of the outer cell wall of *M. tuberculosis* is still under active investigation, although substantial progress has been made in the past decade (reviewed in Brennan and Nikaido, 1995).

In a recent study, the target of ethambutol in *M. smegmatis* was demonstrated to be the arabinosyltransferases and/or other enzymes required in the polymerization of arabinans destined for both arabinogalactan and lipoarabinomannan (Khoo *et al.*, 1996). Mycolic acids are attached to the 5'-hydroxyl groups of the terminal D-arabinose residues of the arabinogalactan polymer, which is in turn attached to peptidoglycan through a phosphodiester link to muramic acid residues of the mycobacterial cell wall (Figure 3; Brennan and Nikaido, 1995).

The cellular target for ethambutol was sought using drug resistance, via target over-expression from a plasmid vector, as a selection tool. This strategy led to the cloning of three complete open reading frames, *embR*, *embA*, and *embB* from *M. avium* (Belanger *et al.*, 1996). Overexpression of *embAB* is associated with high-level ethambutol resistance, suggesting that the *embAB*-encoded arabinosyltransferases are the primary cellular target for ethambutol. Since the protein encoded by the *embR* gene is homologous to known transcriptional activators, and decreased ethambutol resistance is observed when this gene is missing, it was suggested that it modulates the *in vitro* level of arabinosyltransferase activity (Belanger *et al.*, 1996). The *emb* region in *M. tuberculosis* exhibits a different gene organization compared to *M. avium* (Telenti *et al.*, 1997). In *M. tuberculosis*, the *embCAB* cluster is organized as a 10-kb operon encoding proteins with amino acid similarities in the range of 61 to 68%, suggesting a gene duplication event. Secondary structure analysis suggests that the *embCAB* gene products are integral membrane proteins, with 12 putative transmembrane segments, and a C-terminal globular region of approximately 400 amino acids predicted to be of periplasmic location (Figure 10; Telenti *et al.*, 1997).

Resistance to ethambutol has been described in up to 4% of clinical isolates of *M. tuberculosis*, and is prevalent among isolates from patients with multidrug-resistant tuberculosis (Bloch *et al.*,1994). Identification of the *embCAB* genes now permits studies on the molecular basis of ethambutol resistance in mycobacteria. Mutations in *M. tuberculosis* *embCB* genes resulting in M306I or M306V substitutions were identified in 47% of ethambutol-resistant clinical isolates (Telenti *et al.*, 1997). These mutations were not identified in any *M. tuberculosis* susceptible strains. In *M. smegmatis*, low-level resistance was associated with an increased expression of the *embCAB* gene products, and intermediate- and

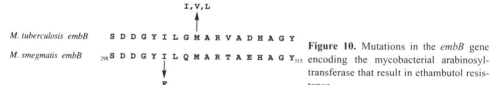

Figure 10. Mutations in the *embB* gene encoding the mycobacterial arabinosyltransferase that result in ethambutol resistance.

high-level resistance was associated with a mutation in the *embB* structural gene resulting in an I303F mutant protein (Telenti *et al.*, 1997). In a subsequent study, it was shown that 69% of ethambutol-resistant clinical isolates of *M. tuberculosis* had mutations in the *embB* gene (Sreevatsan *et al.*, 1997a). Approximately 61% of ethambutol resistance in epidemiologically unassociated organisms could be accounted for by mutations at position 306 of *embB* gene product (M306V, M306L, M306I). Other mutations in the *embB* gene occurred in individual codons, including residues 285 (TTC→TTA, Phe→Leu), 330 (TTC→GTC, Phe→Ala), and 630 (ACC→ATC, Thr→Ile). The mutations at position 306 of *embB* gene are believed to mediate ethambutol resistance (Sreevatsan et al., 1997a). For the remaining 30% of ethambutol-resistant isolates lacking *embB* gene product mutations, alternative mechanisms of resistance must operate, possibly including overexpression of the *embB* gene product shown to mediate drug resistance in *M. smegmatis* (Telenti *et al.*, 1997).

The actual mechanism of action of the drug remains to be determined, although it seems that *embB* gene mutations affect a glycosyltransferase to which ethambutol, believed to act as an arabinose analogue, binds (Maddry *et al.*, 1996). However, owing to the pleiotropic action of ethambutol (Deng *et al.*, 1995), additional genes may be involved in clinical ethambutol resistance. As susceptibility testing to ethambutol remains suboptimally standardized due to the instability of the drug in growth medium (Gangadharam and Gonzales, 1970), automated sequencing and SSCP may be utilized in the future for detection of *embB* mutations to identify ethambutol-resistant strains of *M. tuberculosis*.

Pyrazinamide

The weak antitubercular activity of nicotinamide began a search for more powerful analogs and resulted in the discovery of pyrazinamide (Figure 11). Although shown to have substantial activity in 1952 (Kushner *et al.*, 1952), pyrazinamide was not used extensively in the treatment of tuberculosis until the mid-1980s. Pyrazinamide is now recommended in essentially every combination therapy for the treatment of the disease because of its strong synergistic, and accelerating, effect in combination with isoniazid and rifampicin (Mitchison, 1985; Heifets, 1994). The introduction of pyrazinamide combination chemotherapy allowed treatment to be reduced from 9–12 months to 6 months. It appears to be most effective in the first 2 months of therapy with modest additional incremental effects, and is often discontinued after 2 months of therapy, with continued treatment with other agents (Davidson and Quoc, 1992). The MIC for pyrazinamide varies from 8 to 60 μg/ml depending on the assay method and media (Heifets, 1994). Pyrazinamide does not appear to be bactericidal, even at concentrations significantly greater than its MIC, and its *in vitro* effect is presently termed "sterilizing" (Heifets and Lindholm-Levy, 1992) to distinguish it from the effects of other drugs such as rifampicin. The drug is most active against *M. tuberculosis* at acidic pH values (below 6) but has little, if any, activity at higher pH. Pyrazinamide appears to exhibit its *in vivo* sterilizing activity on the semidor-

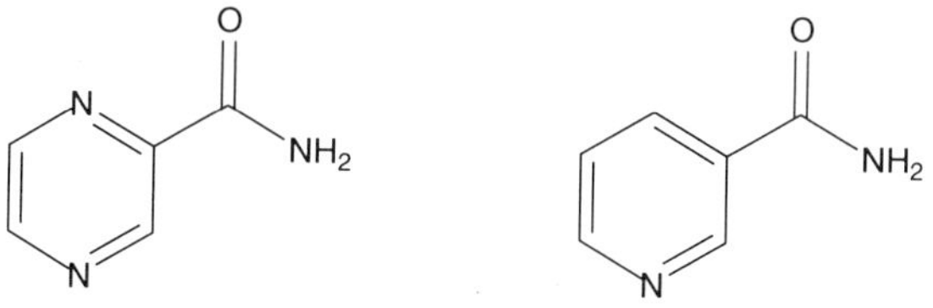

Figure 11. The structures of pyrazinamide and nicotinamide.

mant populations of *M. tuberculosis* in acidic intracellular compartments, such as the macrophage phagolysosomes (Mackaness, 1956). However, the intracellular pH surrounding live *M. tuberculosis* was shown not to be acidic (Crowle *et al.*, 1991). These puzzling experimental observations will require further studies to determine the factors necessary for pyrazinamide activation. Although pyrazinamide is effective against *M. tuberculosis* infection, the compound is not effective in the treatment of other mycobacterial infections, including *M. bovis* and fast-growing mycobacteria.

The precise mechanism of action of pyrazinamide is not known. A definite correlation was found between amidase activity and susceptibility of *M. tuberculosis* to either pyrazinamide or nicotinamide, its presumed physiological substrate (Konno *et al.*, 1967; Butler and Kilburn, 1983). This finding suggests that pyrazinamide, like isoniazid, is a prodrug, transported or diffusing into the organism as a neutral species through the mycobacterial cell wall, and converted into pyrazinoic acid, the presumed active drug form. This proposal is supported by the finding that pyrazinoic acid is active *in vitro* against pyrazinamide- and nicotinamide-resistant strains of *M. tuberculosis*, as well as the naturally resistant *M. bovis*, which lacks pyrazinamidase activity (Konno *et al.*, 1967). Further support for this proposal is the loss of pyrazinamidase activity in strains of *M. tuberculosis* resistant to pyrazinamide (Miller *et al.*, 1995). A series of pyrazinoic acid esters have been shown to exhibit better *in vitro* activity against *M. tuberculosis* than pyrazinamide (Yamamoto *et al.*, 1995), also supporting the view that the acid form is the active component.

The *M. tuberculosis* gene that encodes pyrazinamidase and nicotinamidase activities (*pncA*) has been cloned and sequenced (Scorpio and Zhang, 1996). The *pncA* gene (558bp) encodes a protein of 186 amino acids (20 kDa) with 35% amino acid identity to the *E. coli* nicotinamidase. The *E. coli* gene that encodes pyrazinamidase and nicotinamidase activities (*pncA*) has been cloned, sequenced and shown to be part of an operon with *ansA*, the gene for L-asparaginase I (Frothingham *et al.*, 1996). A remarkable experimental observation was that *M. bovis*, known to lack pyrazinamidase activity, has a *pncA* gene. The defective pyrazinamidase in three *M. bovis* and three *M. bovis* BCG strains studied is due to the same point mutation in the *pncA* gene at position 169 (C→G), which caused the substitution of histidine for aspartic acid at position 57 (Scorpio and Zhang, 1996). This characteristic mutation has been proposed as a marker for the rapid differentiation of *M. bovis* from *M. tuberculosis* (Scorpio *et al.*, 1997). This proposal has been recently challenged, since strains of *M. bovis* with histidine at position 57 in the *pncA* gene product have been identified (Sreevatsan *et al.*, 1997b).

The genetic basis of pyrazinamide resistance, and the correlation between pyrazinamide resistance and *pncA* mutations, has been studied in recent years. Pyrazinamide-resistant strains of *M. tuberculosis*, whose *pncA* gene was amplified by PCR and sequenced, were shown to have primarily missense mutations causing amino acid substitutions but also insertions or small deletions (nonsense mutations), frame shifts, inappropriate stop codons resulting in truncated polypeptides, and upstream mutations (Scorpio *et al.*, 1997a; Sreevatsan et al., 1997b). There appears to be no clear clustering of these mutations along the *pncA* gene (Figure 12; adapted from Sreevatsan *et al.*, 1997b). Sequence analysis of pyrazinamide-resistant strains of *M. tuberculosis* revealed the presence of insertions, deletions and missense mutations in the *pncA* structural gene, as well as a mutation upstream of the start codon of *pncA* (Scorpio *et al.*, 1997a). The upstream mutations may weaken the promoter activity and attenuate pyrazinamidase expression in these mutants. In view of the inconsistent results of pyrazinamide susceptibility testing (Hewlett *et al.*, 1995), the correlation between pyrazinamidase resistance and *pncA* mutations may allow the use of PCR-SSCP technique for rapid detection of pyrazinamide-resistant strains of *M. tuberculosis*.

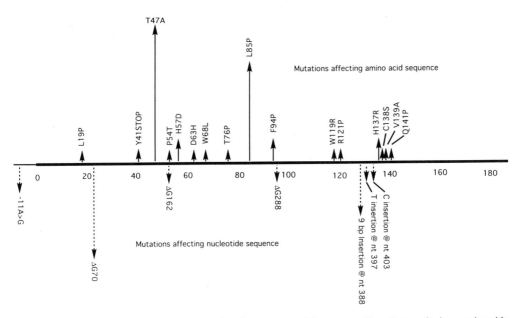

Figure 12. Mutations in the *pncA* gene encoding the mycobacterial pyrazinamidase that results in pyrazinamide resistance. the length of the arrows corresponds to the frequency of the identified mutation.

Transformation studies with a functional *M. tuberculosis pncA* gene showed that the *pncA* mutations found in pyrazinamide-resistant strains are responsible for their defective pyrazinamidase activity and resistance to this drug (Scorpio and Zhang, 1996). It is noteworthy that there was no obvious impairment of the viability of organisms with mutations in the *pncA* gene that result in the loss of pyrazinamidase activity (Sreevatsan *et al.*, 1997b). Although transformation experiments have shown that pyrazinamidase is needed to potentiate pyrazinamide activity (Scorpio and Zhang, 1996), the target of its active derivative, pyrazinoic acid, in *M. tuberculosis* remains to be determined. A combination of genetic and biochemical approaches will be helpful to elucidate the mechanisms of activation and action of this important antitubercular drug.

Fluoroquinolones

The quinolone antibacterials are synthetic derivatives of nalidixic acid (Figure 13), a natural product whose antibacterial action was described more than 30 years ago. The increased activity against Gram-negative rods by the incorporation of a 7-piperazinyl ring

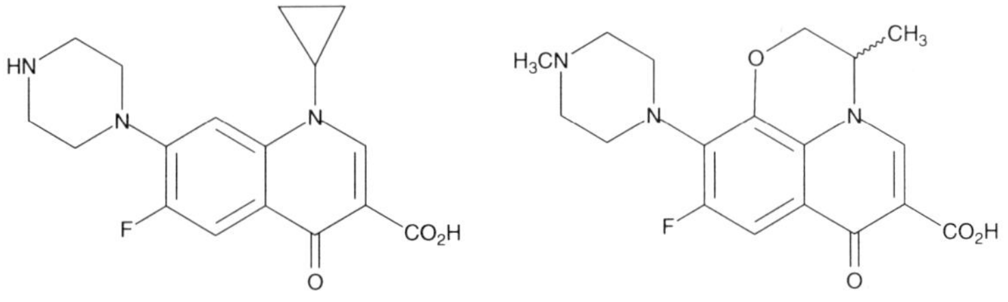

Figure 13. The structures of ciprofloxacin (left) and ofloxacin.

and a 6-fluorine atom on the quinolone nucleus (ciprofloxacin, norfloxacin and pefloxacin) or the 1,8 naphtyridine nucleus (enoxacin) as compared to nalidixic acid gave rise to fluoroquinolones (Bryskier and Chantot, 1995). The antimycobacterial activity of fluoroquinolones was described in 1984 (Gay et al., 1984), and numerous reports of their efficacy have since appeared (reviewed in Leysen et al., 1989; Stratton, 1992; Jacobs, 1995). The most active representatives of fluoroquinolones with antitubercular activity, include ofloxacin, ciprofloxacin, spar-floxacin and levo-floxacin (the S(-) ofloxacin isomer). These compounds are bactericidal against M. tuberculosis, and fluoroquinolones (Klopman et al., 1993, 1993a, 1994; Piersimoni et al., 1992; Truffot-Pernot et al., 1991), such as ciprofloxacin (Figure 13), have MIC's less than 1 µg/ml (Heifets, 1994). Sparfloxacin is more bactericidal against M. tuberculosis in mice than either levofloxacin or ofloxacin (Lounis et al., 1997). There does not appear to be any synergism between fluoroquinolones and other antitubercular drugs (Marinis and Legakis, 1985), and their activity is independent of resistance to other antitubercular drugs. Although not indicated as first-line drug therapy for the treatment of tuberculosis because of their recent introduction, the fluoroquinolones are predominantly prescribed to patients who are infected with multidrug-resistant organisms. In spite of these precautions in the use of fluoroquinolones to treat tuberculosis, fluoroquinolone resistance is emerging via primary resistance mechanisms, as well as via nosocomial infection with fluoroquinolone-resistant organisms (Sullivan et al., 1995; Takiff et al., 1994).

The principal targets of fluoroquinolone action are bacterial type II topoisomerase, including both the bacterial DNA gyrase, which catalyzes the negative supercoiling of closed circular DNA (Wang, 1985), and the highly homologous topoisomerase IV, which deconcatenates the chromosome after DNA replication (Kato et al., 1992; Adams et al., 1992). The ATP-dependent DNA gyrase is a heterotetramer composed of two A and two B subunits (A_2B_2), encoded by the gyrA and gyrB genes, respectively. Topoisomerase IV is an essential enzyme discovered in E. coli and Salmonella typhimurium that plays a role in the segregation or replicated DNA circles (Kato et al., 1990; Springer and Schmid, 1993). The E. coli parC and parE genes, which encode for the two subunits of topoisomerase IV, are homologous to the gyr B (62%) and gyrA (59%) genes, respectively, of M. tuberculosis DNA gyrase (Takiff et al., 1994). Moreover, the regions of gyrB and gyrA involved in quinolone susceptibility are highly conserved in parC and parE. However, the quinolone resistance locus nfxD, which maps on the E. coli chromosome in the region of the genes for the subunits of topoisomerase IV, is recessive to $gyrA^+$ (Soussy et al., 1993). Thus, in E. coli the interaction of quinolones with a sensitive topoisomerase IV may have a less deleterious effect on the bacterial cell than the interactions of quinolones with sensitive DNA gyrase.

Fluoroquinolones bind to DNA gyrase, inhibiting supercoiling and subsequent processes dependent on DNA topology such as replication and transcription. DNA gyrase transiently breaks duplex DNA, with the ends immobilized during the supercoiling reaction. Fluoroquinolones trap a reaction intermediate containing broken DNA, and cell death results when the DNA breaks are released from the gyrase (Chen et al., 1996). The cloning and sequencing of the gyrA and gyrB genes from M. tuberculosis has allowed the quinolone binding site to be identified and the mutations that confer resistance to be mapped (Takiff et al., 1994). These mutations cluster in a small 40 amino acid region amino-terminal to the catalytic tyrosine (Y122 in E. coli) involved in DNA strand scission. In both in vitro-selected ciprofloxacin-resistant strains, and resistant clinical isolates, single-amino acid substitutions at residues 88–94 (equivalent to residues 81–87 in E. coli) were identified in these strains (Figure 14). These single-amino acid substitutions lead to a ca. 10-fold increase in

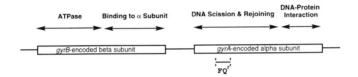

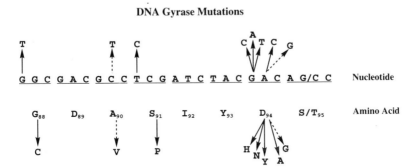

Figure 14. Top: Organization of the mycobacterial *gyrB* and *gyrA* genes. Bottom: mutations in the *gyrA*-encoded mycobacterial DNA gyrase subunit that result in ciprofloxacin resistance.

the MIC for ciprofloxacin (Wolucka *et al.*, 1994). Some fluoroquinolone-resistant clinical isolates of *M. tuberculosis* lack mutations in the *gyrA* gene, suggesting other mechanisms of resistance (Xu *et al.*, 1996). In other bacteria, fluoroquinolone resistance is the result of mutations in *gyrA* and in also in the *gyrB*, *norA*, and *parC* genes (Chen *et al.*, 1996; Ferrero *et al.*, 1994), although these latter mutations have not been identified in fluoroquinolone-resistant *M. tuberculosis*.

In a parallel study, mutations in the *gyrA* gene of *M. smegmatis* were obtained by selection for ofloxacin resistance (Revel *et al.*, 1994). Two amino acid substitutions were observed in these studies, A83V and D87G (equivalent to A90V and D94G in *M. tuberculosis*), which could account for low level resistance, comparable to the levels of resistance observed in *M. tuberculosis*. However, a second round of selection at higher ofloxacin levels yielded double mutants that displayed high-level resistance to fluoroquinolones. These double mutants contained substitutions at both positions 90 and 94, A90V/D94G (*M. tuberculosis* numbering), suggesting that the accumulation of specific mutations in the presumptive quinolone binding site had cumulative effects on the MIC for quinolones (Revel *et al.*, 1994). These results suggest that fluoroquinolone susceptibility must be continuously monitored in the treated patient population to prevent low-level fluoroquinolone-resistant strains from acquiring additional mutations that will result in high-level resistance.

More recently, the *lfrA*-encoded efflux pump of *M. smegmatis* has been shown to confer low-level fluoroquinolone resistance and to increase the frequency of mutations to higher-level resistance (Takiff *et al.*, 1996). The *lfrA* gene product belongs to a family of membrane efflux pumps termed the major facilitators, which transport drugs out of the bacteria via proton antiport. No mutations have been detected in the *lfrA* gene of fluoroquinolone-resistant *M. smegmatis* strains, but increased expression of plasmid-encoded *lfrA* may allow survival of bacteria with single mutations resulting in low level fluoroquinolone resistance. Subsequent drug treatment results in selection for a second mutation conferring increased resistance (Takiff *et al.*, 1996).

RESISTANCE TO SECOND-LINE ANTITUBERCULAR DRUGS

Cycloserine

In 1956, D-cycloserine (D-4-amino-isoxazolidone, Figure 15) was reported to have a broad germicidal spectrum which included not only Gram-positive and Gram-negative bacteria but also protozoa, viruses and tubercle bacilli (Weiss, 1956). D-Amino acids, especially D-alanine, D-glutamate, and D,L-diaminopimelate, are important components of all bacterial cell walls, including those of mycobacteria. As a structural analog of D-alanine, D-cycloserine inhibits *E. coli* L-alanine racemase and D-alanyl-D-alanine synthetase (Neuhaus and Lynch, 1964; Lambert and Neuhaus, 1972). The biosynthesis of the mycolyl-arabinogalactan-peptidoglycan complex is inhibited by D-cycloserine in *M. tuberculosis* (David *et al.*, 1970). Biochemical studies suggested that D-alanyl-D-alanine synthetase is one of the targets of the drug in mycobacteria (David *et al.*, 1969).

Resistance to D-cycloserine in *M. tuberculosis* has been attributed to mutations in the gene encoding the D-alanyl-D-alanine synthetase (David, 1971), although no biochemical or molecular evidence was provided in support of the proposed hypothesis. More recently, a molecular genetic analysis of D-cycloserine resistance in mycobacteria has led to the identification of one of the drug targets, and the mechanism of resistance, in *Mycobacterium smegmatis* (Cáceres *et al.*, 1997). The D-alanine racemase is encoded by the *alrA* gene, which was shown to be necessary and sufficient to confer D-cycloserine resistance in mc^{2}155 *M. smegmatis*. The predicted 41-kDa polypeptide chain has 66% amino acid identity to the homologous protein in *M. tuberculosis*. Amino acid sequence alignments reveal the presence of both a pyridoxal phosphate binding domain, and a conserved lysine residue responsible for Schiff base formation with the pyridoxal phosphate. The D-cycloserine-resistance phenotype is due to the overexpression of the wild-type *alrA* gene product and not to a mutation in the structural gene. The overexpression of the enzyme results from a single mutation (T→G) in the promoter region of *alrA* gene (Cáceres *et al.*, 1997).

Para-Aminosalicylic Acid

Para-aminosalicylic acid is a structural analog of para-aminobenzoic acid (Figure 16). Its use is reserved for patients with multi-drug resistant *M. tuberculosis* infection due to the high incidence of adverse effects. Para-aminosalicylic acid produces only an inhibitory effect in *M. tuberculosis*, and its MIC's were reported to be from 1.0 µg/ml to 10.0 µg/ml depending on the type of medium and inoculum size (Heifets, 1994). Para-aminosalicylic acid seems to act like the sulfonamides in inhibiting the biosynthesis of folate cofactors (Winder, 1982). This drug may also inhibits the synthesis of mycobactin, leading to reduced iron uptake by mycobacteria (Ratledge and Brown, 1972). The half life of para-aminosalicylic acid is about 1 hour, undergoing acetylation to its inactive metabolite, acetyl-para-aminosalicylic

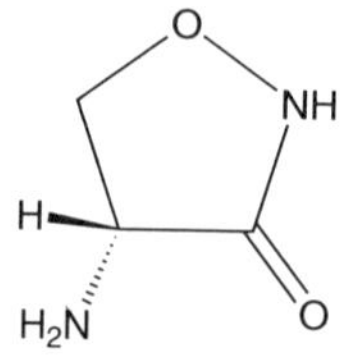

Figure 15. The structure of cycloserine.

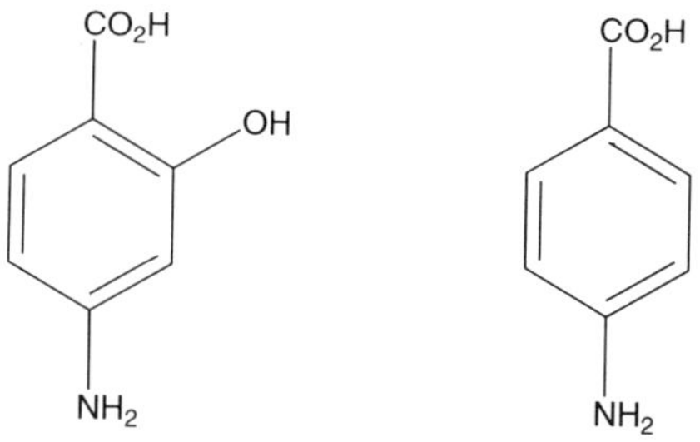

Figure 16. The structures of para-aminosalicylic and para-aminobenzoic acids.

acid. Resistance develops rapidly when the drug is used alone, but when used in combination with other agents, resistance is delayed or prevented. There is no evidence of cross resistance with other antitubercular drugs (Hobby *et al.*, 1974). Primary resistance of *M. tuberculosis* to para-aminosalicylic acid (6%) and acquired resistance (12%) are alarmingly high in some developing countries (Sifuentes-Osornio *et al.*, 1995).

Ethionamide

The discovery of the potent antitubercular activity of isoniazid was followed by a search for structural analogs, of which ethionamide (Figure 17) was found to be the most potent. Ethionamide is presently assumed to have a similar mechanism of action to isoniazid; inhibition of mycolic acid synthesis (Winder, 1982). The *inhA*-encoded enoyl reductase, which is the target for isoniazid, may also be a target of ethionamide (Banerjee *et al.*, 1994). Nevertheless, there are some significant differences in their activation mechanisms (Johnsson *et al.*, 1995). Ethionamide, like isoniazid, is a prodrug that is metabolized to its *S*-oxide which is capable of undergoing addition reactions to nucleophilic protein side chains. Whereas mutations in the enoyl reductase generate resistance to both isoniazid and ethionamide (Banerjee *et al.*, 1994), isoniazid-resistant strains containing mutations in the catalase-peroxidase gene remain susceptible to ethionamide. A second enzyme that activates ethionamide must be present in mycobacteria to convert this prodrug into a form capable of binding to, and presumably inhibiting, the *inhA*-encoded enoyl reductase (Quémard *et al.*, 1995).

RESISTANCE TO OTHER ANTITUBERCULAR DRUGS

Cyclic Peptides (Tuberactinomycin Family)

The tuberactinomycins are a group of basic cyclic peptide antibiotics. Viomycin and capreomycin (Figure 18) are members of this group, which show potent bacteriostatic activity against mycobacteria (Sutton *et al.*, 1966). Capreomycin is a mixture of four active

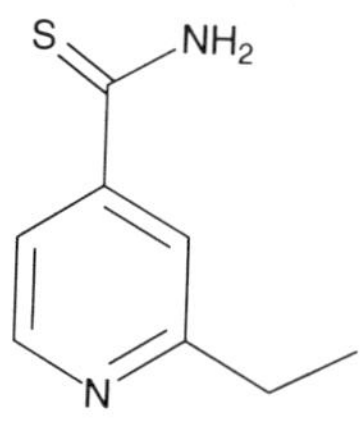

Figure 17. The structure of ethionamide.

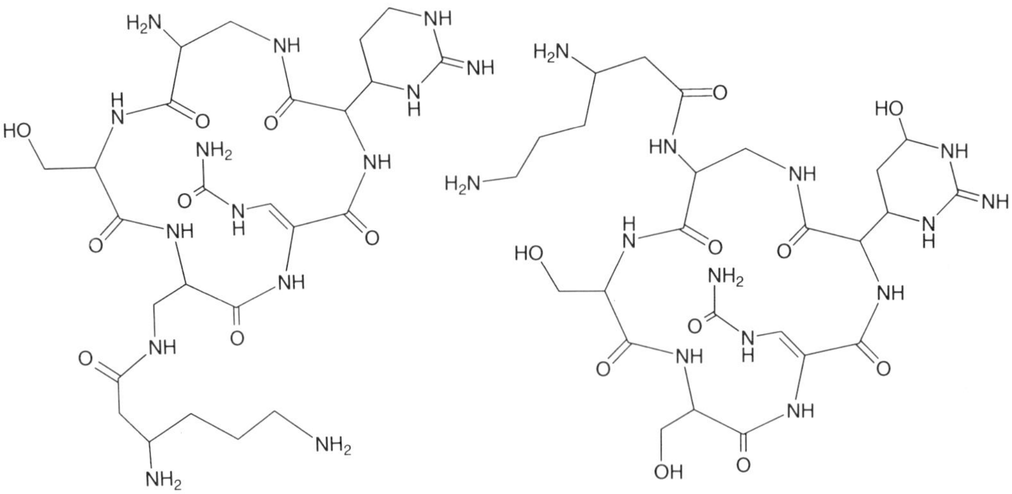

Figure 18. The structures of capreomycin (left) and viomycin.

compounds, capreomycin IA, IB, IIA, and IIB. Tuberactinomycins are potent inhibitors of bacterial translation, inhibiting both the initiation and elongation steps (Liou and Tanaka, 1976). Inhibition of translocation occurs by sequestration of peptidyl-tRNA in the ribosomal A-site (Modolell and Vázquez, 1977). Viomycin inhibits ribosomal subunit dissociation by binding to both ribosomal subunits, and the sites of interaction has been mapped to residues U913 and G914 in the 23S rRNA (Moazed and Noller, 1987a). *In vitro* transcription and self-splicing studies show that tuberactinomycins inhibit the self-splicing reaction of group I intron RNA and interact with the G-binding site (Wank *et al.*, 1994).

Clinical viomycin-resistant strains of *M. tuberculosis* have increased resistance to capreomycin, especially in strains that were also resistant to streptomycin (Verbist and Gyselen, 1964). Since viomycin-resistant strains are also resistant to kanamycin (Choi *et al.*, 1979), it is likely that viomycin acts at a site on the 16S rRNA that overlaps with the binding site for aminoglycosides. Accordingly, mutations in the *vicA* (50S subunit) and *vicC* (30S subunit corresponding to *E. coli* S12) genes of *M. smegmatis* give only low level resistance to viomycin and capreomycin, but high level resistance is observed when one or the other of these mutations is accompanied by streptomycin-resistance mutations (Winder, 1982). The recent report of a clinical isolate of *M. tuberculosis* resistant to isoniazid and capreomycin (Al Jarad *et al.*, 1994) is particularly alarming, since capreomycin is reserved for drug therapy of multi-drug resistant organisms.

FUTURE STUDIES AND SOLUTIONS

The challenge to the scientific community is to eliminate the comparative lack of modern biochemical and genetic information about mycobacteria in general. *M. tuberculosis*, in particular, is not an organism whose large scale culture is achievable in any but a handful of laboratories. The recent development of strains of the nonpathogenic, fast-growing *M. smegmatis* that can be genetically manipulated (Shinnick *et al.*, 1995; Snapper *et al.*, 1990) has allowed classical genetic studies to be performed in this non-pathogenic organism. These approaches have clarified the mechanism of action of, and resistance to, rifampicin (Levin and Hatfull, 1993), isoniazid and ethionamide (Banerjee *et al.*, 1994), ethambutol (Telenti *et al.*, 1997), and D-cycloserine (Cáceres *et al.*, 1997). PCR-based techniques and genetic manipulations of *M. bovis* and *M. tuberculosis* have allowed the identification of mechanism of resistance to, and mechanism of action of, pyrazinamide (Scorpio and Zhang, 1997). The biochemical transformations occurring in mycobacteria during the acquisition of drug resistance are generally inferred, rather than demonstrated, and tremendous progress should be made in this area in the next decade.

The serendipitous discovery of isoniazid, ethionamide, and ethambutol has now provided clues into critical and unique biosynthetic pathways in mycobacteria. The chemical simplicity of these molecules, and a decade of synthetic endeavors after their initial discovery, suggests that more potent analogs, prepared by classic organic synthesis or novel combinatorial synthetic methods, will be hard to find. Given what is now known about the mechanism of action of isoniazid, the discovery of homologues that are both actively accumulated and oxidatively activated, and still inhibit long chain fatty acid elongation processes involved in outer envelope biosynthesis, seems unlikely. However, as the mechanism of action of these drugs is clarified, and their molecular targets are biochemically and structurally characterized, more rational mechanism-based and structure-based approaches to inhibitor design will be possible. The synthesis and clinical evaluation of any lead compound is a long and expensive process, and the worldwide distribution of tuberculosis in the developing nations may discourage such investments.

An understanding of the biochemistry of the unique cell wall lipids should provide a rational basis for seeking drugs targeted at the biosynthesis of these lipids. The synthesis of ethylenic and cyclopropanated mycolic acids involves fatty acid elongation, desaturation, cyclopropanation of the double bond and a Claisen-type condensation (Figure 19;

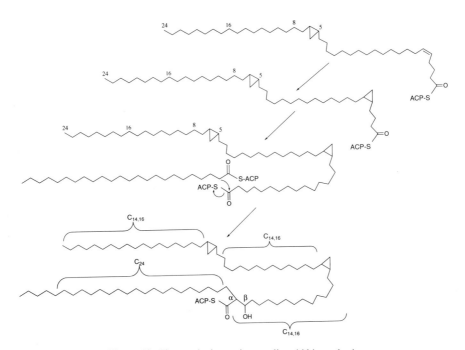

Figure 19. The terminal steps in mycolic acid biosynthesis.

Besra and Chatterjee, 1994). The *M. tuberculosis cma1* and *cma2* gene products have been shown to cyclopropanate the distal and proximal double bond, respectively, of mycolic acids (Yuan *et al.*, 1995; George *et al.*, 1995). Subsequently, cyclopropanation was shown to alter fluidity and permeability of the mycobacterial cell wall (Liu *et al.*, 1996). More recently, the *mm1–4* genes have been shown to encode for methyl transferases involved in methoxylation of the methoxymycolates series (Figure 2) found in *M. tuberculosis* (Yuan and Barry, 1996). Studies of the biosynthetic pathways of methyl-branched fatty acids, phthiocerol and phenolphthiocerol have unveiled new genes and their products (Kolattukudy *et al.*, 1997).

Alternative solutions that should also be examined include the revaluation of existing antibacterials. The example of fluoroquinolone inhibitors of DNA gyrase was discussed above. A second example could include the β-lactam inhibitors of peptidoglycan biosynthesis. Mycobacteria are naturally insensitive to β-lactams, because of their extremely hydrophobic cell wall (Jarlier *et al.*, 1991) and an active β-lactamase (Fattorini *et al.*, 1992; Zhang *et al.*, 1992). However, the presence of a penicillin-binding protein, which possesses transpeptidase activity, has been demonstrated in *M. smegmatis* (Basu et al., 1992). Accordingly, the combined administration of β-lactams and β-lactamase inhibitors has recently been shown to be effective in inhibiting the growth of mycobacteria (Prabhakaran *et al.*, 1992, 1993; Zhang *et al.*, 1992). Given their oral availability and favorable toxicology profile, the thousands of β-lactams that have been synthesized seem worthy of re-examination, in combination with inhibitors of mycobacterial β-lactamases (Blanchard, 1996). Acquired beta-lactam resistance in *M. smegmatis* has been shown to arise from a combination of decreased affinities of high-molecular-weight penicillin-binding protein (PBP 1) for β-lactams and reduced cell wall permeability (Murkhopadhyay and Chakrabarti, 1997).

The activity of nitroimidazoles such as metronidazole (Ashtekar *et al.*, 1993; Wayne and Sramek, 1994) against dormant populations of *M. tuberculosis*, which are poorly treated in present drug regiments, represents a potential new chemotherapeutic addition. More recently, a fluoroquinolone derivative (CG 5501) has been shown to have *in vitro* antibacterial activity against sensitive and multi-resistant strains of *Mycobacterium tuberculosis* (Wise *et al.*, 1997). Another example is the synergistic effect of current antitubercular drugs used in combination with poloxamer surfactant CRL8131 (Jagannath *et al.*, 1995). Inhibitors of cell wall biosynthesis, such as ethambutol, not only are potential antimycobacterial agents but also increase mycobacterial susceptibility to other antimicrobial agents (Rastogi *et al.*, 1990). Utilization of antisense oligodeoxynucleotide phosphorothioates to inhibit the expression of proteins essential for cellular growth, in combination with ethambutol results in the inhibition of drug-resistant *M. smegmatis* (Rapaport *et al.*, 1996). Combination therapy could therefore be exploited further. An alternative approach has been to improve drug delivery vehicles using isoniazid and rifampicin encapsulated in liposomes with enhanced affinity towards lung tissue, which would reduce *in vivo* toxicity and allow for higher concentrations of antitubercular drugs to be prescribed (Deol and Khuller, 1997). An exciting new development is the restoration of antibiotic sensitivity to resistant strains of *E. coli* by external guide sequences (EGS) of RNA nucleotides (Guerrier-Takada *et al.*, 1997). EGSs form complexes with the mRNAs encoded by genes responsible for drug resistance, and these complexes are recognized as substrates by endoribonuclease RNase P which cleaves and inactivates the targeted mRNA, thereby rendering the host cells drug-susceptible. Whether or not such approaches can be applied to *M. tuberculosis* remains to be seen. Ultimately, the best solution to the problems with tuberculosis chemotherapy and the explosion of multi-drug resistance is patient surveillance and treatment compliance by directly observed therapy.

REFERENCES

Adams, D.E., Shekhtman, E.M., Zechiedrich, E.L., Schmid, M.B., and Cozzarelli, N.R., 1992, The role of topoisomerase IV in partitioning bacterial replicons and the structure of catenated intermediates in DNA replication. *Cell* 71:277.

Al Jarad, N., Parastatides, S., Paul, E.A., Sheldon, C.D., Gaya, H., Rudd, R.M., and Empey, D.W., 1994, Characteristics of patients with drug resistant and drug sensitive tuberculosis in East London between 1984 and 1992. *Thorax* 49:808.

Allen, P.N., and Noller, H.F., 1989, Mutations in ribosomal S4 and S12 influence the higher order structure of 16S ribosomal RNA. *J. Mol. Biol.* 208:457.

Ashtekar, D.R., Costa-Pereira, R., Nagrajan, K., Vishvanathan, N., Bhatt, A.D., and Rittel, W., 1993, In vitro and in vivo activities of the nitroimidazole CGI 17341 against *Mycobacterium tuberculosis. Antimicrob. Agents Chemother.* 37:183.

Baldock, C., Rafferty, J.B., Sedelnikova, S.E., Baker, P.J.., Stuitje, A.R., Slabas, A.R., Hawkes, T.R., and Rice, D.W., 1996, A mechanism of drug action revealed by structural studies of enoyl reductase. *Science* 274:2107.

Banerjee A, Dubnau E, Quémard A, Balasubramanian, V., Um, K.S., Wilson, T., Collins, D., de Lisle, G., and Jacobs, W.R.Jr., 1994, *inhA*, a gene encoding a target for isoniazid and ethionamide in *Mycobacterium tuberculosis. Science* 263:227.

Basso, L.A., Zheng, R., and Blanchard, J.S., 1996, Kinetics of inactivation of WT and C243S mutant of *Mycobacterium tuberculosis* enoyl reductase by activated isoniazid. *J. Am. Chem. Soc.* 118:11301.

Basu, J., Chattopadhyay, R., Kundu, M., and Chakrabarti, P., 1992, Purification and partial characterization of a penicillin-binding protein from *Mycobacterium smegmatis. J. Bacteriol.* 174:4829.

Bax, R.P., 1997, Antibiotic resistance: a view from the pharmaceutical industry. *Clin. Infect. Dis.* 24:S151.

Belanger, A.E., Besra, G.S., Ford, M.E., Mikusová, K., Belisle, J.T., Brennan, P.J., and Inamine, J.M., 1996, The *embAB* genes of *Mycobacterium avium* encode an arabinosyl transferase involved in cell wall arabinan biosynthesis that is the target for the antimycobacterial drug ethambutol. *Proc. Natl. Acad. Sci. USA* 93:11919.

Benveniste, R., and Davies, J., 1973, Mechanisms of antibiotic resistance in bacteria. *Annu. Rev. Biochem.* 42:471.

Bergler, H., Högenauer, G., and Turnowsky, F., 1992, Sequences of the *envM* gene and two mutated alleles in *Escherichia coli. J. Biol. Chem.* 269:5493.

Bergler H., Wallner P., Ebeling A., Leitinger, B., Fuchsbichler, S., Aschauer, H., Kollenz, G., Högenauer, G., and Turnowsky, F., 1994, Protein envM is the NADH-dependent enoyl-ACP reductase (fabI) of *Escherichia coli. J. Biol. Chem.* 269:5493.

Berstein J., Lott W.A., Steinberg B.A., and Yale H.L., 1952, Chemotherapy of experimental tuberculosis. *Am. Rev. Tuberc.* 65:357.

Besra, G.S., and Chatterjee, D., 1994, Lipids and carbohydrates of *Mycobacterium tuberculosis*, in: *Tuberculosis. Pathogenesis, Protection, and Control*, B.R. Bloom, ed., Ameican Society for Microbiology, Washington D.C.

Blanchard, J.S., 1996, Molecular mechanisms of drug resistance in *Mycobacterium tuberculosis. Annu. Rev. Biochem.* 65:215.

Bloch, A.B., Cauthen, G.M., Onorato, I.M., Dansbury, K.G., Kelly, G.D., Driver, C.R., and Snider, D.E., 1994, Nationwide survey of drug-resistant tuberculosis in the United States. *J. Am. Med. Assoc.* 271:665.

Bloom, B.R., and Murray, C.J.L., 1992, Tuberculosis: commentary on a reemergent killer. *Science* 257:1055.

Brennan, P.J., and Nikaido, H., 1995, The envelope of mycobacteria. *Annu. Rev. Biochem.* 64:29.

Bryskier, A., and Chantot, J.F., 1995, Classification and structure-activity relationships of fluoroquinolones. *Drugs* 49:16.

Butler, W.R., and Kilburn, J.O., 1983, Susceptibility of *Mycobacterium tuberculosis* to pyrazinamide and its relationship to pyrazinamidase activity. *Antimicrob. Agents Chemother.* 24:600.

Cáceres, N.E., Harris, N.B., Wellehan, J.F., Feng, Z., Kapur, V., and Barletta, R.G., 1997, Overexpression of the D-alanine racemase gene confers resistance to D-cycloserine in *Mycobacterium smegmatis. J. Bacteriol.* 179:5046.

Canetti, G., 1965, The J. Burns Amberson lecture: present aspects of bacterial resistance in tuberculosis. *Am. Rev. Resp. Dis.* 92:687.

Casadevall, A., 1996, Crisis in infectious diseases: time for a new paradigm? *Clin. Infect. Dis.* 23:790.

Chen, C.R., Malik, M., Snyder, M., and Drlica, K., 1996, DNA gyrase and topoisomerase IV on the bacterial chromosome: quinolone-induced DNA cleavage. *J. Mol. Biol.* 258:627.

Choi, E.C., Misumi, M., Nishimura, T., Tanaka, N., Nomoto, S., Teshima, T., and Shiba, T., 1979, Viomycin resistance: alterations of either ribosomal subunit affect the binding of the antibiotic to the pair subunit and the entire ribosome becomes resistant to the drug. *Biochem. Biophys. Res. Commun.* 87:904.

Clemens, D.L., 1996, Characterization of the *Mycobacterium tuberculosis* phagosome. *Trends Microbiol.* 4:113.

Cockerill, F.R., Uhl, J.R., Temesgen, Z., Zhang, Y., Stockman, L., Roberts, G.D., Williams, D.L., and Kline, B.C., 1995, Rapid identification of a point mutation of the Mycobacterium tuberculosis catalase-peroxidase (*katG*) gene associated with isoniazid resistance. *J. Infect. Dis.* 171:240–245.

Cohn, D.L., Bustreo, F., and Raviglione, M.C., 1997, Drug-resistant tuberculosis: review of the worldwide situation and the WHO/IUATLD global survaillance project. *Clin. Infect. Dis.* 24:S121.

Cole, S.T., 1994, *Mycobacterium tuberculosis*: drug-resistance mechanisms. *Trends Microbiol.* 2:411.

Coleman, K., Athalye, M., Clancey, A., Davison, M., Payne, D.J., Perry, C.R., and Chopra, I., 1994, Bacterial resistance mechanisms as targets. *J. Antimicrob. Chemother.* 33:1091.

Cooksey, R.C., Morlock, G.P., McQueen, A., Glickman, S.E., and Crawford, J.T., 1996, Characterization of streptomycin resistance mechanisms among *Mycobacterium tuberculosis* isolates from patients in New York City. *Antimicrob. Agents Chemother.* 40:1186.

Crowle, A.J., Dahl, R., Ross, E., and May, M.H., 1991, Evidence that vesicles containing living, virulent *Mycobacterium tuberculosis* or *M. avium* in cultured human macrophages are not acidic. *Infect. Immun.* 59:1823.

David, H. L., 1971, Resistance to D-cycloserine in the tubercle bacilli: mutation rate and transport of alanine in parental cells and drug-resistant mutants. *Appl. Microbiol.* 21:888.

David, H. L., 1980, Drug Resistance to *M. tuberculosis* and other Mycobacteria. *Clin. Chest. Med.* 11:227.

David, H.L., Goldman, D.S., and Takayama, K., 1970, Inhibition of the synthesis of wax D peptidoglycolipid of *Mycobacterium tuberculosis* by D-cycloserine. *Infect. Immun.* 1:74.

David, H.L., Takayama, K., and Goldman, D.S., 1969, Susceptibility of mycobacterial D-alanyl-D-alanine synthetase to D-cycloserine. *Am. Rev. Respir. Dis.* 100:579.

Davidson, P.T., and Quoc, L.H., 1992, Drug treatment of tuberculosis. *Drugs* 43:651.

Deng, L., Mikusová, K., Robuck, K.G., Scherman, M., Brennan, P.J., and McNeil, M.R., 1995, Recognition of multiple effects of ethambutol on metabolism of mycobacterial cell envelope. *Antimicrob. Agents Chemother.* 39:694.

Deol, P., and Khuller, G.K., 1997, Lung specific stealth liposomes: stability, biodistribution and toxicity of liposomal antitubercular drugs in mice. *Biochim. Biophys. Acta.* 1334:161.

Dessen A., Quémard A., Blanchard J.S., Jacobs W.R.Jr., and Sacchettini J.C., 1995, Crystal structure and function of the isoniazid target of *Mycobacterium tubertculosis*. *Science* 267:1638.

Dhandayuthapani, S., Zhang, Y., Mudd, M.H., and Deretic, V., 1996, Oxidative stress response and its role in sensitivity to isoniazid in mycobacteria: characterization and inducibility of *ahpC* by peroxides in *Mycobacterium smegmatis* and lack of expression in *M. aurum* and *M. tuberculosis*. *J. Bacteriol.* 178:3641.

Dickinson, J.M., and Mitchison, D.A., 1981, Experimental models to explain the high sterilizing activity of rifampin in the chemotherapy of tuberculosis. *Am. Rev. Respir. Dis.* 123:367.

Donnabella, M.V., Martiniuk, F., Kinney, D., Bacerdo, M., Bonk, S., et al., 1994, Isolation of the gene for the β subunit of RNA polymerase from rifampicin-resistant *Mycobacterium tuberculosis* and identification of new mutations. *Am. J. Respir. Cell Mol. Biol.* 11:639.

Douglass, J., and Steyn, L.M., 1993, A ribosomal gene mutation in streptomycin-resistant *Mycobacterium tuberculosis* isolates. *J. Infect. Dis.* 167:1505.

Dutt, A. K., and Stead W., 1997, The treatment of tuberculosis. *Dis. Month* 43:247.

Fattorini, L., Orefici, G., Jin, S.H., Scardaci, G., Amicosante, G., Franceschini, N., and Chopra, I., 1992, Resistance to β-Lactams in Mycobacterium fortuitum. *Antimicrob. Agents Chemother.* 36:1068.

Ferrero, L., Cameron, B., Manse, B., Lagneaux, D., Crouzet, J., Famechon, A., and Blanche, F., 1994, Cloning and primary structure of *Staphylococcus aureus* DNA topoisomerase IV: a primary target of fluoroquinolones. *Mol. Microbiol.* 13:641.

Finken, M., Kirschner, P., Meier, A., Wrede, A., and Böttger, E.C., 1993, Molecular basis of streptomycin resistance in *Mycobacterium tuberculosis*: alterations of the ribosomal protein S12 gene and point mutations within a functional 16S ribosomal RNA pseudoknot. *Mol. Microbiol.* 9:1239.

Fischl, M.A., Daikos, G.L., Uttamchandani, R.B., Poblete, R.B., Moreno, J.N., Reyes, R.R., Boota, A.M., Thompson, L.M., Cleary, T.J., Oldham, S.A., Saldana, M.J., and Lai, S., 1992, Clinical presentation and outcome of patients with HIV infection and tuberculosis caused by multiple-drug-resistant bacilli. *Ann. Intern. Med.* 117:184.

Frieden, T.R., Sterling, T., Pablos-Mendez, A, Kilburn, J.O., Cauthen, J.O., and Dooley, S.W., 1993, The emergence of drug-resistant tuberculosis in New York City. *N. Engl. J. Med.* 328:521.

Frothingham, R., Meeker-O'Connel, W.A., Talbot, E.A.S., George, J.W., and Kreuzer, K.N., 1996, Identification, cloning, and expression of the *Escherichia coli* pyrazinamidase and nicotinamidase gene, *pncA*. *Antimicrob. Agents Chemother.* 40:1426.

Gangadharam, P.R., and Gonzales, E.R., 1970, Influence of the medium on the *in vitro* susceptibility of *Mycobacterium tuberculosis* to ethambutol. *Am. Rev. Resp. Dis.* 102:653.

Gay, J.D., DeYoung, D.R., and Roberts, G.D., 1984, *In vitro* activities of norfloxacin and ciprofloxacin against *Mycobacterium tuberculosis*, *M. avium* complex, *M. chelonei*, *M. fortuitum*, and *M. kansasii*. *Antimicrob. Agents Chemother.* 26:94.

George, K.M., Yuan, Y., Sherman, D.R., Sherman, D.R., and Barry, III,C.E., 1995, The biosysnthesis of cyclopropanated mycolic acids in *Mycobacterium tuberculosis*. Identification and functional analysis of CMAS-2. *J. Biol. Chem.* 45:27292.

Ghuysen, M.M., 1994, Molecular structures of penicillin binding proteins and β-lactamases. *Trends Microbiol.* 2:372.

Goble, M., Iseman, M.D., Madsen, L.A., Waite, D., Ackerson, L., and Horsburgh C.R., 1993, Treatment of 171 patients with pulmonary tuberculosis resistant to isoniazid and rifampicin. *N. Engl. J. Med.* 328:527.

Grosset, J., 1980, Bacteriologic basis of short course chemotherapy for tuberculosis. *Clin. Chest Med.* 1:231.

Guerrier-Takada, C., Salavati, R., and Altman, S., 1997, Phenotypic conversion of drug-resistant bacteria to drug sensitivity. *Proc. Natl. Acad. Sci. USA* 94:8468.

Heifets, L.B., 1994, Antimycobacterial drugs. *Semin. Respir. Infect.* 9:84.

Heifets, L.B., and Lindholm-Levy, P.J., 1989, Comparison of bactericidal activities of streptomycin, amikacin, kanamycin, and capreomycin against *Mycobacterium avium* and *M. tuberculosis*. *Antimicrob. Agents Chemother.* 33:1298.

Heifets, L.B., and Lindholm-Levy, P.J., 1992, Pyrazinamide sterilizing activity *in vitro* against semidormant *Mycobacterium tuberculosis* bacterial populations. *Am. Rev. Respir. Dis.* 145:1223.

Heifets, L.B., Lindholm-Levy, P.J., and Flory, M.A., 1990, Bactericidal activity in vitro of various rifamycins against *Mycobacterium avium* and *Mycobacterium tuberculosis*. *Am. Rev. Respir. Dis.* 141:626.

Hewlett, D., Horn, D.L., and Alfalla, C., 1995, Drug-resistant tuberculosis: inconsistent results of pyrazinamide susceptibility testing. *J. Am. Med. Assoc.* 273:916.

Heym, B., Alzari, P.M., Honore, N., and Cole, S.T., 1995, Missense mutations in the catalase-peroxidase gene, *katG*, are associated with isoniazid resistance in *Mycobacterium tuberculosis*. *Mol. Microbiol.* 15:235.

Heym, B., and Cole, S.T., 1992, Isolation and characterization of isoniazid-resistant mutants of *Mycobacterium smegmatis* and *M. aurum*. *Res. Microbiol.* 143:721.

Heym, B., Honoré, N., Truffot-Pernot, C.,Banerjee, A., Schurra, C., Jacobs, W.R.Jr., van Embden, J.D.A., Grosset, J.H., and Cole, S.T., 1994, Implications of multidrug resistance for the future of short-course chemotherapy of tuberculosis: a molecular study. *Lancet* 344:293.

Hiriyanna, K.T., and Ramakrishnan, T., 1986, Deoxyribonucleic acid replication time in *Mycobacterium tuberculosis* H37 Rv. *Arch. Microbiol.* 144:105.

Hobby, G., Johnson, P.M., and Boytar-Papirnyik, V., 1974, Primary drug resistance: a continuing study of drug resistance in tuberculosis in a veteran population within the United States. X. September 1970 to September 1973. *Am. Rev. Respir. Dis.* 110:95.

Honoré, N., and Cole, S.T., 1993, Molecular basis of rifampin resistance in *Mycobacterium leprae*. *Antimicrob. Agents Chemother.* 37:414.

Honoré, N., and Cole, S.T., 1994, Streptomycin resistance in mycobacteria. *Antimicrob. Agents Chemother.* 38:238.

Huebner, R.E., and Castro, K.G., 1995, The changing face of tuberculosis. *Annu. Rev. Med.* 46:47.

Jacobs, M.R., 1995, Activity of quinolones against mycobacteria. *Drugs* 49(Suppl. 2):67.

Jagannath, C., Allaudeen, H.S., and Hunter, R.L., 1995, Activities of poloxamer CRL8131 against *Mycobacterium tuberculosis in vitro* and *in vivo*. *Antimicrob. Agents Chemother.* 39:1349.

Jarlier, V.L., Gutmann, L., Nikaido, H., 1991, Interplay of cell wall barrier and β-lactamase activity determines high resistance to β-lactam antibiotics in *Mycobacterium chelonae*. *Antimicrob. Agents Chemother.* 35:1937.

Jarlier, V., and Nikaido, H., 1994, Mycobacterial cell wall: structure and role in natural resistance to antibiotics. *FEMS Microbiol. Lett.* 123:11.

Johnsson, K., and Schultz, P.G., 1994, Mechanistic studies of the oxidation of isoniazid by the catalase peroxidase from *Mycobacterium tuberculosis*. *J. Am. Chem. Soc.* 116:7425.

Johnsson, K., King, D.S., and Schultz, P.G., 1995, Studies on the mechanism of action of isoniazid and ethionamide in the chemotherapy of tuberculosis. *J. Am. Chem. Soc.* 117:5009.

Kapur, V., Li, L.L., Iordanescu, S., Hamrick, M.R., Wanger, A., Kreiswirth, B.N., and Musser, J.M., 1994, Characterization by automated DNA sequencing of mutations in the gene (*rpoB*) encoding the RNA polymerase β subunit in rifampin-resistant *Mycobacterium tuberculosis* strains from New York City and Texas. *J. Clin. Microbiol.* 32:1095.

Kapur, V., Li, L.L., Hamrick, M.R., Plikaytis, B.B., Shinnick, T.M., Telenti, A., Jacobs, W.R.Jr., Banerjee, A.B., Cole, S., Yuen, K.Y., Clarridge, J.E., Kreiswirth, B.N., and Musser, J.M., 1995, Rapid mycobacterium species assignment and unambigous identification of mutations associated with anti-microbial resistance in *Mycobacterium tuberculosis* by automated DNA sequencing. *Arch. Pathol. Lab. Med.* 119:131.

Kato, J-I., Nishimura, Y., Imamura, R., Niki, H., Hiraga, S., and Suzuki, H., 1990, New topoisomerase essential for chromosome segregation in *E. coli. Cell* 63:393.

Kato, J-I., Suzuki, H., and Ikeda, H., 1992, Purification and characterization of DNA topoisomerase IV in *Escherichia coli. J. Biol. Chem.* 267:25676.

Kelley, C.L., Rouse, D.A., and Morris, S.L., 1997 Analysis of *ahpC* gene mutatiions in isoniazid-resistant clinical isolates of *Mycobacterium tuberculosis. Antimicrob. Agents Chemother.* 41:2057.

Kessler, R.E., 1997, Perspectives on chemotherapeutic approaches to antibiotic-resistant bacteria. *Clin. Infect. Dis.* 24:S146.

Khoo, K.-H., Douglas, E., Azadi, P., Inamine, J.M., Besra, G.S., Mikusová, K., Brennan, P.J., and Chatterjee, D., 1996, Truncated structural variants of lipoarabinomannan in ethambutol drug-resistant strains of *Mycobacterium smegmatis. J. Biol. Chem.* 271:28682.

Kilburn, J.O., and Takayama, K., 1981, Effects of ethambutol on accumulation and secretion of trehalose mycolates and free mycolic acid in *Mycobacterium smegmatis. Antimicrob. Agents Chemother.* 20:401.

Klopman, G., Wang, S., Jacobs, M.R., Bajaksouzian, S., Edmonds, K., and Ellner, J.J., 1993, Anti-*Mycobacterium avium* activity of quinolones: *in vitro* activities. *Antimicrob. Agents Chemother.* 37:1799.

Klopman, G., Wang, S., Jacobs, M.R., and Ellner, J. J., 1993a, Anti-*Mycobacterium avium* activity of quinolones: structure-activity relationship studies. *Antimicrob. Agents Chemother.* 37:1807.

Klopman, G., Li,, J.Y., Wang, S., Pearson, A.J., Chang, K., Jacobs, M.R., Bajaksouzian, S., and Ellner, J.J., 1994, *In vitro* anti-*Mycobacterium avium* activities of quinolones: predicted active structures and mechanistic considerations. *Antimicrob. Agents Chemother.* 38:1794.

Koch, R., 1932, Die aetiologie der tuberculose, *Am. Rev. Tuberc.* 25:285–323. [Translated from the original 1882 article by Berna Pinner and Max Pinner.]

Kolattukudy, P.E., Fernandes, N.D., Azad, A.K., Fitzmaurice, A.M., and Sirakova, T.D., 1997, Biochemistry and molecular genetics of cell-wall lipid biosynthesis in mycobacteria. *Mol. Microbiol.* 24:263.

Konno, K., Feldmann, F., and McDermott, W., 1967, Pyrazinamide susceptibility and amidase activity of tubercle bacilli. *Am. Rev. Resp. Dis.* 95:461.

Kritski, A.L., Marques, M.J.O., Rabahi, M.F., Vieira, M.A.M.S., Werneck-Barroso, E., Carvalho, C.E.S., Andrade, G.N., Bravo-de-Souza, R., Andrade, L.M., Gontijo, P.P., and Riley, L.W., 1996, Transmission of tuberculosis to close contacts of patients with multidrug-resistant tuberculosis. *Am. J. Respir. Crit. Care Med.* 153:331.

Kushner, S., Dalalian, H., Sanjurjo, J.L., Bach, F.L., Safir, S.R., Smith, V.K.Jr., and Williams, J.H., 1952, Experimental chemotherapy of tuberculosis. II. The synthesis of pyrazinamides and related compounds. *J. Am. Chem. Soc.* 74:3617.

Lambert, M.P., and Neuhaus, F.C., 1972, Mechanism of D-cycloserine action: alanine racemase from *Escherichia coli* W. *J. Bacteriol.* 110:978.

Levin, M.E., and Hatfull, G.F., 1993, *Mycobacterium smegmatis* RNA polymerase: DNA supercoiling, action of rifampicin and mechanism of rifampicin resistance. *Mol. Microbiol.* 8:277.

Leysen, D.C., Haemers, A., and Pattyn, S.R., 1989, Mycobacteria and the new quinolones. *Antimicrob. Agents Chemother.* 33:1.

Liou, Y.F., and Tanaka, N., 1976, Dual actions of viomycin on the ribosomal functions. *Biochem. Biophys. Res. Commun.* 71:477.

Liu, J., Barry, C.E., Besra, G.S., and Nikaido, H., 1996, Mycolic acid structure determines the fluidity of the mycobacterial cell wall. *J. Biol. Chem.* 47:29545.

Lounis, N., Ji, B., Truffot-Pernot, C., and Grosset, J., 1997, Which aminoglycoside or fluroquinolone is more active against *Mycobacterium tuberculosis* in mice? *Antimicrob. Agents Chemother.* 41:607.

Mackaness, G.B., 1956, The intracellular activation of pyrazinamide and nicotinamide. *Am. Rev. Tuberc.* 74:718.

Maddry, J.A., Suling, W.J., and Reynolds, R.C., 1996, Glycosyl transferases as targets for inhibition of cell wall synthesis in *M. tuberculosis* and *M. avium. Res. Microbiol.* 147:106.

Marinis, E., and Legakis, N.J., 1985, *In vitro* activity of ciprofloxacin against clinical isolates of mycobacteria resistant to antimycobacterial drugs. *J. Antimicrob. Chemother.* 16:527.

Meier, A., Kirschner, P., Bange, F.C., Vogel U., and Böttger, E.C., 1994, Genetic alterations in streptomycin-resistant *Mycobacterium tuberculosis*: mapping of mutations conferring resistance. *Antimicrob. Agents Chemother.* 38:228.

Meier, A., Sander, P., Schaper, K.J., Scholz, M., and Böttger, E.C., 1996, Correlation of molecular resistance mechanisms and phenotypic resistance levels in streptomycin-resistant *Mycobacterium tuberculosis*. *Antimicrob. Agents Chemother.* 40:2452.

Middlebrook, G., 1952, Sterilization of tubercle bacilli by isonicotinic acid hydrazide and the incidence of variants resistant to the drug *in vitro*. *Am. Rev. Tuberc.* 65:765.

Middlebrook, G., 1954, Isoniazid-resistance and catalase activity of tubercle bacilli. *Am. Rev. Tuberc.* 69:471.

Middlebrook, G., Cohn, M.L., and Schaefer, W.B., 1954, Studies on isoniazid and tubercle bacilli. *Am. Rev. Tuberc.* 70:852.

Miller, L.P., Crawford, J.T., and Shinnick, T.M., 1994, The *rpoB* gene of *Mycobacterium tuberculosis*. *Antimicrob. Agents Chemother.* 38:805.

Miller, M.A., Thibert, L., Desjardins, F., Siddiqi, S.H., and Dascal, A., 1995, Testing of susceptibility of *Mycobacterium tuberculosis* to pyrazinamide: comparison of Bactec method with pyrazinamidase assay. *J. Clin. Microbiol.* 33:2468.

Mitchison, D.A., 1985, The action of antituberculosis drugs in short-course chemotherapy.*Tubercle* 66:219.

Moazed, D., and Noller, H.F., 1987, Interaction of antibiotics with functional sites in 16S ribosomal RNA. *Nature* 327:389.

Moazed, D., and Noller, H.F., 1987a, Chloramphenicol, erythromycin, carbomycin and vernamycin B protect overlapping sites in the peptidyl transferase region of 23S ribosomal RNA. *Biochimie* 69:879.

Modolell, J., and Vázquez, D., 1977, The inhibition of ribosomal translocation by viomycin. *Eur. J. Biochem.* 81:491.

Montandon, P.E., Wagner, R., and Stutz, E., 1986, *E. coli* ribosomes with a C912 to U base change in the 16S rRNA are streptomycin resistant. *EMBO J.* 5:3705.

Morris, S., Bai, G.H., Suffys, P., Portillo-Gomez, L., Fairchock, M., and Rouse, D., 1995, Molecular mechanisms of multiple drug resistance in clinical isolates of *Mycobacterium tuberculosis*. *J. Infect. Dis.* 171:954.

Mukhopadhyay, S., and Chakrabarti, P., 1997, Altered permeability and β-lactam resistance in a mutant of *Mycobacterium smegmatis*. *Antimicrob. Agents Chemother.* 41:1721.

Musser, J.M., Kapur, V., Williams, D.L., Kreiswirth, B.N., Soolingen, D.V., van Embden, J.D.A., 1996, Characterization of the catalase-peroxidase gene (*katG*) and *inhA* locus in isoniazid-resistant and -susceptible strains of *Mycobacterium tuberculosis* by automated DNA sequencing: restricted array of mutations associated with drug resistance. *J. Infect. Dis.* 173:196.

Nair, J., Rouse, D.A., Bai, G.H., and Morris, S.L., 1993, The *rpsL* gene and streptomycin resistance in single and multiple drug-resistant strains of *Mycobacterium tuberculosis*. *Mol. Microbiol.* 10:521.

Nash, K.A., Gaytan, A., and Inderlied, C.B., 1997, Detection of rifampin resistance in *Mycobacterium tuberculosis* by use of a rapid, simple, and specific RNA/RNA mismatch assay. *J. Infect. Dis.* 176:533.

Neuhaus, F.C., and Lynch, J.L., 1964, The enzymatic synthesis of D-alanyl-D-alanine. III. On the inhibition of D-alanyl-D-alanine synthetase by the antibiotic D-cycloserine. *Biochemistry* 3:471.

Noller, H.F., 1984, Structure of ribosomal RNA. *Annu. Rev. Biochem.* 53:119.

Ohno, H., Koga, H., Kohno, S., Tashiro, T., and Hara, K., 1996, Relationship between rifampin MICs for and *rpoB* mutations of *Mycobacterium tuberculosis* strains isolated in Japan. *Antimicrob. Agents Chemother.* 40:1053.

Piersimoni, C., Morbiducci, V., Bornigia, S., DeSio, G., and Scalise, G., 1992, *In vitro* activity of the new quinolone lomefloxacin against *Mycobacterium tuberculosis*. *Am. Rev. Respir. Dis.* 146:1445.

Prabhakaran, K., Harris, E.B., Randhawa, B., and Hastings, R.C., 1992, Reversal of drug resistance in *Mycobacterium leprae* by ampicillin/sulbactam. *Microbios* 72:137–142.

Prabhakaran, K., Harris, E.B., Randhawa, B., Adams, L.B., Williams, D.L., and Hastings, R.C., 1993, Use of β-lactam/β-lactamase-inhibitor combinations as antimycrobacterial agents. *Microbios* 76:251.

Quémard, A., Sacchettini, J.C., Dessen ,A., Vilcheze,, C., Bittman, R., Jacobs, W.R.Jr., and Blanchard, J.S., 1995, Enzymatic characterization of the target for isoniazid in *Mycobacterium tuberculosis*. *Biochemistry* 34:8235.

Quémard, A.., Dessen, A., Sugantino, M., Jacobs, W.R.Jr., Sacchettini, J.C., and Blanchard, J.S., 1996, Binding of catalase-peroxidase-activated isoniazid to wild-type and mutant *Mycobacterium tuberculosis* enoyl-ACP reductases. *J. Am. Chem. Soc.* 118:1561.

Rapaport, E., Levina, A., Metelev, V., and Zamecnik, P., 1996, Antimycobacterial activities of antisense oligodeoxynucleotide phosphorothioates in drug-resistant strains. *Proc. Natl. Acad. Sci. USA* 93:709.

Rastogi, N., Goh, K.S., and David, H.L., 1990, Enhancement of drug susceptibility of *Mycobacterium avium* by inhibitors of cell envelope synthesis. *Antimicrob. Agents Chemother.* 34:759.

Ratledge, C., and Brown, K.A., 1972, Inhibition of mycobactin formation in *Mycobacterium smegmatis* by *p*-aminosalicylate. A new proposal for the mode of action of *p*-aminosalicylate. *Am. Rev. Resp. Dis.* 106:774.

Revel, V., Cambau, E., Jarlier, V., and Sougakoff, W., 1994, Characterization of mutations in *Mycobacterium smegmatis* involved in resistance to fluoroquinolones. *Antimicrob. Agents Chemother.* 38:1991.

Ristow, M., Möhlig, M., Rifai, M., Schatz, H., Feldmann, K., and Pfeiffer, A., 1995, New isoniazid/ethionamide resistance gene mutation and screening for multidrug-resistant *Mycobacterium tuberculosis* strains. *Lancet* 346:502.

Rozwarski, D.A., Grant, G.A., Barton, D.H.R., Jacobs, W.R. and Sacchettini, J.C., 1998, Modification of the NADH of the isoniazid target (InhA) from *Mycobacterium tuberculosis*. *Science* 279:98.

Sareen, M., and Khuller, G.K., 1990 Cell wall and membrane changes associated with ethambutol resistance in *Mycobacterium tuberculosis* H$_{37}$Ra. *Antimicrob. Agents Chemother.* 34:1773.

Schatz, A., and Waksman, S.A., 1944, Effect of streptomycin and other antibiotic substances upon *Mycobacterium tuberculosis* and related organisms. *Proc. Soc. Exp. Biol. Med.* 57:244.

Scorpio, A., Collins, D.M., Whipple, D., Cave, D., Bates, J., and Zhang, Y., 1997, Rapid differentiation of bovine and human tubercle bacilli based on a characteristic mutation in the bovine pyrazinamidase gene. *J. Clin. Microbiol.* 35:106.

Scorpio, A., Lindholm-Levy, P., Heifets, L., Gilman, R., Siddiqi, S., Cynamon, M., and Zhang, Y., 1997a, Characterization of *pncA* mutations in pyrazinamide-resistant *Mycobacterium tuberculosis*. *Antimicrob. Agents Chemother.* 41:540.

Scorpio, A., and Zhang, Y., 1996, Mutation in *pncA*, a gene encoding pyrazinamidase/nicotinamidase, cause resistance to the antituberculous drug pyrazinamide in tubercle bacilli. *Nature Med.* 2:662.

Sherman, D.R., Mdluli, K., Hickey, M.J., Arain, T.M., Morris, S.L., Barry, C.E., and Stover, C.K., 1996, Compensatory *ahpC* gene expression in isoniazid-resistant *Mycobacterium tuberculosis*. *Science* 272:1641.

Shinnick, T.M., King, C.H., and Quinn, F.D., 1995, Molecular biology, virulence, and pathogenicity of Mycobacteria. *Am. J. Med. Sci.* 309:92.

Shoeb, H.A., Bowman, B.U., Ottolenghi, A.C., and Merola, A.J., 1985, Peroxidase-mediated oxidation of isoniazid. *Antimicrob. Agents Chemother.* 27:399.

Sifuentes-Osornio, J., Ponce-de-Leon, L.A., Camacho-Mezquita, F.E., Bobadilla-del-Valle, J.M., Infante-Suarez. M.L., Ramirez-Fernandez, N., Hernandez-Gomez, L., and Nelson, A.M., 1995, Resistance of *Mycobacterium tuberculosis* in mexican patients. *Revista de Investigacion Clinica.* 47:273.

Silver, L., and Bostian, K., 1990, Screening of natural products for antimicrobial agents. *Eur. J. Clin. Microbiol. Infect. Dis.* 9:455.

Snapper, S.B., Melton, R.E., Mustafa, S., Kieser, T., Jacobs, W.R.Jr., 1990, Isolation and characterization of efficient plasmid transformation mutants of *Mycobacterium smegmatis*. *Mol. Microbiol.* 4:1911.

Soussy, C.J., Wolfson, J.S., Ng, E.Y., and Hooper, D.C., 1993, Limitations of plasmid complementation test for determination of quinolone resistance due to changes in the gyrase A protein and identification of conditional quinolone resistance locus. *Antimicrob. Agents Chemother.* 37:2588.

Sreevatsan, S., Pan, X., Stockbauer, K.E., Williams, D.L., Kreiswirth, B.N., and Musser, J.M., 1996, Characterization of *rpsL* and *rrs* mutations in streptomycin-resistant *Mycobacterium tuberculosis* isolates from diverse geographic localities. *Antimicrob. Agents Chemother.* 40:1024.

Springer, A.L., and Schmid, M.B., 1993, Molecular characterization of the *Salmonella typhimurium parE* gene. *Nucl. Acids Res.* 21:1805.

Sreevatsan, S., Pan, X., Zhang, Y., Deretic, V., and Musser, J.M., 1997, Analysis of the *oxyR-ahpC* region in isoniazid-resistant and -susceptible *Mycobacterium tuberculosis* complex organisms recovered from diseased humans and animals in diverse localities. *Antimicrob. Agents Chemother.* 41:600.

Sreevatsan, S., Stockbauer, K.E., Pan, X., Kreiswirth, B.N., Moghazeh, S.L., Jacobs, W.R.Jr., Telenti, A., and Musser, J.M., 1997a, Ethambutol resistance in *Mycobacterium tuberculosis*: critical role of *embB* mutations. *Antimicrob. Agents Chemother.* 41:1677.

Sreevatsan, S., Pan, X., Zhang, Y., Kreiswirth, B.N., and Musser, J.M. (1997b) Mutations associated with pyrazinamide resistance in *pncA* of *Mycobacterium tuberculosis* complex organisms. *Antimicrob. Agents Chemother.* 41:636.

Stratton, C., 1992, Fluoroquinolone antibiotics: properties of the class and individual agents. *Clin. Ther.* 14:348.

Stratton, M.A. and Reed, M.T., 1986, Short-course drug therapy for tuberculosis. *Clin. Pharm.* 5:977.

Sullivan, E.A., Kreiswirth, B.N., Palumbo, L., Kapur, V., Musser, J.M., Ebrahimzadeh, A., and Frieden, T.R., 1995, *Lancet* 345:1148.

Sutton, W.B., Gordee, R.S., Wick, W.E., and Stanfield, L., 1966, *In vitro* and *in vivo* laboratory studies of the antituberculous activity of capreomycin. *Ann. N. Y. Acad. Sci.* 135:947.

Takayama, K., Armstrong, E.L., Kunugi, K.A., and Kilburn, J.O., 1979, Inhibition by ethambutol of mycolic acid transfer into the cell wall of *Mycobacterium smegmatis*. *Antimicrob. Agents Chemother.* 16:240.

Takiff, H.E., Salazar, L., Guerrero, C., Philipp, W., Huang, W.M., Kreiswirth, B., Cole, S.T., Jacobs, W.R., and Telenti, A., 1994, Cloning and nucleotide sequence of *Mycobacterium tuberculosis gyrA* and *gyrB* genes and detection of quinolone resistance mutations. *Antimicrob. Agents Chemother.* 38:773.

Takiff, H.E., Cimino, M., Musso, M.C., Weisbrod, T., Martinez, R., Delgado, M.B., Salazar, L., Bloom, B.R., and Jacobs, W.R.Jr., 1996, Efflux pump of the proton antiporter family confers low-level fluoroquinolone resistance in *Mycobacterium smegmatis*. *Proc. Natl. Acad. Sci. USA* 93:362.

Taniguchi, H., Aramaki, H., Nikaido, Y., Mizuguchi, Y., Nakamura, M., Koga, T., and Yoshida, S., 1996, Rifampicin resistance and mutation of the *rpoB* gene in *Mycobacterium tuberculosis*. *FEMS Microbiol. Lett.* 144:103.

Telenti, A., Imboden, P., Marchesi, F., Lowrie, D., Cole, S., Colston, M.J., Matter, L., Schopfer, K., and Bodmer, T., 1993, Detection of rifampicin-resistance mutations in *Mycobacterium tuberculosis*. *Lancet* 341:647.

Telenti, A., Philipp, W.J., Sreevatsan, S., Bernasconi, C., Stockbauer, K.E., Wieles, B., Musser, J.M., and Jacobs, W.R., 1997, The *emb* operon, a gene cluster of *Mycobacterium tuberculosis* involved in resistance to ethambutol. *Nature Med.* 3:567.

Thomas, J.P., Baughn, C.O., Wilkinson, R.G., and Shepherd, R.G., 1961, A new synthetic compound with antituberculous activity in mice: ethambutol (dextro-2,2'-(ethylenediimino)-di-1-butanol). *Am. Rev. Respir. Dis.* 83:891.

Truffot-Pernot, C., Ji, B., and Grosset, J., 1991, Activities of pefloxacin and ofloxacin against mycobacteria: *in vitro* and mouse experiments. *Tubercle* 72:57.

Verbist, L., and Gyselen, A., 1964, Capreomycin susceptibility of strains resistant to streptomycin and/or viomycin. *Am. Rev. Resp. Dis.* 90:640.

Wallace, R.J., Hull, S.I., Bobey, D.G., Price, K.E., Swenson, J.M., Steele, L.C., and Christensen, L., 1985, Mutational resistance as the mechanism of acquired drug resistance to aminoglycosides and antibacterial agents in *Mycobacterium fortuitum* and *Mycobacterium chelonei*. *Am. Rev. Respir. Dis.* 132:409.

Wang, J.C., 1985, DNA topoisomerases. *Ann. Rev. Biochem.* 54:665.

Wank, H., Rogers, J., Davies, J., and Schroeder, R., 1994, Peptide antibiotics of the tuberactinomycin family as inhibitors of group I intron RNA splicing. *J. Mol. Biol.* 236:1001.

Wayne, L.G., and Sramek, H.A., 1994, Metronidazole is bactericidal to dormant cells of *Mycobacterium tuberculosis*. *Antimicrob. Agents Chemother.* 38:2054.

Weis, S.E., Slocum, P.C., Blais, F.X., King, B., Nunn, M., Matney, G.B., Gomez, E., and Foresman, B.H., 1994, The effect of directly observed therapy on the rates of drug resistance and relapse in tuberculosis. *N. Engl. J. Med.* 330:1179.

Weiss, C., 1956, Some new antibiotics: penicillin V, cycloserine and candicidin. *J. Albert Einstein Med. Cent.* 4:66.

Weltman, A.C., and Rose, D.N., 1994, Tuberculosis susceptibility patterns: predictors of multidrug resistance, and implications for initial therapeutic regimens at a New York City hospital. *Arch. Intern. Med.* 154:2161.

Williams, D.L., Waguespack, C., Eisenach, K., Crawford, J.T., Portaels, F., Salfinger, M., Nolan, C.M., Abe, C., Sticht-Groh, V., and Gillis, T.P., 1994, Characterization of rifampin resistance in pathogenic Mycobacteria. *Antimicrob. Agents Chemother.* 38:2380.

Wilson, T.M., and Collins, D.M., 1996, *ahpC*, a gene involved in isoniazid resistance of the *Mycobacterium tuberculosis* complex. *Mol. Microbiol.* 19:1025.

Winder, F.G., 1960, Catalase and peroxidase in mycobacteria. *Am. Rev. Respir. Dis.* 81:68.

Winder, F.G., 1982, Mode of action of the antimycobacterial agents and associated aspects of the molecular biology of the mycobacteria, in: *The Biology of the Mycobacteria*, C. Ratledge, and J. Stanford, eds., Academic Press, New York.

Wise, R., Brenwald, N.P., Andrews, J.M., and Boswell, C.G., 1997, The activity of the methylpiperazinyl fluoroquinolone CG 5501: a comparison with other fluoroquinolones. *J. Antimicrob. Chemother.* 39:447.

Woese, C.R., and Gutell, R.R., 1989, Evidence for several higher order structural elements in ribosomal RNA. *Proc. Natl. Acad. Sci. USA* 86:3119.

Wolucka, B.A., McNeil, M.R., de Hoffmann, E., Chojnacki, T., Brennan, P.J., 1994, Recognition of the lipid intermediate for arabinogalactan/arabinomannan biosynthesis and its relation to the mode of action of ethambutol on Mycobacteria. *J. Biol. Chem.* 269:23328.

Woodley, C.L., Kilburn, J.O., David, H.L., and Silcox, V.A., 1972, Susceptibility of Mycobacteria to rifampin. *Antimicrob. Agents Chemother.* 2:245.

Xu, C., Kreiswirth, B. N., Sreevatsan, S., Musser, J.M., and Drlica, K., 1996, Fluoroquinolone resistance associated with specific gyrase mutations in clinical isolates of multidrug-resistant *Mycobacterium tuberculosis*. *J. Infect. Dis.* 174:1127.

Yamamoto, S., Toida, I., Watanabe, N., and Ura, T., 1995, *In vitro* antimycobacterial activities of pyrazinamide analogs. *Antimicrob. Agents Chemother.* 39:2088.

Young, D. B., Marshall, B., and Smet K.D., 1996, The return of the resistant microbes, in: *The Diagnostic Challenge*, E. P. Fischer and S. Klose, eds., Boehringer Mannheim GmbH, Mannheim.

Yuan, Y., and Barry,C.E., 1996, A common mechanism for the biosynthesis of methoxy and cyclopropyl mycolic acids in *Mycobacterium tuberculosis*. *Proc. Natl. Acad. Sci. USA* 93:12828.

Yuan, Y., Lee, R.E., Besra, G.S., Belisle, J.T., and Barry,C.E., 1995, Identification of a gene involved in the biosynthesis of cyclopropanated mycolic acids in *Mycobacterium tuberculosis*. *Proc. Natl. Acad. Sci. USA* 92:6630.

Zabinski, R.F., and Blanchard, J.S., 1997, The requirement for manganese and oxygen in the isoniazid-dependent inactivation of *Mycobacterium tuberculosis* enoyl reductase. *J. Am. Chem. Soc.* 119:2331.

Zhang, Y., Garbe, T., Young, D., 1993, Transformation with *katG* restores isoniazid-sensitivity in *Mycobacterium tuberculosis* isolates resistant to a range of drug concentrations. *Mol. Microbiol.* 8:521.

Zhang, Y., Heym, B., Allen, Bryan, Young, D., and Cole, S., 1992, The catalase-peroxidase gene and isoniazid resistance of *Mycobacterium tuberculosis*. *Nature* 358:591.

Zhang, Y., Steingrube, V.A., and Wallace, R.J.Jr., 1992, Beta-lactamase inhibitors and the inducibility of the beta-lactamase of *Mycobacterium tuberculosis*. *Am. Rev. Respir. Dis.* 145:657.

8

STRUCTURE AND FUNCTION OF MULTIDRUG TRANSPORTERS

Hendrik W. van Veen[*] and Wil N. Konings

Department of Microbiology
Groningen Biomolecular Sciences and Biotechnology Institute
University of Groningen
Kerklaan 30, NL-9751 NN Haren, The Netherlands

INTRODUCTION

Toxic compounds have always been part of the natural environment in which microorganisms dwell. The development of strategies for life in this habitat has been crucial for survival of the cell. As a result, microorganisms have developed versatile mechanisms to resist antibiotics and other cytotoxic drugs. Examples are the enzymatic degradation or inactivation of drugs (Davies, 1994), and the alteration of drug targets (Spratt, 1994). In addition, microorganisms possess membrane proteins which catalyze transmembrane drug transport, and hence, are able to overcome cell cytotoxicity by lowering the cytoplasmic drug concentration (Lewis, 1994; Balzi and Goffeau, 1994; Borst and Ouellette, 1995). Some of these drug transporters are fairly specific for a given drug or class of drugs, but the so-called multidrug transporters have specificity for compounds with very different chemical structures and cellular targets. Microbial multidrug transporters can be amplified in drug resistant pathogenic microorganisms, and can shift their drug profiles, making them a menace to drug treatment. Multidrug transporters are also found in mammals, in which they are a cause of multidrug resistance of tumor cells. The structure and function of multidrug transporters is conserved from bacteria to man. On the basis of bioenergetic and structural criteria, multidrug transport systems can be divided into two major classes. Secondary transporters mediate the extrusion of drugs from the cell in a coupled exchange with ions (Paulsen et al., 1996a). ATP-binding cassette [ABC] transporters utilize the release of phosphate bond-energy by ATP hydrolysis, to pump drugs out of the cell (Higgins, 1992). This chapter represents a comprehensive review in which we will summarize the

---

[*] E-mail: h.w.van.veen@biol.rug.nl

Resolving the Antibiotic Paradox, edited by Rosen and Mobashery.
Kluwer Academic / Plenum Publishers, New York, 1998.

current state of knowledge on three major aspects of drug efflux-based multidrug resistance in pro- and eukaryotic cells: [i] the functional and structural similarities among secondary and ABC-type multidrug transporters, [ii] the molecular mechanism of these transporters, and [iii] their potential physiological role.

SECONDARY MULTIDRUG TRANSPORTERS

The number of secondary multidrug transporters discovered in pro- and eukaryotic cells is vast and rapidly expanding. Secondary multidrug transporters have been detected in pathogenic yeasts such as *Candida albicans* [caMDR1p] (Ben-Yaacov *et al.*, 1994), and pathogenic bacteria such as methicillin-resistant *Staphylococcus aureus* [QacC] (Littlejohn *et al.*, 1992), *Mycobacterium smegmatis* [LfrA] (Liu *et al.*, 1997), and *Neisseria gonorrhoeae* [MtrD] (Hagman *et al.*, 1995). Secondary multidrug transporters have also been detected in mammals, such as in rat kidney cells [OCT1] (Gründemann *et al.*, 1995).

Computer-based sequence analyses have revealed that secondary drug transporters belong to one of three distinct families of transport proteins: the Major Facilitator Superfamily [MFS] (Marger and Saier, 1993), the Resistance-Nodulation-Cell Division [RND] family (Saier *et al.*, 1994), and the Small Multidrug Resistance (SMR) family (Paulsen *et al.*, 1996b) (Table 1). Bacterial examples of each type of secondary drug transporter, *Lactococcus lactis* LmrP [MFS family] (Bolhuis *et al.*, 1995), *S. aureus* QacC [SMR family] (Littlejohn *et al.*, 1992), and *Pseudomonas aeruginosa* MexB [RND family] (Poole *et al.*, 1993), are presented schematically in Figure 1. LmrP and QacC have specificity for an exceptionally wide range of amphiphilic, cationic drugs including antibiotics, quaternary ammonium compounds, aromatic dyes, and phosphonium ions. MexB confers resistance to amphiphilic anionic compounds such as antibiotics, basic dyes and detergents. In Gram-negative bacteria, transport of drugs from the interior of the cell to the external medium requires the translocation of solutes across the cytoplasmic and outer membrane. Therefore, some drug transporters [*e.g.*, MexB] in such organisms are found in association with an accessory protein which spans the periplasmic space and interacts with a porin in the

Table 1. Examples of secondary multidrug transporters

Transporter family	Protein	Organism	Accession no.[1]
MFS family[2]	caMDR1p	*Candida albicans*	SW P28873
	LmrP	*Lactococcus lactis*	GB X89779
	Bmr	*Bacillus subtilis*	SW P33449
	NorA	*Staphylococcus aureus*	SW P21191
	QacA	*Staphylococcus aureus*	EM X56628
	EmrB	*Escherichia coli*	SW P27304
RND family[3]	AcrB	*Escherichia coli*	EM U00734
	MexB	*Pseudomonas aeruginosa*	GB L11616
	MtrD	*Neisseria gonorrhoeae*	SW P43505
SMR family[4]	QacC	*Staphylococcus aureus*	SW P14319
	QacE	*Klebsiella aerogenes*	PR S25583
	EmrE	*Escherichia coli*	SW P23895

[1] Accession number: GB, Genbank; SW, SwissProt; EM, EMBL; PR, PIR.
[2] Major Facilitator Superfamily (Marger and Saier, 1993).
[3] Resistance-Nodulation-Cell Division family (Saier *et al.*, 1994).
[4] Small Multidrug Resistance family (Paulsen *et al.*, 1996b).

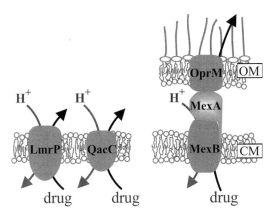

Figure 1. Schematic presentation of representative secondary multidrug transporters in prokaryotes. LmrP in *Lactococcus lactis* [Major Facilitator Superfamily], QacC in *Staphylococcus aureus* [Small Multidrug Resistance family] and MexB in *Pseudomonas aeruginosa* [Resistance-Nodulation-Cell Division family] are driven by the proton motive force which is present across the cytoplasmic membrane [CM]. MexB is associated with the accessory protein MexA [Membrane Fusion Protein family] and the outer membrane porin OprM. These additional proteins enable the MexB-mediated transport of drugs across the outer membrane [OM] in the Gram-negative bacterium.

outer membrane. These auxiliary proteins belong to the Membrane Fusion Protein family (Saier *et al.*, 1994) and Outer Membrane Factor family (Dinh *et al.*, 1994).

Energetics of Drug Transport

Bacterial secondary transporters are located in the cytoplasmic membrane, across which usually a proton motive force [interior negative and alkaline] exists. Based on [i] the structural similarity between secondary drug transport proteins and known proton motive force-dependent transport systems, and [ii] the sensitivity of drug transport to agents that dissipate the proton motive force, it is assumed that secondary drug transporters function as drug/proton antiporters. The direct involvement of the proton motive force as driving force was demonstrated for the *E. coli* tetracycline transporter TetA(B) [MFS family], which mediates an electroneutral exchange reaction of a metal^{2+}-tetracycline^{1-} complex and one proton (Yamaguchi *et al.*, 1991), and *L. lactis* LmrP [MFS family] (Bolhuis *et al.*, 1996a) and *E. coli* EmrE [SMR family] (Yerushalmi *et al.*, 1995) which both mediate an electrogenic drug/nH^{+} antiport reaction [n 2].

Structure-Function Relationships

Analysis of the topography of secondary drug transporters suggest the presence of either 12 or 14 membrane-spanning segments in members of the MFS family, and 12 membrane-spanning segments in members of the RND family. The transmembrane segments are most likely in α-helical configuration, and are connected by hydrophilic loops protruding into the cytoplasm or periplasmic space. The structure of TetA(B) has been studied most extensively, by limited proteolysis (Eckert and Beck, 1989), site-directed antibody binding (Yamaguchi *et al.*, 1990), PhoA-fusion analysis (Allard and Bertrand, 1992), and site-directed chemical labeling (Kimura *et al.*, 1997). A relatively large cytoplasmic loop in the middle of the protein separates TetA(B) in an N- and C-terminal half, each containing 6 transmembrane segments. Both halves are evolutionary related, presumably by a gene duplication event, and are well conserved among TetA proteins of various classes (Rubin et al., 1990). The N- and C-terminal halves of TetA(B) represent separate domains in the drug transporter (Curiale and Levy, 1982). The functional interaction between these domains is suggested by [i] the intragenic complementation between mutations in the first and second halves of the tetA(B) gene (McNicholas et al., 1995), [ii] the ability of hybrid tetracycline efflux transporters containing N- and C-terminal halves of different classes of tetracycline efflux proteins to confer resistance (Rubin and Levy, 1990) and [iii] the functional reconstitution of tetracycline resistance upon co-expression of the N- and C-terminal halves of TetA(B) as separate polypeptides (Rubin and Levy, 1991). Members of the SMR family contain 4 putative transmembrane α-helices. This topological model has recently been confirmed for QacC by genetic fusion using alkaline phosphatase and β-galactosidase as reporters of subcellular localization (Paulsen et al., 1995), and for E. coli EmrE by transmission fourier-transform infrared spectroscopy (Arkin et al., 1996). In view of the 12 transmembrane models proposed for members of the MFS and RND families, members of the SMR family may function as a homotrimer.

Multiple alignment of the amino acid sequences of the MFS family members reveals the presence of two conserved sequence motifs that are located at similar positions within the putative secondary structure of the proteins. Motif A [GXXXDRXGR(K/R)] is found in many members of the MFS family (Marger and Saier, 1993) and is present in the cytoplasmic loop between transmembrane segment 2 and 3. Motif A may be of structural importance by mediating opening and closing of the translocation pathway. Motif B [GXXXGXXGG], the drug extrusion consensus sequence, is found at the end of transmembrane segment 5, and is typical for LmrP and other drug export systems of the Major Facilitator superfamily (Griffith et al., 1992; Bolhuis et al., 1995). At present, the role of motif B in drug recognition or binding is unclear.

It has been suggested that amino residues within transmembrane segments of the human multidrug resistance P-glycoprotein MDR1 (Pgp) play a role in drug specificity (Gottesman et al., 1995). Observations on secondary drug transporters are consistent with this notion. The MFS members QacA and QacB in S. aureus are homologous proteins [98% identical amino acid residues]. QacB confers resistance to monovalent organic cations but differs from QacA by conferring no resistance to the divalent organic cations pentamidine isethionate and propamidine isethionate. This phenotypic difference between QacA and QacB is solely due to the presence of the acidic Asp[323] within the putative transmembrane segment 10 of the QacA protein, but of the neutral Ala[323] in QacB (Paulsen et al., 1996c). The ability of the MFS member Bmr in Bacillus subtilis to interact with reserpine and other drugs is strongly affected by substitutions of Val[286] (Ahmed et al., 1993), and of Phe[143] or Phe[306] (Klyachko et al., 1997), which are located within transmembrane segments. Thus, both charged and aromatic residues located within the phospholipid bilayer appear to interact with drugs and may be involved in drug recognition or binding. Interestingly, it has been shown that quaternary ammonium compounds and other cations can bind to the face of the aromatic ring structures of tyrosine, phenylalanine or tryptophan residues in the hydrophobic environment of the membrane (Dougherty, 1996).

ABC-TYPE MULTIDRUG TRANSPORTERS

Transport proteins belonging to the ABC transporter superfamily are involved in the tolerance to a wide diversity of cytotoxic agents in both prokaryotes and eukaryotes (Higgins, 1992). Included in this superfamily are the Pgp (Gottesman and Pastan, 1993) and human multidrug resistance-associated protein MRP1 [MRP] (Cole *et al.*, 1992) plasma membrane transporters, which catalyse the extrusion of anti-tumor drugs during the chemotherapy of cancer cells. Based on [i] the alignment analysis of amino acid residues that comprise the nucleotide binding domain[s] of ABC proteins, [ii] protein topology, and [iii] transport mechanism, the ABC transporter superfamily can be divided into two major clusters: the Pgp cluster and MRP cluster.

Pgp Cluster

Members of the Pgp cluster play an important role in microbial resistance to neutral or positively charged, amphiphilic drugs (Table 2). These transporters function in human pathogens such as the malaria parasite *Plasmodium faliciparum* [pfMDR1] (Wilson *et al.*, 1989), the *Entamoeba histolytica* [ehPgp] protozoan responsible for human amoebiasis (Descoteaux *et al.*, 1992), or the *Leishmania donovani* [ldMDR1] protozoan responsible for visceral leishmaniasis (Henderson *et al.*, 1992). In addition, infections in immunodeficiency patients are often related to Cdr1p, an ABC transporter which confers antifungal resistance in the pathogenic yeast *Candida albicans* (Prasad *et al.*, 1995). ABC proteins in the non-pathogenic *Saccharomyces cerevisiae* include the multidrug transporters Pdr5p (Balzi *et al.*, 1994) and Snq2p (Decottignies *et al.*, 1995). Pgp cluster members have also been identified in bacteria. In *Streptomyces* strains, dedicated transporters such as DrrAB (Guilfoile and Hutchinson, 1991) mediate the excretion of specific antibiotics to ensure self-resistance to the antibiotics that they produce. A true prokaryotic multidrug transporter with significant sequence identity to Pgp in both the ABC and membrane domains has been found in *L. lactis* [LmrA] (van Veen *et al.*, 1996) (Fig. 2).

Like Pgp, some ABC transporters in microorganisms are expressed as single multifunctional polypeptides containing two homologous halves, each with an ABC domain and a membrane domain. The membrane domain is usually composed of 6 putative α-helical transmembrane segments. Other ABC proteins, such as lactococcal LmrA and *Escherichia coli* α-hemolysine transporter HlyB (Felmlee *et al.*, 1985), have half the size of Pgp with only a single transmembrane domain and ABC domain (Fig. 2). The notion that two of these half-molecules must cooperate to the formation of a single transporter is, amongst others, supported by the observation that the independent expression of each half

Table 2. Examples of ABC[1]-type multidrug transporters

	Protein	Organism	Accession no.[2]
Pgp cluster	pfMDR1	*Plasmodium falciparum*	GB A32547
	ehPgp	*Entamoeba histolytica*	GB M88599
	ldMDR1	*Leishmania donovani*	GB L01572
	Cdr1p	*Candida albicans*	GB X77589
	Pdr5p	*Saccharomyces cerevisiae*	GB L19922
	Snq2p	*Saccharomyces cerevisiae*	GB Z48008
	LmrA	*Lactococcus lactis*	GB U63741
MRP cluster	Ycf1p	*Saccharomyces cerevisiae*	GB Z48179
	Yor1p	*Saccharomyces cerevisiae*	GB Z73066
	ltPgpA	*Leishmania tarentolae*	GB A34207
	ceMRP1	*Caenorhabditis elegans*	EM 466260

[1]ATP-binding cassette superfamily (Higgins, 1992).
[2]Accession number: GB, Genbank; EM, EMBL.

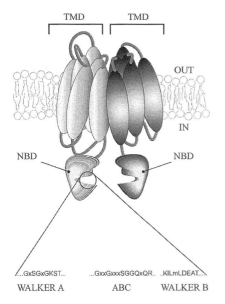

Figure 2. Secondary structure model of a homodimer of the ABC-type multidrug transporter LmrA of *Lactococcus lactis*. LmrA is predicted to contain a transmembrane domain (TMD) with 6 transmembrane α-helices (depicted as ellipses), and a nucleotide-binding domain (NBD) with the ABC signature and Walker A/B sequences. The most conserved residues in these sequence motifs are indicated. The structure of LmrA is very similar to that of the mammalian multidrug resistance P-glycoprotein (Pgp). Pgp contains two covalently linked homologous halves, each with 6 transmembrane segments and an ATP-binding domain. In view of the twelve-transmembrane model proposed for Pgp, LmrA may function as a homodimeric complex. OUT and IN refer to the outside and inside of the cytoplasmic membrane, respectively.

of the *a*-mating pheromone transporter Ste6p in yeast cells does not yield a functional transporter, while simultaneous expression of both halves does (Berkower amd Michaelis, 1991). In drug transporters such as DrrAB, the two membrane domains are fused into a single polypeptide which is associated with a second polypeptide containing the two ABC domains.

Interestingly, the sequence conservation between LmrA and Pgp includes particular regions [*e.g.*, the first cytoplasmic loop and the region comprising transmembrane segments V and VI] that have been implicated as determinants of drug recognition and binding by Pgp. LmrA also shares significant sequence identity with the hop-resistance protein HorA in *Lactobacillus brevis* (Sami *et al.*, 1997) and ABC proteins in *Bacillus subtilis*, *Staphylococcus aureus*, *Escherichia coli*, *Helicobacter pylori*, *Haemophilus influenzae*, and *Mycoplasma genitalium* (Fig. 3).

MRP Cluster

Members of the MRP cluster contain an N-terminal membrane-bound domain consisting of 4 putative α-helical transmembrane segments, which is followed by two homologous halves each with 6 putative α-helical transmembrane segments and an ABC domain (Deeley and Cole, 1997). Like MRP, MRP homologs in microorganisms mediate the extrusion of a wide variety of organic anions, such as carboxyfluorescein derivatives, taurocholate, bis(glutathionate)- cadmium and other glutathione S-conjugates. The best characterized members of this cluster include: (i) the yeast cadmium factor [Ycf1] (Li *et al.*, 1996; 1997) and Yor1 protein (Cui *et al.*, 1996) in *S. cerevisiae*, (ii) transporters associated with heavy metal resistance in *Leishmania* species [lmPgpA] (Callahan and Beverley, 1991; Grondin *et al.*, 1997) and the nematode *Caenorhabditis elegans* [ceMRP1] (Broeks *et al.*, 1996), and (iii) the bile acid transporter Bat1p in *S. cerevisiae* (Ortiz *et al.*, 1997) (Table 2). The BCECF (2',7'-bis-(2-carboxyethyl)-5(and 6)-carboxyfluorescein) transporter in *L. lactis* may be the first prokaryotic example of this cluster (Molenaar *et al.*, 1992).

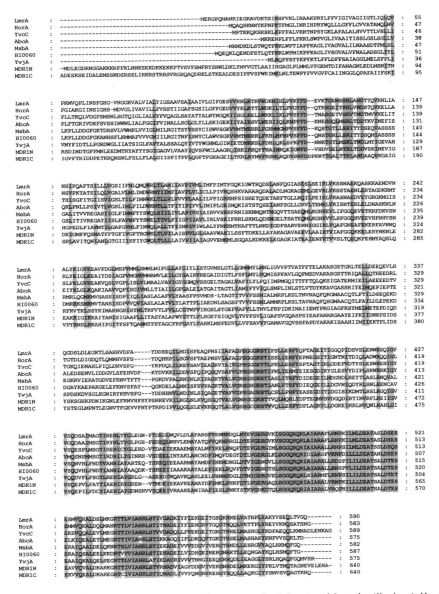

Figure 3. Comparison of the amino acid sequence of *Lactococcus lactis* LmrA and *Lactobacillus brevis* HorA, *Bacillus subtilis* YvcC and YwjA, *Staphylococcus aureus* AbcA, *Escherichia coli* MsbA, *Haemophilus influenzae* HI0060 and the N- and C-terminal half of the human multidrug resistance P-glycoprotein (Pgp). MDR1-N and MDR1-C represent amino acid residues 1 to 640 and 641 to 1280 of Pgp, respectively. The last residue in each row is numbered. A dark background indicates conserved residues in 7 or more individual proteins. (-) Gaps introduced to optimize the alignment.

Structure-Function Relationships

The effects of amino acid substitutions on the substrate specificity of ABC-type multidrug transporters has been studied most extensively using Pgp. In general, Pgp mutants can be classified into three groups. The first group is of mutations Gly141-to-Val, Gly185-to-Val, and Gly187-to-Val, and others, all in the first cytoplasmic loop (Choi *et al.*, 1988;

Kioka *et al.*, 1989; Kwan and Gros, 1998); Gly228-to-Val in the second cytoplasmic loop (Loo and Clarke, 1994a); Gly812-to-Val and Gly830-to-Val in transmembrane segment 4 (Loo and Clarke, 1994a); Phe335-to-Ala and Val338-to-Ala in transmembrane segment 6 (Loo and Clarke, 1993a; 1994b). These mutations increase the ability of Pgp to confer resistance to colchicine and doxorubicin, and decrease the ability of Pgp to confer resistance to vinblastine. The second group consists of mutations Pro223-to-Ala in transmembrane segment 4 (Loo and Clarke, 1993b); Gly341-to-Val in transmembrane segment 6 (Loo and Clarke, 1994b); Pro866-to-Ala in transmembrane segment 10 (Loo and Clarke, 1993b); Phe978-to-Ala in transmembrane segment 12 (Loo and Clarke, 1993a); Ser939-to-Phe, Tyr949-to-Ala, and Phe953-to-Ala in transmembrane segment 11 of mouse mdr1 (Hanna *et al.*, 1996; Kajiji *et al.*. 1993); and Ser941-to-Phe in transmembrane segment 11 of mouse mdr3 (Gros *et al.*, 1991). These mutations decrease the ability of Pgp to confer resistance to colchicine and doxorubicin, and increase or do not affect the ability of Pgp to confer resistance to vinblastine. Interestingly, Pgp mutants with amino acid substitutions at position 61 in transmembrane segment 1 fall into the first or the second group of mutants, depending on the size of the side chain (Taguchi *et al.*, 1997). Hence, this transmembrane segment is also important in substrate specificity. The third group of mutations that affect substrate specificity of Pgp fall in the ATP-binding domains: Lys536-to-Arg in the ABC signature sequence, and mutations at positions 522–525 and 578 near the Walker B region of the N-terminal ATP-binding domain (Hoof *et al.*, 1994; Beaudet and Gros, 1995). In summary, amino acid substitutions which affect the substrate specificity of Pgp are found scattered throughout the molecule in transmembrane domains, cytoplasmic loops and ATP binding domains.

A limited set of chimeric Pgp proteins has been constructed using mammalian P-glycoproteins, such as human MDR2, as partner protein to identify proteins segments and amino acids in Pgp implicated in drug recognition (Currier *et al.*, 1992; Dhir and Gros, 1992; Zhang *et al.*, 1995a). Human MDR2 (often called MDR3), a phosphatidylcholine-specific translocase in the bile canicular membrane of hepatocytes, shares about 77% identity with Pgp. However, overexpression of human MDR2 or mouse mdr2 in drug-sensitive cells does not confer MDR (Smit *et al.*, 1993; Smith *et al.*, 1994). Greenberger and coworkers have replaced regions with the greatest sequence diversity between Pgp and MDR2, from transmembrane segment 10 to the C-terminus of Pgp, by the corresponding sequences from MDR2 (Zhang *et al.*, 1995a). Only a replacement limited to transmembrane segment 12 of both protein results in a functional hybrid Pgp, which was markedly impaired in conferring resistance to actinomycinD, vincristine, and doxorubicin, but not to colchicine. The drug resistance phenotype was associated with an impaired ability to photoaffinity label the hybrid protein with iodoaryl azidoprazosin. Thus, amino acids within transmembrane segment 12 may compose part of a drug binding pocket of Pgp and are in close proximity to a photoaffinity drug-labeling domain.

Taken together, a number of amino acid substitutions in Pgp have been found to affect the drug specificity of the protein, but particular domains in Pgp involved in drug recognition, binding and translocation have not yet been identified.

Functional Complementation

The structural similarity between ABC-type drug transporters can result in functional similarity as the mouse Pgp-homolog mdr3 (Raymond *et al.*, 1992) and *Plasmodium* pfMdr1 (Volkman *et al.*, 1995) can complement yeast Ste6p, thus restoring mating in a *ste6* sterile yeast strain. Likewise, MRP can functionally complement the Ycf1 protein in a *ycf1* cadmium-sensitive strain of *S. cerevisiae* (Tommasini *et al.*, 1996), and partially complement Ste6p in the sterile *ste6* null mutant of this organism (Ruetz *et al.*, 1996). The functional substitution of one ABC-type drug transporter by another is not only confined to eukaryotic transport proteins. Bacterial LmrA was able to functionally complement human Pgp in human lung fibroblast cells (van Veen *et al.*, 1998). Surprisingly, LmrA was targetted to the plasma membrane. The pharmacological characteristics of LmrA and Pgp-expressing lung fibroblasts were very similar, and the affinities of both proteins for vinblastine and magnesium-ATP indistinguishable. Blockers of P-glycoprotein-mediated multidrug resistance also inhibited LmrA-dependent drug resistance. Kinetic analysis of drug dissociation from LmrA expressed in plasma membranes of insect cells, revealed the presence of two allosterically-linked drug binding sites indistinguishable from those of P-glycoprotein (van Veen *et al.*, 1998; Martin *et al.*, 1997).The remarkable conservation of function between ABC-type drug transporters suggests a fundamental molecular mechanism of these proteins in pro- and eukaryotic cells.

MOLECULAR MECHANISM

Several transport models have been postulated for Pgp and LmrA pump function to explain the broad specificity for chemically unrelated compounds. Drug translocation may involve substrate transport from the cytoplasm to the exterior (conventional transport hypothesis, Altenberg *et al.*, 1994) which would require an enormous flexibility of an 'enzyme-like' substrate recognition site. Alternatively, the multidrug transporters could recognize the lipophilic drugs by their physical property to intercalate into the lipid bilayer, and transport drugs from the lipid bilayer to the exterior (vacuum cleaner hypothesis, Raviv *et al.*, 1990), or from the inner leaflet to the outer leaflet of the lipid bilayer (flippase hypothesis, Higgins and Gottesman, 1992). A property common to all known Pgp and LmrA substrates is their ability to intercalate between the phospholipids of biological membranes. This notion has led to the suggestion that these transporters recognize substrates within the membrane (Gottesman and Pastan, 1993; Bolhuis *et al.*, 1996a, b). Drug recognition within the membrane is supported by a number of observations: (i) photoaffinity analogs of Pgp-substrates label Pgp predominantly in or near the transmembrane helices 4–6, and 11–12 (Greenberger, 1993; Morris *et al.*, 1994; Germann, 1996), (ii) point mutations resulting in the alteration in drug specificity of Pgp are frequently found in transmembrane helices (Gottesman *et al.*, 1995), (iii) acetoxymethyl esters of several fluorescent probes accumulate less in Pgp or LmrA-expressing cells, despite the fact that the ester moieties are rapidly cleaved by intracellular esterases and the resulting carboxylates are not substrates for Pgp and LmrA (Homolya *et al.* 1993; Bolhuis *et al.*, 1996b), (iv) the kinetics of ATP-dependent transport of Hoechst 33342 by Pgp and of TMA-DPH by LmrA in membrane vesicles is consistent with transport of the compounds from the inner, but not from the outer leaflet of the lipid bilayer (Bolhuis *et al.*, 1996b; Shapiro and Ling, 1997a, b). Interestingly, these latter observations have also been made for the secondary lactococcal multidrug transporter LmrP (Bolhuis *et al.*, 1996a). Thus, a main determinant of specificity would be the ability of a substrate to be intercalated into the lipid bilayer.

This transport mechanism is likely to be a more general mechanism for ABC transporters with hydrophobic substrates. The human *MDR2* gene-encoded P-glycoprotein transports phosphatidylcholine from the cytoplasmic leaflet of the bile canicular membrane of hepatocytes into the bile (Smit *et al.*, 1993; Ruetz and Gros, 1994). In addition, the *E. coli* α-hemolysine transporter HlyB most likely binds the transport signal sequence of α-hemolysine, when the signal sequence forms an amphiphilic helix that binds to the cytoplasmic leaflet of the plasma membrane (Zhang *et al.*, 1995b; Sheps *et al.*, 1995).

PHYSIOLOGICAL ROLE

It has been proposed that Pgp participates in the protection of human cells against hydrophobic xenobiotics by active excretion of these compounds from the membrane into bile, urine, or the intestinal lumen, preventing their accumulation in critical organs such as the brain (Schinkel *et al.* 1994). Likewise, a defense function can be envisaged for multidrug transporters in microorganisms. These organisms encounter numerous hydrophobic compounds in their habitat which will accumulate in phospholipid bilayers (for review, see Sikkema *et al.*, 1995). It is noteworthy that the natural environment of enteric microorganisms is enriched in bile salts and fatty acids, and that these compounds are substrate for various multidrug transporters (Ma *et al.*, 1995; Thanassi *et al.*, 1997). In addition, some microbial multidrug transporters may play a role in the transport of an endogenous substrates, such as lipids (Smit *et al.*, 1993; Ruetz and Gros, 1994; van Helvoort *et al.*, 1996; Bosch *et al.*, 1997), pheromones (Alloing *et al.*, 1996; Perego, 1997), or lipid-linked precursors of peptidoglycan (for review, see Höltje, 1998) or other extracellular biopolymers, which remains to be established.

ACKNOWLEDGMENTS

We would like to thank Chris Higgins and collegues for stimulating discussions. Research in the authors laboratory was supported by the Biotechnology program of the Commission of the European Communities, and by the Dutch Cancer Society. H.W.V.V. is a fellow of the Royal Netherlands Academy of Arts and Sciences.

REFERENCES

Ahmed, M., Borsch, C.M., Neyfakh, A.A., and Schuldiner, S., 1993, Mutants of the *Bacillus subtilis* multidrug transporter Bmr with altered sensitivity to the antihypertensive alkaloid reserpine, *J. Biol. Chem.* 268:11086.

Allard, J.D., and Bertrand, K.P., 1992, Membrane topology of the pBR322 tetracycline resistance protein, *J. Biol. Chem.* 267:17809.

Alloing, G., Granadel, C., Morrison, D.A., and Claverys, J.-P., 1996, Competence pheromone, oligopeptide permease, and induction of competence in *Streptococcus pneumoniae, Mol. Microbiol.* 21:471.

Altenberg, G.A., Vanoye, C.G., Horton, J.K., and Reuss, L., 1994, Unidirectional fluxes of rhodamine 123 in multidrug resistant cells: Evidence against direct extrusion from the plasma membrane, *Proc. Natl. Acad. Sci. USA* 91:4654.

Arkin, I.T., Russ, W.P., Lebendiker, M., and Schuldiner, S., 1996, Determining the secondary structure and orientation of EmrE, a multidrug transporter, indicates a transmembrane four-helix bundle, *Biochemistry* 35:7233.

Balzi, E., and Goffeau, A., 1994, Genetics and biochemistry of yeast multidrug resistance, *Biochim. Biophys. Acta* 1187:152.

Balzi, E., Wang, M., Leterme, S., van Dijk, L., and Goffeau, A., 1994, Pdr5, a novel yeast multidrug resistance conferring transporter controlled by the transcription regulator Pdr1, *J. Biol. Chem.* 269:2206.

Beaudet, L., and Gros, P., 1995, Functional dissection of P-glycoprotein nucleotide-binding domains in chimeric and mutant proteins, *J. Biol. Chem.* 270:17159.

Ben-Yaacov, R., Knoller, S., Caldwell, G.A., Becker, J.M., and Klotin, Y., 1994, *Candida albicans* gene encoding resistance to benomyl and methotrexate is a multidrug resistance gene, *Antimicrob. Agents Chemother.* 38:648.

Berkower, C., and Michaelis, S., 1991, Mutational analysis of the yeast a-factor transporter STE6, a member of the ATP binding cassette (ABC) protein superfamily, *EMBO J.* 10:3777.

Bolhuis, H., Poelarends, G., van Veen, H.W., Poolman, B., Driessen, A.J.M., and Konings, W.N., 1995, Thelactococcal *lmrP* gene encodes a proton motive force-dependent drug transporter, *J. Biol. Chem.* 270:26092.

Bolhuis, H., van Veen, H.W., Brands, J.R., Putman, M., Poolman, B., Driessen, A.J.M., and Konings, W.N., 1996a, Energetics and mechanism of drug transport mediated by the lactococcal MDR transporter LmrP, *J. Biol. Chem.* 271:24123.

Bolhuis, H., van Veen, H.W., Molenaar, D., Poolman, B., Driessen, A.J.M., and Konings, W.N., 1996b, Multidrug resistance in *Lactococcus lactis*: evidence for ATP-dependent drug extrusion from the inner leaflet of the cytoplasmic membrane, *EMBO J.* 15:4239.

Borst, P., and Ouellette, M., 1995, New mechanisms of drug resistance in parasitic protozoa, *Annu. Rev.Microbiol.* 49:427.

Bosch, I., Dunussi-Joannopoulos, K., Wu, R.-L., Furlong, S.T., Croop, J., 1997, Phosphatidylcholine and phosphatidylethanolamine behave as substrates of the human MDR1 P-glycoprotein, *Biochemistry* 36:5685.

Broeks, A., Gerrard, B., Allikmets, R., Dean, M., and Plasterk, R.H.A., 1996, Homologues of the human multidrugresistance genes *MRP* and *MDR* contribute to heavy metal resistance in the soil nematode *Caenorhabditis elegans*, *EMBO J.* 15:6132.

Callahan, H.L., and Beverley, S.M., 1991, Heavy metal resistance: a new role of P-glycoproteins in *Leishmania*, *J. Biol. Chem.* 266:18427.

Choi, K., Chen, C., Kriegler, M., and Roninson, I.B., 1988, An altered pattern of cross-resistance in multidrug- resistant human cells results from spontaneaous mutations in the *mdr1* (P-glycoprotein) gene, *Cell* 53:519.

Cole, S.P.C., Bhardwaj, G., Gerlach, J.H., Mackie, J.E., Grant, C.E., Almquist, K.C., Stewart, A.J., Kurz, E.U., Duncan, A.M.V., and Deeley, R.G., 1992, Overexpression of a transporter gene in a multidrug-resistant human lung cancer cell line, *Science* 258:1650.

Cui, Z., Hirata, D., Tsuchiya, E., Osada, H., and Miyakawa, T., 1996, The multidrug resistance-associated protein (MRP) subfamily (Yrs1/Yor1) of *Saccharomyces cerevisiae* is important for the tolerance to a broad rang of organic anions, *J. Biol. Chem.* 271:14712.

Curiale, M., and Levy, S.B., 1982, Two complementation groups mediate tetracycline resistance determined by Tn10, *J. Bacteriol.* 151:209.

Currier, S.J., Kane, S.E., Willingham, M.C., Cardarelli, C.O., Pastan, I., and Gottesman, M.M., 1992, Identification of residues in the first cytoplasmic loop of P-glycoprotein involved in the function of chimeric human *MDR1-MDR2* transporters, *J. Biol. Chem.* 267:25153.

Davies, J., 1994, Inactivation of antibiotics and the dissemination of resistance genes, *Science* 264:375.

Decottignies, A., Lambert, L., Catty, P., Degand, H., Epping, E.A., Moye-Rowley, W.S., Balzi, E., and Goffeau, A., 1995, Identification and characterization of Snq2, a new multidrug ATP binding cassette transporter of the yeast plasma membrane, *J. Biol. Chem.* 270:18150.

Deeley, R.G., and Cole, S.P.C., 1997, Function, evolution and structure of multidrug resistance protein (MRP), *Sem. Cancer Biol.* 8:193.

Descoteaux, S., Ayala, P., Orozco, E., and Samuelson, J., 1992, Primary sequences of two P-glycoprotein genes in *Entamoeba histolytica*, *Mol. Biochem. Parasitol.* 54:201.

Dhir, R., and Gros, P., 1992, Functional analysis of chimeric proteins constructed by exchanging homologous domains of two P-glycoproteins conferring distinct drug resistance profiles. *Biochemistry* 31:6103.

Dinh, T., Paulsen, I.T., and Saier, M.H., 1994, A family of extracytoplasmic proteins that allow transport of large molecules across the outer membranes of gram-negative bacteria, *J. Bacteriol.* 176:3825.

Dougherty, D.A., 1996, Cation-" interactions in chemistry and biology: a new view of benzene, Phe, Tyr, and Trp, *Science* 271:163.

Eckert, B., and Beck, C.F., 1989, Topology of the transposon Tn10-encoded tetracycline resistance protein within the inner membrane of *Escherichia coli*, *J. Biol. Chem.* 264:11663.

Felmlee, T., Pellett, S., and Welch, R.A., 1985, Nucleotide sequence of an *Escherichia coli* chromosomal hemolysin, *J. Bacteriol.* 163:94.

Germann, U.A., 1996, P-glycoprotein - a mediator of multidrug resistance in tumour cells, Eur. J. Cancer 32A: 927.

Gottesman, M.M., and Pastan, I., 1993, Biochemistry of multidrug resistance mediated by the multidrug transporter, *Annu. Rev. Biochem.* 62:385.

Gottesman, M.M., Hrycyna, C.A., Schoenlein, P.V., Germann, U.A., Pastan, I. , 1995, Genetic analysis of the multidrug transporter, *Annu. Rev. Genet.* 29:607.

Greenberger, L.M., 1993, Major photoaffinity drug labeling sites for iodoaryl azidoprazosin in P-glycoprotein are within, or imeediately C-terminal to, transmembrane domain 6 and 12, *J. Biol. Chem.* 268:11417.

Griffith, J.K., Baker, M.E., Rouch, D.A., Page, M.G.P., Skurray, R.A., Paulsen, I.T., Chater, K.F., Baldwin, S.A., and Henderson, P.J.F., 1992, Membrane transport proteins: implications of sequence comparisons, *Curr. Opinion. Cell Biol.* 4:684.

Grondin, K., Haimeur, A., Mukhopadhyay, R., Rosen, B.P., Ouelette, M., 1997, Co-amplification of of the γ-glutamylcysteine synthetase gene *gsh1* and of the ABC transporter gene *pgpA* in arsenite-resistant*Leishmania tarentolae. EMBO J.* 16:3057.

Gros, P., Dhir, R., Croop, J., and Talbot, F., 1991, A single amino acid substitution strongly modulates the activity and substrate specificity of the mouse mdr1 and mdr3 drug efflux pumps, *Proc. Natl. Acad. Sci. USA* 88: 7289.

Gründemann, D., Gorboulev, V., Gambaryan, S., Veyhl, M., and Koepsell., H., 1994, Drug excretion mediated by a new prototype of polyspecific transporter, *Nature* 372:549.

Guilfoile, P.G., and Hutchinson, C.R., 1991, A bacterial analog of the *mdr* gene of mammalian tumour cells is present in *Streptomyces peuceticus*, the producer of daunorubicin and doxorubicin, *Proc. Natl. Acad. Sci. USA* 88:8553.

Hagman, K.E., Pan, W., Spratt, B.G., Balthazar, J.T., Judd, R.C., and Shafer, W.M., 1995, Resistance of *Neisseria gonorrhoeae* to antimicrobial agents is modulated by the *mtrRCDE* efflux system, *Microbiology* 141:611.

Hanna, M., Brault, M., Kwan, T., Kast, C., and Gros, P., 1996, Mutagenesis of transmembrane domain 11 of P-glycoprotein by alanine scanning, *Biochemistry* 35:3625.

Henderson, D.M., Sifri, C.D., Rodgers, M., Wirth, D.F., Hendrickson, N., and Ullman, B., 1992, Multidrug resistance in *Leishmania donovani* is conferred by amplification of a gene homologous to the mammalian*mdr1* gene, *Mol. Cell. Biol.* 12:2855.

Higgins, C.F., 1992, ABC transporters: from microorganisms to man, *Annu. Rev. Cell Biol.* 8:67.

Higgins, C.F., and Gottesman, M.M., 1992, Is the multidrug transporter a flippase?, *Trends Biochem. Sci.* 17:18.

Höltje, J.-V., 1998, Growth of the stress-bearing and shape-maintaining murein sacculus of *Escherichia coli, Microbiol. Mol. Biol. Rev.* 62:181.

Homolya, L., Holló, Z., Germann, U.A., Pastan, I., Gottesman, M.M., and Sarkadi, B., 1993, Fluorescent cellular indicators are extruded by the multidrug resistance protein, J. Biol. Chem. 268:21493.

Hoof, T., Demmer, A., Hadam, M.R., Riordan, J.R., and Tümmler, B., 1994, Cystic fibrosis-type mutational analysis in the ATP-binding cassette transporter of P-glycoprotein, *J. Biol. Chem.* 269:20575.

Kajiji, S., Talbot, F., Grizzuti, K., Dyke-Philips, V.V., Agresti, M., Safa, A.R., and Gros, P., 1993, Functional analysis of P-glycoprotein mutants identifies predicted transmembrane domain 11 as a putative drug binding site, *Biochemistry* 32:4185.

Kimura, T., Ohnuma, M., and Sawai, T., and Yamaguchi, A., 1997, Membrane topology of the transposon 10- encoded metal-tetracycline/H^+ antiporter as studied by site-directed chemical labeling, *J. Biol. Chem.*272: 580.

Kioka, N., Tsubota, J., Kakehi, Y., Komano, T., Gottesman, M.M., Pastan, I., and Ueda, K., 1989, P-glycoprotein gene (MDR1) cDNA from human adrenal: normal P-glycoprotein carries Gly-185 with an altered pattern of multidrug resistance, *Biochem. Biophys. Res. Commun.* 162:224.

Klyachko, K.A., Schuldiner, S., and Neyfakh, A.A., 1997, Mutations affecting substrate specificity of the *Bacillus subtilis* multidrug transporter Bmr, *J. Bacteriol.* 179:2189.

Kwan, T., and Gros, P., 1998, Mutational analysis of the P-glycoprotein first intracellular loop and flanking transmembrane domains, *Biochemistry*, 37:3337.

Lewis, K., 1994, Multidrug resistance pumps in bacteria: variations on a theme, *Trends Biochem. Sci.* 19:119.

Li, Z.-S., Szczypka, M., Lu, Y.-P., Thiele, D.J., and Rea, P.A., 1996, The yeast cadmium factor protein (Ycf1) is a vacuolar glutathione *S*-conjugate pump, *J. Biol. Chem.* 271:6509.

Li, Z.-S., Lu, Y.-P., Zhen, R.-G., Szczypka, M., Thiele, D.J., and Rea, P.A., 1997, A new pathway for cadmium sequestration in *Saccharomyces cerevisiae*: YCF-1 catalyzed transport of bis(glutathionato)cadmium, *Proc. Natl. Acad. Sci. USA* 94:42.

Littlejohn, T.G., Paulsen, I.T., Gillespie, M.T., Tennent, J.M., Midgley, M., Jones, I.G., Purewal, A.S., and Skurray, R.A., 1992, Substrate specificity and energetics of antiseptic and disinfectant resistance in *Staphylo- coccus aureus, FEMS Microbiol. Lett.* 95:259.

Liu, J., Takiff, H.E., and Nikaido, H., 1997, Active efflux of fluoroquinolones in *Mycobacterium smegmatis* mediated by LfrA, a multidrug efflux pump, *J. Bacteriol.* 178:3791.

Loo, T.W., and Clarke, D.M., 1993a, Functional consequences of phenylalanine mutations in the predicted transmembrane domains of P-glycoprotein, *J. Biol. Chem.* 268:19965.

Loo, T.W., and Clarke, D.M., 1993b, Functional consequences of proline mutations in the transmembrane domain of P-glycoprotein, *J. Biol. Chem.* 268:3143.

Loo, T.W., and Clarke, D.M., 1994a, Functional consequences of glycine mutation in the predicted cytoplasmic loops of P-glycoprotein, *J. Biol. Chem.* 269:7243.

Loo, T.W., and Clarke, D.M., 1994b, Mutation of amino acids located in predicted transmembrane domain segment 6 (TM6) modulate the activity and substrate specificity of human P-glycoprotein, *Biochemistry* 33: 14049.

Ma, D., Cook, D.N., Alberti, M., Pon, N.G., Nikaido, H., and Hearst, J.E., 1995, Genes *acrA* and *acrB* encode a stress-induced efflux system of *Escherichia coli*, *Mol. Microbiol.* 16:45.

Marger, M., and Saier, M.H., 1993, A major superfamily of transmembrane facilitators that catalyse uniport, symport and antiport, *Trends Biochem. Sci.* 18:13.

Martin, C., Berridge, G., Higgins, C.F., and Callaghan, R., 1997, The multidrug resistance reversal agent SR33557 and modulation of vinca alkaloid binding to P-glycoprotein by an allosteric interaction, *Br. J. Pharmacol.* 122:765.

McNicholas, P., McGlynn, M., Guay, G.G., and Rothstein, D.M., 1995, Genetic analysis suggests functional interactions between the N- and C-terminal domains of the TetA(C) efflux pump encoded by pBR322, *J. Bacteriol.* 177:5355.

Molenaar, D., Bolhuis, H., Abee, T., Poolman, B., and Konings, W.N., 1992, The efflux of a fluorescent probe is catalyzed by an ATP-driven extrusion system in *Lactococcus lactis*, *J. Bacteriol.* 174:3118.

Morris, D.I., Greenberger, L.M., Bruggeman, E.P., Cardarelli, C., Gottesman, M.M., Pastan, I., and Seamon, K.B., 1994, Localization of the forskolin labeling sites for both halves of P-glycoprotein: similarity of the sites labeled by forskolin and prazosin, *Mol. Pharmacol.* 46:329.

Ortiz, D.F., St. Pierre, M.V., Abdulmessih, A., and Arias, I.M., 1997, A yeast ATP-binding cassette-type protein mediating ATP-dependent bile acid transport, *J. Biol. Chem.* 272:15358.

Paulsen, I.T., Brown, M.H., Dunstan, S.J., and Skurray, R.A., 1995, Molecular characterization of the staphylococcal multidrug resistance export protein QacC, *J. Bacteriol.* 177:2827.

Paulsen, I.T., Brown, M.H., and Skurray, R.A., 1996a, Proton-dependent multidrug efflux systems, *Microbiol. Rev.* 60:575.

Paulsen, I.T., Skurray, R.A., Tam, R., Saier, M.H., Turner, R.J., Weiner, J.H., Goldberg, E.B., and Grinius, L.L., 1996b, The SMR family: a novel family of multidrug efflux proteins involved with the efflux of lipophilic drugs, *Mol. Microbiol.* 19:1167.

Paulsen, I.T., Brown, M.H., Littlejohn, T.G., Mitchell, B.A., and Skurray, R.A., 1996c, Multidrug resistance proteins QacA and QacB from *Staphylococcus aureus*: membrane topology and identification of residues involved in substrate specificity, *Proc. Natl. Acad. Sci. USA* 93:3630.

Perego, M., 1997, A peptide export-import control circuit modulating bacterial development regulates protein phosphatases of the phosphorelay, *Proc. Natl. Acad. Sci. USA* 94:8612.

Poole, K., Krebes, K., McNally, C., and Neshat, S., 1993, Multiple antibiotic resistance in *Pseudomonas aeruginosa* evidence for involvement of an efflux operon, *J. Bacteriol.* 175:7363.

Prasad, R., de Wergifosse, P., Goffeau, A., and Balzi, E., 1995, Molecular cloning and characterization of a novel gene of *Candida albicans* conferring multiple resistance to drugs and antifungals, *Curr. Genet.* 27: 320.

Raviv, Y., Pollard, H.B., Bruggeman, E.P., Pastan, I., and Gottesman, M.M., 1990, Photosensitized labeling of a functional multidrug transporter in living drug resistant tumor cells, *J. Biol. Chem.* 265:3975.

Raymond, M., Gros, P., Whiteway, M., and Thomas, D.Y., 1992, Functional complementation of Yeast *ste6* by a mammalian multidrug resistance *mdr* gene, *Science* 256:232.

Rubin, R.A., and Levy, S.B., 1990, Interdomain hybrid Tet proteins confer tetracycline resistance only when derived from more closely related members of the *tet* gene family, *J. Bacteriol.* 172:2303.

Rubin, R.A., and Levy, S.B., 1991, Domains of Tet protein interact productively to mediate tetracycline resistance when present of separate polypeptides, *J. Bacteriol.* 173:4503.

Rubin, R.A., Levy, S.B., Heinrikson, R.L., and Kezdy, F.S., 1990, Gene duplication in the evolution of the two complementing domains of gram-negative tetracycline efflux proteins, *Gene* 87:7.

Ruetz, S., and Gros, P., 1994, Phosphatidylcholine translocase: a physiological role for the *mdr2* gene, *Cell* 77: 1071.

Ruetz, S., Brault, M., Kast, C., Hemenway, C., Heitmans, J., Grant, C.E., Cole, S.P.C., Deeley, R.G., and Gros, P., 1996, Functional expression of the multidrug resistance-associated protein in the yeast *Saccharomyces cerevisiae*, *J. Biol. Chem.* 271:4154

Saier, M.H., Tam, R., Reizer, A., and Reizer, J., 1994, Two novel families of bacterial membrane proteins concerned with nodulation, cell division and transport, *Mol. Microbiol.* 11:841.

Sami, M., Yamashita, H., Hirono, T., Kadoruka, H., Kitamoto, K., Yoda, K., and Yamasaki, M., 1997, Hop resistant *Lactobacillus brevis* contains a novel plasmid harboring a multidrug resistance-like gene, *J. Fermen. Bioengineer.* 84, 1.

Schinkel, A.H., Smit, J.J., van Tellingen, O., Beijnen, J.H., Wagenaar, E., van Deemter, L., Mol, C.A.A.M., van der Valk, M.A., Robanus-Maandag, E.C., te Riele, H.P.J., Berns, A.J.M., and Borst, P., 1994, Disruption of the mouse *mdr1a* P-glycoprotein gene leads to a deficiency in the blood-brain barrier and to increased sensitivity to drugs, *Cell* 77:491.

Shapiro, A.B., and Ling, V., 1997a, P-glycoprotein-mediated Hoechst 33342 transport out of the lipid bilayer, *Eur. J. Biochem.* 250:115.

Shapiro, A.B., and Ling, V., 1997b, Extraction of Hoechst 33342 from the cytoplamsic leaflet of the plasma membrane by P-glycoprotein, *Eur. J. Biochem.* 250:122.

Sheps, J.A., Cheung, I., and Ling, V., 1995, Hemolysin transport in *Escherichia coli*: point mutations in HlyB compensate for a deletion in the predicted amphiphilic helix regions of the HlyA signal, *J. Biol. Chem.* 270: 14829.

Sikkema, J., de Bont, J., and Poolman, B., 1995, Mechanisms of membrane toxicity of hydrocarbons, *Microbiol. Rev.* 59:201.

Smit, J.J.M., Schinkel, A.H., Oude Elferink, R.P.J., Groen, A.K., Wagenaar, E., van Deemter, L., Mol, C.A.A.M., Ottenhoff, R., van der Lugt, N.M.T., van Roon, M.A., van der Valk, M.A., Offerhaus, G.J.A., Berns, A.J.M., and Borst, P., 1993, Homozygous disruption of the murine mdr2 P-glycoprotein gene leads to a complete absence of phospholipid from bile an to liver disease, *Cell* 75:451.

Smith, A.J., Timmermans-Hereijgers, J.L.P.M., Roelofsen, B., Wirtz, K.W.A., van Blitterswijk, W.J., Smit, J.J.M., Schinkel, A.H., and Borst, P., 1994, The human MDR3 P-glycprotein promotes translocation of phosphatidyl choline through the plasma membrane of fibroblasts from transgenic mice, *FEBS Lett.* 354:263.

Spratt, B.G., 1994, Resistance to antibiotics mediated by target alterations, *Science* 264:388.

Taguchi, Y., Kino, K., Morishima, M., Komano, T., Kane, S.E., and Ueda, K., 1997, Amino acid substitutions in the first transmembrane domain (TM1) of P-glycoprotein alter substrate specificity, *Biochemistry*, 36:8883.

Thanassi, D.G., Cheng, L.W., and Nikaido, H., 1997, Active efflux of bile salts by *Escherichia coli, J. Bacteriol.* 179:2512.

Tommasini, R., Evers, R., Vogt, E., Mornett, C., Zaman, G.J.R., Schinkel, A.H., Borst, P., and Martinoia, E., 1996, The human multidrug resistance-associated protein functionally complements the yeast cadmium resistance factor 1, *Proc. Natl. Acad. Sci. USA* 93:6743.

van Helvoort, A., Smith, A.J., Sprong, H., Fritzsche, I., Schinkel, A.H., Borst, P., and van Meer, G., 1996, MDR1 P-glycoprotein is a lipid translocase of broad specificity, while MDR3 P-glycoprotein specifically translocates phosphatidylcholine, *Cell* 87:507.

van Veen, H.W., Venema, K., Bolhuis, H., Oussenko, I., Kok, J., Poolman, B., Driessen, A.J.M., and Konings, W.N., 1996, Multidrug resistance mediated by a bacterial homolog of the human multidrug transporter MDR1, *Proc. Natl. Acad. Sci. USA* 93:10668.

van Veen, H.W., Callaghan, R., Soceneantu, L., Sardini, A., Konings, W.N., and Higgins, C.F., 1998, A bacterial antibiotic resistance gene that complements the human multidrug resistance P-glycoprotein gene, *Nature* 391:291.

Volkman, S.K., Cowman, A.F., and Wirth, D.F., 1995, Functional complementation of the *ste6* gene of *Saccharomyces cerevisiae* with the *pfmdr1* gene of *Plasmodium falciparum, Proc. Natl. Acad. Sci. USA* 92:8921.

Wilson, C.M., Serrano, A.E., Wasley, A., Bogenschutz, M.P., Shankar, A.H., and Wirth, D.F., 1989, Amplification of a gene related to mammalian mdr genes in drug-resistant *Plasmodium falciparum, Science* 244:1184.

Yamaguchi, A., Adachi, K., and Sawai, T., 1990, Orientation of the carboxyl terminus of the transposon Tn10-encoded tetracycline resistance protein, *FEBS Lett.* 265:17.

Yamaguchi, A., Iwasaki-Ohba, Y., Ono, N., Kaneko-Ohdera, M., and Sawai, T., 1991, Stoichiometry of metal-tetracycline/H^+ antiport mediated by transposon Tn10-encoded tetracycline resistance protein, *FEBS Lett.*282:415.

Yerushalmi, H., Lebendiker, M., and Schuldiner, S., 1995, EmrE, an *Escherichia coli* 12-kDa multidrug transporter, exchanges toxic cations and H^+ and is soluble in organic solvents, *J. Biol. Chem.* 270:6856.

Zhang, X., Collins, K.I., and Greenberger, L.M., 1995, Functional evidence that transmembrane 12 and the loop between transmembrane 11 and 12 form part of the drug-binding domain in P-glycoprotein encoded by MDR1, *J. Biol. Chem.* 270:5441.

Zhang, F., Yin, Y., Arrowsmith, C.H. and Ling, V., 1995, Secretion and circular dichroism analysis of the C-terminal signal peptides of HlyA and LktA, *Biochemistry* 34, 4193.

9

METALLOID RESISTANCE MECHANISMS

Rita Mukhopadhyay, Jiaxin Li, Hiranmoy Bhattacharjee, and Barry P. Rosen

Department of Biochemistry and Molecular Biology
Wayne State University
School of Medicine
Detroit, Michigan 48201

INTRODUCTION

Transport systems are intimately involved in both drug action and resistance. The targets of most drugs are intracellular, requiring the existence of drug uptake systems. The most common mechanism of resistance to drugs and antibiotics is through the expression of genes for extrusion systems that reduce the intracellular concentration to subtoxic levels[1]. The treatment of clinical drug and antibiotic resistance requires knowledge of the routes of entry and exit of the drugs and of the molecular mechanisms by which transport occur. In addition, the systems for resistances are often regulated at several levels, including transcriptionally and allosterically[2].

The mechanisms and regulation of metal resistances share many features with drug and antibiotic resistances and serve as excellent models for clinically related resistances. Bacterial metal resistances evolved originally as a response to exposure to natural sources and were more common than antibiotic resistances before the wide-spread use of antibiotics[3]. Toxic metal ions are ubiquitous in the environment, both from natural sources and from their use in agriculture, animal husbandry and industry[4]. In eubacteria, both chromosomal and plasmid-mediated resistances to inorganic salts, such as arsenate, arsenite, antimony, lead, cadmium, zinc, bismuth and mercury have been previously reported[5].

Arsenicals and antimonials were among the first chemotherapeutic agents used to treat infectious diseases; nearly a century ago Paul Ehrlich introduced into clinical use his *silver bullet,* Salvarsan, for the treatment of syphilis and trypanosomal diseases. For his development of chemotherapeutic arsenical drugs Ehrlich was awarded the Nobel Prize in 1908. Ehrlich was not only the father of modern antimicrobial chemotherapy but also the discoverer of drug resistance. He noted that resistance rapidly arose in previously arsenic sensitive cells and postulated that arsenicals must be taken up by cells via a cell surface arsenical receptor in order to be effective. He proposed that organisms became resistant because they no longer accumulated the arsenical drug! This chapter will review resis-

Resolving the Antibiotic Paradox, edited by Rosen and Mobashery.
Kluwer Academic / Plenum Publishers, New York, 1998.

tance to the toxic metalloids arsenic and antimony in eukaryotes and prokaryotes where, in every case active extrusion of the metalloids is related to resistance.

Drug resistance in parasitic protozoa has become an increasing threat to antimicrobial chemotherapy. Aromatic arsenicals or antimony-containing drugs such as pentostam (sodium stibogluconate) are still the first line of drugs in the treatment of trypanosomiasis and leishmaniasis. All organisms, from bacteria to protozoan parasites to *Homo sapiens* have resistance mechanisms to the metalloids arsenic and antimony.

RESISTANCE TO METALLOID-CONTAINING ANTIPARASITIC DRUGS IN TRYPANOSOMATIDS

Trypanosomes

Resistance to melarsoprol (Fig. 1) and other arsenical drugs in *Trypanosoma* has been observed both in strains selected under laboratory conditions and in clinical isolates refractory to arsenicals[6]. To understand the mechanism of resistance it is necessary to understand the site of action of these oxyanions. For a long time all of the glycolytic kinases of trypanosomes have been suggested as the primary target[7]. More recently, trypanothione (TSH), a kinetoplastid-specific diglutathione-spermidine conjugate (Fig. 2), has been a center of attraction. Trypanothione is the most abundant thiol in this group of parasitic protozoa for maintaining an intracellular reducing environment[8]. The secondary targets are trypanothione reductase (TR)[8] and lipoic acid[9]. Resistant cells contain less lipoic acid (Fig. 2), which suggests that they may be involved in the transport of arsenicals. However resistance was not associated with the level of intracellular trypanothione, glutathione (Fig. 2) or related compounds. The properties of TRs isolated from resistant and sensitive cell lines were identical, suggesting that the primary or secondary targets are not involved in resistance. The recent identification of substantial amounts of ovothiol (4-mercaptohistidine) (Fig. 2) in *Crithidia fasciculata*[10] and *Leishmania donovani*[11] raises the possibility that there are other thiol containing targets for arsenicals.

Trypanosomes resistant to melarsoprol are cross-resistant to diamidines[6, 12], and the resistant strains accumulate less diamidine[13]. These results suggest that melaminophenyl arsenicals and diamidines may be transported by the same route. Carter and Fairlamb[14] found only adenosine and adenine prevented lysis of *Trypanosoma brucei* by melarsen ox-

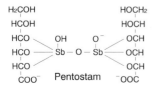

Figure 1. Structure of metalloid-containing antiparasitic drugs. Melarsoprol (left) contains As(III). Pentostam (right) contains Sb(V).

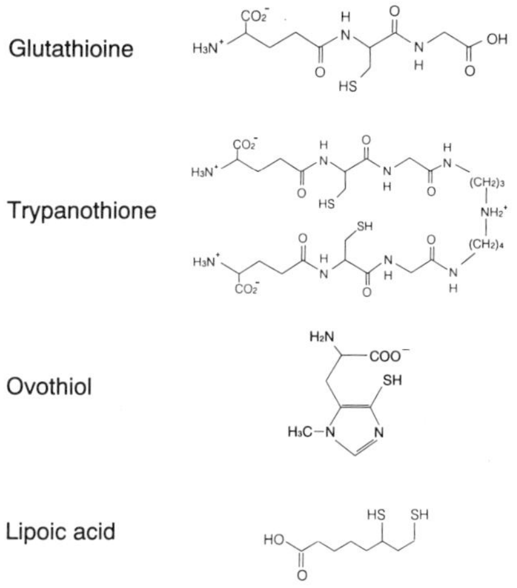

Glutathioine

Trypanothione

Ovothiol

Lipoic acid

Figure 2. Structure of intracellular thiols in protozoan parasites.

ide. Wild type trypanosomes have two high affinity transport systems for adenosine. One of the two, the P2 transporter, also transports melamine based arsenicals. Trypanosomes resistant to melarsen oxide lack this P2 transport system, suggesting that the resistance is due to a defect in uptake[14]. This illustrates an instance in which resistance ensues from a mutation in the route of uptake of a drug, just as Ehrlich had proposed for salvarsan resistance nearly a century ago.

Leishmania

The mode of action of drugs containing arsenicals and antimonials in *Leishmania spp.* is poorly understood, but is thought to have more than one component. Croft *et al.*[15] proposed that pentavalent antimony derivatives are metabolized *in vivo* into trivalent antimonials that may be the active form of the drug. Thus clinical resistance to pentavalent antimonial-containing drugs such as pentostam (Fig. 1) may have the same biochemical basis as resistance to As(III) or Sb(III) in strains selected *in vitro*. Pentostam-resistant clones of *Leishmania* exhibited a five-fold lower intracellular accumulation of [^{125}Sb]pentostam and specific binding of pentostam to a protein similar in mass to the drug resistance protein P-glycoprotein[16]. In *L. tarentolae* and *L. major* resistance to arsenite correlated with amplification of the genes *ltpgpA* and *lmpgpA*, respectively, that encode similar P-glycoprotein homologues[17]. In *L. tarentolae* four different types of arsenite resistant mutants were isolated[18]. All four classes showed resistance to high concentrations of arsenite and low intracellular accumulation of ^{73}AsO$_2^-$ [19]. However, only two had detectable amplification of the *ltpgpA* gene. Partial revertants of mutants that initially showed *ltpgpA* gene amplification but had lost the amplicons during growth in absence of selective pressure were isolated. These partial revertants retained arsenite resistance and accumulated 100-fold less ^{73}AsO$_2^-$ than the wild type. Transfection of wild type cells with *ltpgpA* or *lmpgpA* confer only a low level (two-four fold) of resistance to arsenite and, at least in *L. tarentolae*, showed no alteration in the level of ^{73}AsO$_2^-$ accumulation in the cell. However, mutation of the putative ATP binding site of the *ltpgpA* gene resulted in loss of resistance in the transfectants[20]. Thus, while *pgpA* amplification gives a slight increase in metalloid resistance, reduced accumulation and high level resistance does not correlate with *pgpA*.[19, 21]

In contrast to melarsoprol resistance in African trypanosomes, pentostam resistance in *Leishmania* does not appear to be a defect in uptake. Acquisition or amplification of genes for efflux systems is a more common mechanism of resistance than loss of an uptake system[1]. First, the reduction in accumulation of arsenite in resistant mutants could be reversed to wild type levels by treatment with the uncoupler 2,4-dinitrophenol, suggesting that the lack of uptake is an active process and not simply the loss of an uptake system[19]. Second, from the results of studies with everted membrane vesicle preparations, it is clear that the apparent reduction in accumulation was actually due to rapid efflux of the metalloid from the resistant cells[22]. Transport of $^{73}AsO_2^-$ into everted membrane vesicles was an ATP-dependent process insensitive to uncouplers, indicating that the pump is an arsenite-translocating ATPase. Transport also required the presence of a reductant such as GSH. Initially it was hypothesized that $^{73}As(III)$ was transported as a thiol complex[22]. However, the presence of an As-thiol complex could not be demonstrated inside of the vesicles, nor was co-transport of ^{73}As and [^3H]GSH observed (S. Dey, R. Mukhopadhyay and B. P. Rosen, unpublished). Moreover, the non-thiol reductant tris-(2-carboxyethyl)phosphine (TCEP) could replace thiols (R. Mukhopadhyay and B. P. Rosen, unpublished). Thus, while reduction is required for transport, the nature of the transported species is still an open question, as discussed in more detail below.

Disruption of both alleles of *pgpA* had no effect on the accumulation of $^{73}AsO_2^-$ in membrane vesicles, supporting the previous conclusion that this efflux system is not related to *pgpA*[20]. However, the activity of this arsenite translocating ATPase was similar in everted membrane vesicles isolated from either resistant or sensitive isolates, suggesting that the pump is not the rate limiting step in resistance[23]. Since GSH[23] and many physiological and non-physiological thiols (R. Mukhopadhyay and B. P. Rosen, unpublished) facilitate accumulation of $^{73}AsO_2^-$ in the everted membrane vesicles, it was reasonable to examine the levels of intracellular thiols in sensitive and resistant strains. The resistant mutants were found to greatly overproduce the intracellular thiol trypanothione, and produced increased amounts of GSH and cysteine[24]. There was a correlation between the intracellular concentration of TSH and resistance. There are several possible mechanisms for this effect. First, increased intracellular thiol can result in sequestration of metalloid as the $As(GS)_3$ or $As(TS)$ complex, which, by itself, may provide some degree of resistance. Second, the thiol complex may be the metalloid-containing species recognized by the pump. Even if the As-thiol complex is not the transported species, the metalloid binding site on the cytoplasmic side of the pump could be specific for the thiol conjugate. From inhibitor studies it can be predicted that the pump has a critical vicinal thiol pair required for activity (R. Mukhopadhyay and B. P. Rosen, unpublished). This suggests a model in which As(III) is transferred from As(TS) to a vicinal thiol pair on the pump, followed by extrusion of As(III) as free arsenite and oxidation of the thiol pair to a disulfide (Fig. 3). Reductant would be required at three steps in the overall process: reduction of As(V) to As(III), conjugation of As(III) to the thiol, and reduction of the cystine disulfide to regenerate the active pump.

Thus rate of synthesis of thiols may be the limiting factor in resistance. In resistant strains there are several loci that are amplified[25]. One of these loci was first observed as part of a 50 kb linear amplicon derived from a 800 kb chromosome[18]. Characterization of this amplicon revealed that it encodes the catalytic subunit of γ-glutamylcysteine synthetase (γ-GCS), the rate limiting enzyme in GSH biosynthesis (Fig. 4)[26]. The heavy

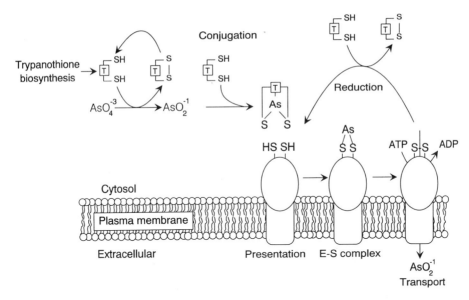

Figure 3. Model of arsenical/antimonial resistance in *Leishmania.* The first step is reduction of Sb(V)/As(V) to Sb(III)/As(III) by trypanothione. The second step is conjugation of the reduced semimetal to trypanothione. It is not known if these two steps are enzyme catalyzed. The trypanothione-As(III) conjugate is recognized by the pump (presentation). In a thiol-exchange reaction As(III) is transferred to a vicinal thiol pair on the pump (E-S complex formation). As(III) is transported across the membrane and released as free arsenite, with the vicinal thiols on the pump forming a disulfide. The oxidized pump is reduced by another molecule trypanothione. Extrusion by the ATP-coupled As-thiol pump lowers the intracellular concentration of metalloid to subtoxic levels. Due to relatively low amounts of intracellular thiols in metalloid-sensitive cells, the limiting step in resistance is proposed to be formation of the As-trypanothione conjugate rather than the amount of pump.

subunit of γ-GCS (*gsh1*) is overexpressed in the arsenite resistant mutants. Transfection of *gsh1* alone in the wild type strains of *L. tarentolae* was sufficient to produce comparable levels of TSH observed in the resistant mutants. Interestingly, however, this was not sufficient to confer resistance to arsenite. In contrast, transfection of *gsh1* into the revertant conferred resistance, indicating that the *gsh1* gene product is necessary but not sufficient for resistance. The levels of the polyamines putrescine and spermidine were also found to be increased in the resistant mutants. Since trypanothione is composed of two GSH molecules joined by a spermidine moiety (Fig 2), it is reasonable that increased TSH biosynthesis would require increased amounts of both GSH and spermidine. The rate limiting enzyme in spermidine biosynthesis is ornithine decarboxylase (ODC). The steady state level of the mRNA for ODC and ODC activity was found to be increased, although not as a result of gene amplification[27]. Modulation of thiol or polyamine levels using specific γ-GCS or ODC inhibitors was shown to sensitize resistant mutants to metalloids. In addition, co-transfection of the *pgpA* gene with *gsh1* produced synergistic resistance. Although the role of *pgpA* in arsenite resistance is still unclear, Papadopoulou *et al.* (1996)[21] hypothesized that *pgpA* gene product is a pump that transports As-thiol conjugates into intracellular compartments. Thus high level resistance is the result of multiple factors - amplification of the genes for the rate limiting steps in biosynthesis of intracellular thiols, amplification of the *pgpA* gene leading to increased sequestration of As(III), and increased As(III) extrusion from cells by a plasma membrane arsenite-translocating ATPase.

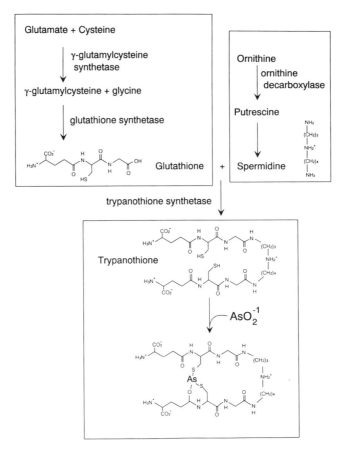

Figure 4. Amplification of the trypanothione biosynthetic pathway produces metalloid resistance in *Leishmania.* Trypanothione is synthesized by condensation of two glutathiones and one spermidine. The rate limiting step in glutathione biosynthesis is catalyzed by the enzyme γ-glutamylcysteine synthetase, the product of the *gsh1* gene, which is amplified during selection for metalloid resistance. The rate limiting step in spermidine biosynthesis is catalyzed by ornithine decarboxylase (ODC). The amount of mRNA for ODC is increased during selection for metalloid resistance, although the mechanism is uncertain.

RESISTANCE TO ARSENIC AND ANTIMONY IN OTHER EUKARYOTES

A stable and inducible resistance to arsenite and antimonite has been reported in Chinese hamster cell lines[28]. Compared to wild type cells, resistant cell lines exhibited reduced intracellular accumulation of $^{73}AsO_2^-$ [29]. Decreased accumulation could be the result of loss of activity of an uptake system, or increased activity of an extrusion system. A hypersensitive mutant accumulated higher levels of $^{73}AsO_2^-$. A similar resistance to arsenite was selected in Chinese hamster ovary cell lines[30]. Resistance was due to increased efflux of the arsenic, leading to low intracellular accumulation[31]. An elevated level of the class II isozyme of glutathione-S-transferase (GST-II) in the cell also correlated with resistance and active extrusion. Inhibitors of GST, such as cibacron blue or ethacrinic acid, decreased resistance to arsenite. Re-elevation of GST activity by treatment with sodium arsenite, cadmium acetate or zinc sulfate resulted in recovery of arsenite resistance[30].

These results have led to the suggestion that As(III) is extruded as a glutathione conjugate[31]. Although arsenate (As(V)) can be reduced nonenzymatically by GSH to form arsenite (As(III)), and arsenite nonenzymatically forms the $As(GS)_3$ conjugate with excess GSH[32, 33], there are no data correlating nonenzymatic conjugation with arsenite detoxification. The elevation of GST-II activity in resistant cell lines suggests that an enzyme is required to increase the rate of conjugation, and that formation of the conjugate, which may be the substrate of the pump, is rate limiting for extrusion and hence for resistance in animal cells.

Guyrasics et al.[34] reported that biliary excretion of arsenic is dependent on hepatobiliary transport of glutathione and also suggested transport of arsenic as a glutathione conjugate. Efflux of GS-conjugates has been observed in vesicles from rat heart and liver[35]. This system is most likely an isoform of the multidrug resistance associated protein (MRP), a MgATP-dependent efflux pump for GS-conjugates. Its physiological role may be extrusion of xenobiotics such as aflatoxin B1 and release of substances such as leukotrienes. Overexpression of human MRP has been shown to confer resistance to arsenicals and antimonials[36]. Prior to excretion into the medium, arsenate is reduced to arsenite by eukaryotic cells[29]. Although there are no direct data demonstrating coupled transport of As(III) and GSH, the report by Zaman et al.[37] provides indirect support. A lung carcinoma cell line transformed with a cDNA encoding MRP was depleted of intracellular glutathione by treatment with DL-buthionine (S,R)-sulfoximine. The cells, which were resistant to drugs such as daunorubicin and vincristine, became sensitive following depletion of GSH. MRP-expressing cells extrude daunorubicin, and GSH depletion decreased efflux. The GSH-depleted cells were incubated with [^{35}S]cysteine, which was incorporated into GSH. Addition of arsenite accelerated efflux of [^{35}S]glutathione, which was found in the medium as the oxidized GSSG form. Even though no complex of arsenite and glutathione was found in the medium, the results support the hypothesis that MRP functions as a carrier for $As(GS)_3$.

Metalloid resistance has been demonstrated in fungi. Recently, three contiguous genes ACR1, ACR2 and ACR3, located on chromosome XVI, were identified as involved in resistance to arsenic compounds in the yeast *Saccharomyces cerevisiae*[38, 39]. The hypothetical product of the ACR1 gene is structurally related to the transcriptional regulatory proteins encoded by the YAP1 and YAP2 genes from *S. cerevisiae* and the *pap1* gene from *S. pombe*. Although the overexpression of ACR1 alone did not produce resistance to arsenicals, the presence of this gene together with ACR2 and ACR3 on a multicopy plasmid considerably increased the level of arsenite resistance. A strain in which ACR1 was disrupted was hypersensitive to both arsenite and arsenate and could be complemented with a multicopy plasmid containing the ACR3 gene. Thus ACR1 is most likely the transcriptional regulator of ACR3 or other gene(s) involved in arsenical resistance in yeast. Overexpression of ACR3 increased arsenite resistance, and disruption of ACR3 produced hypersensitivity. The ACR3 gene product is predicted to be a membrane protein of 404 residues (45,846 Da), suggesting that it functions as an arsenite transporter that removes metalloid from the cytosol, producing resistance. ACR3 is similar in size and function to the ArsB arsenite transporter (429 residues, 45,598 Da) of bacteria (see below). However, as discussed below, ArsB and ACR3 share no apparent sequence similarity. Expression of ACR2 on a multicopy plasmid led to a slight increase in arsenate resistance, and, in addition, resistance to high concentrations of arsenate was observed only when the ACR2 and ACR3 gene together were overexpressed on a multicopy plasmid. These results indicate that ACR2 is involved in resistance to arsenate but not arsenite. As described below, in bacteria the ArsC arsenate reductase is required for reduction of As(V) to As(III), which is then extruded from cells. Since ArsC (141 residues, 15,830 Da) and the ACR2 gene product (130 residues, 14,882 Da) are similar in size and are both required for arsenate resistance, the latter may also be an arsenate reductase. However, the sequences of the two proteins show no similarity and could either be separated from a common ancestor long ago enough to allow for complete divergence of primary sequence or may be the products of independent evolution.

METALLOID RESISTANCE IN PROKARYOTES

Metalloid Uptake

To understand drug action, it is necessary to know the routes of drug entry into cells. Although high level resistance in prokaryotes is most commonly associated with active extrusion systems[1, 5], mutations in the genes for the uptake system can also produce resistance. Cells of *E. coli* normally have a moderate level resistance to metalloids produced by expression of a chromosomal *ars* operon, and disruption of this operon resulted in a metalloid hypersensitive strain[40]. To discover the route of entry of metalloids, Sanders *et al.*[41] mutagenized this hypersensitive strain by transposon mutagenesis, selecting for metalloid resistance. An antimonite-resistant mutant was isolated, and the transposon was shown to be in the *glpF* gene. GlpF is a polyol transporter responsible for the non-energy dependent transport of glycerol and larger polyols and is a homolog of the water channel aquaporin. Thus it is likely that the GlpF is the major route of entry of antimonite into cells of *E. coli*. However, the *glpF* disruption was still sensitive to arsenite. This may mean that GlpF does not transport arsenite or that there is a second system that also transports arsenite. If there are two systems that both transport arsenite, then a mutation in only one would not prevent arsenite entry and not produce resistance. The known substrates of GlpF are all uncharged organic alcohols. That GlpF could transport antimonite is somewhat surprising and suggests that there is a species of Sb(III) that resembles a polyol. The solution chemistry of Sb(III) is largely uncharacterized. However, species such as $(HO)_2Sb-O-Sb(OH)_2$ or $(HO)_2Sb-Sb(OH)_2$ are not inconsistent with the properties of trivalent antimony. Since the pKa's of these species would be predicted to be high, they would be present as largely uncharged molecules. Thus, this is a case where molecular genetics suggests that the solution structure of a drug may be quite different from the expected form.

Metalloid Extrusion

The metal and metalloid containing salts to which bacterial resistances have been reported include arsenate, arsenite, antimony, lead, cadmium, zinc, silver, copper, bismuth and mercury[5, 42]. The determinants for these resistances are on transmissible plasmids, transposons and chromosomes. Perhaps as a result of the application of arsenic-containing compounds as antimicrobials, feed supplements and herbicides, resistance to metalloids have been found in both gram-positive and gram-negative bacteria.

An ever-growing number of arsenic and antimony resistance determinants, designated *ars* operon, have been reported in bacteria. These operons consist of either three (*arsRBC*) or five (*arsRDABC*) genes (Fig. 5). *Staphylococcus* plasmids pI258[43] and pSX267[44] and *E. coli*[45] *ars* operons belong to the three gene category, whereas the *E. coli* plasmids R773[46] and R46[47] and plasmid pKW301 of *Acidiphilium multivorum*[48] to the five

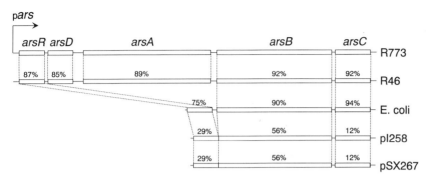

Figure 5. Bacterial ars operons. Shown from top to bottom are the five-gene and three-gene *ars* operons from *E. coli* plasmids R773 and R46, the chromosome of *E. coli* and streptococcal plasmids pI258 and pSX267. The direction of transcription is indicated by the arrow. Genes are indicated by boxes, with the intergenic spaces as single lines.

gene category. In either category, resistance results from the active extrusion of oxyanions[49, 50]. The conjugative plasmid R773-borne resistance has been most extensively studied and will be described in detail.

Among the five genes of R773, *arsR* and *arsD* encode two metalloregulatory proteins[51, 52]. The products of *arsA* and *arsB* genes form an ATP-driven oxyanion pump[53]. ArsA functions as the catalytic subunit of the pump[54], while ArsB is the membrane anchor for ArsA and forms the anion-conducting pathway[22, 55]. The *arsC* gene encodes a reductase that catalyzes reduction of As(V) to As(III), expanding the range of resistance to include pentavalent arsenicals[56, 57].

ArsA: The Catalytic Subunit of the Ars Pump. Analysis of the predicted amino acid sequence of the 63 kDa ArsA (583 residues) indicated that the protein originated from homologous N-terminal (A1) half and C-terminal (A2) half by an ancestral gene duplication and fusion[46] (Fig. 6A). Each half of ArsA contains a consensus sequence for the phosphate binding loop (P-loop or Walker A motif) of a nucleotide binding site[58]. Although functionally a peripheral membrane protein, when overexpressed, ArsA can be purified from the cytosol of *E. coli* cells[59]. As predicted from the *in vivo* energetics and the protein sequence, purified ArsA is an As(III)/Sb(III)-stimulated ATPase[54, 59], where the metalloid serves as an allosteric activator[60, 61].

ArsA is evolutionarily unrelated to other known classes of ion-translocating ATPases[62], although it has structural and functional similarities to members of the ABC (<u>A</u>TP <u>b</u>inding <u>c</u>assette) superfamily. For example, most ABC transporters have duplicated nucleotide binding sites. Many are complexes of peripheral ATPase subunits and integral membrane proteins, although others such as P-glycoprotein are single polypeptides that contain both catalytic and membrane domains. Thus elucidation of the mechanism of ArsA catalysis may be applicable to the mechanism of ABC transporters. Do both A1 and A2 Walker A consensus sites in ArsA bind ATP? Is there interaction of the sites? Are both catalytic? These and other questions have been investigated by a variety of genetic, biochemical and biophysical approaches.

From the increase in fluorescence of the labeled ATP analogue 2',3'-O-(2,4,6-trinitrophenylcyclohexadienylidene)adenosine-5'-triphosphate (TNP-ATP) upon interaction with wild type ArsA, it was shown that both sites bind nucleotide[63]. Substitutions of resi-

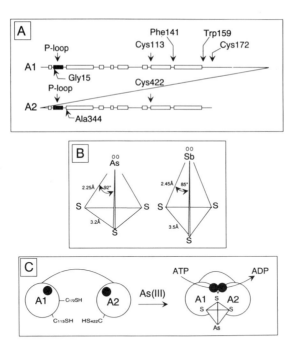

Figure 6. Metalloregulation of the ArsA ATPase. **Top:** The 583 amino acid residue ArsA protein consists of two homologous halves, N-terminal A1 and C-terminal A2. The aligned boxes in the two halves indicate the regions of greatest sequence similarity. Each half has a consensus sequence for the binding site of phosphoryl groups of ATP (P-loop). The location of Gly15 in the A1 P-loop and Ala344 near the A2 P-loop, three cysteine residues in the allosteric binding site, and Phe141 and Trp159, the residues used for spectroscopic probes of catalysis, are indicated. **Middle:** The structure of the soft metal-thiol complex in ArsA is postulated from the bond angles and distances found by crystallographic analysis of small molecules containing As-S or Sb-S bonds. This trigonal pyramidal structure contains three sulfur thiolates liganded to As(III) or Sb(III), with the metal at the apex. In ArsA the three sulfurs are the thiolates of Cys113, Cys172 and Cys422. **Bottom:** ArsA ATPase activity is allosterically regulated by binding of the As(III) or Sb(III) to the allosteric site. This is hypothesized to bring the A1 and A2 into contact to make a catalytic site at the interface between the two ATP binding sites.

dues in either site resulted in loss of arsenite resistance and inactivation of ATPase activity[64–66]. The purified proteins also lost the ability to bind TNP-ATP at the substituted site but could still bind nucleotide at the intact site[63]. Thus loss of binding at either site inactivated the enzyme, demonstrating that both are required for catalysis.

ATP binding could also be assayed by photoactivation of the bound nucleotide with ultraviolet radiation, resulting in adduct formation between the adenine ring of ATP and ArsA. From analysis of peptides crosslinked with α-[^{32}P]ATP, a short sequence in the linker region connecting the A1 and A2 halves of the protein was inferred to be in contact with the adenine ring[67]. The nucleotide bound in the A1 site most likely formed the photoadduct with α-[^{32}P]ATP. Thus, this assay measures binding to only the A1 site, raising the possibility that the two sites have different properties. To examine the role of the two sites in more detail, ArsA was modified with the ATP analogue 5-p-fluorosulfonylbenzoyladenosine (FSBA), which forms a covalent adduct with ArsA[68]. To determine which site bound FSBA, ArsA was partially digested with trypsin. The initial rapid cleavage occurred in the linker region at Arg290, generating a 32 kDa N-terminal fragment and a 27 kDa C-terminal fragment. The 32 kDa peptide was relatively resistant to further treatment, sug-

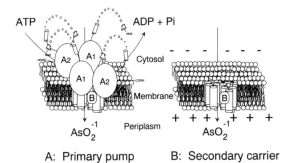

A: Primary pump B: Secondary carrier

Figure 7. Dual energetics of the Ars transporter. **A:** The complex of ArsA and ArsB forms an oxyanion-translocating ATPase that catalyzes extrusion of arsenite or antimonite. The stoichiometery of the complex is hypothesized to be two subunits of ArsA and one ArsB. The primary sequence of the two P-loops of the nucleotide binding domains in the A1 and A2 halves of each ArsA are shown. The complex is an obligatory ATP-coupled pump that is unable to utilize $\Delta\psi$. **B:** ArsB functions as a $\Delta\psi$–driven carrier protein in the absence of ArsA, transporting the arsenite (antimonite) anion, with energy derived from the proton pumping respiratory chain or F_0F_1 ATPase.

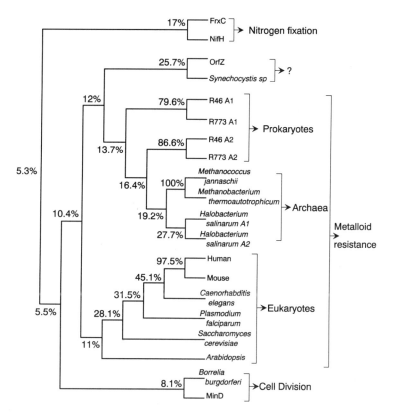

Figure 8. Phylogenetic relationship of ArsA homologues from prokaryotes, archaea and eukaryotes. The dendogram was made using DNasis (Hitachi). The calculated matching percentages are indicated at each branch point.

gesting a compact conformation. The 27 kDa fragment was more sensitive to further trypsin digestion. Using an antibody to FSBA it was shown that ATP analogue preferentially bound at the A2 site in the presence or absence of the antimonite, the allosteric activator. In contrast, it appeared that ATP itself preferentially bound to the A1 site and would bind to the A2 site only in the presence of antimonite. This has lead to the proposal that the A1 site binds ATP with high affinity ATP site, whereas the A2 site binds with low affinity. The allosteric activator increases the affinity at the A2 site, producing catalytic cooperativity. Thus, the anion binding acts as a switch in regulating ATP binding to A2 and hence the ATPase activity of ArsA.

From a combination of genetic and molecular biological analyses it appears that the A1 and A2 ATP binding sites functionally interact with each other. Two mutated *arsA* genes, one with an amino acid substitution in the A1 site and the second with a substitution in the A2 site, complemented each other when expressed from compatible plasmids[69]. In those experiments cells containing either single mutant gene did not confer arsenite resistance, but when the two mutant genes were co-expressed, the cells were resistant. This suggests that two inactive ArsAs, one with a defective A1 ATP binding site and the other with a defective A2 site, can form an active ATPase complex. This suggestion was further confirmed by biochemical reconstitution experiments[70]. Individually expressed peptides corresponding to the A1 and A2 halves were purified. Alone neither had catalytic activity, nor was a mixture of the A1 and A2 polypeptides active. However, if denatured and refolded together, the resulting complex exhibited metalloid-stimulated ATPase activity. The results of recent studies utilizing intragenic suppression further supported the model of interacting A1 and A2 ATP-binding sites[66]. A G15C substitution in the A1 ATP binding site resulted in a defective ArsA and reduced arsenite resistance (Fig. 6A). This mutant *arsA* gene was then chemically mutagenized, and arsenite resistant strains selected. One mutant had both the original G15C substitution in the A1 site and another alteration, A344V. The second substitution was adjacent to the A2 ATP binding site. Subsequently, Gly15 and Ala344 were each changed to variety of residues representing negatively charged, positively charged, neutral, polar, or aromatic amino acids, and steric limitations on the interaction of ArsA ATP binding sites were observed. The smaller the residue at 15, the higher the arsenite resistance and ATPase activity; on the contrary, the larger the residue at 344, the better the suppression effect to G15C or G15R. These data again support the idea of the proximity and interaction of ATP binding sites of the ArsA[71].

Data from crosslinking experiments and light scattering suggested that ArsA is functionally a homodimer[72]. Since the results from both intergenic and intragenic complementation support the concept of interacting A1 and A2 ATP binding sites, we have hypothesized that there are two actively catalytic sites in an ArsA dimer, each formed by a pair of interacting A1 and A2 ATP binding sites. This concept is similar to the mechanism of the H^+-translocating F_1-ATPase, in which the catalytic site on the β subunit has residues contributed from the α subunit[73]. Since ArsA appears to be a functional homodimer, there are two possibilities for interaction of A1 and A2 ATP binding sites: intra- or intersubunit interactions. Intersubunit interaction was tested by mixing of purified inactive and active ArsAs. The assumption was that formation of a dimer between active and inactive subunits would decrease the overall activity of the mixture, that is, the inactive subunit would "poison" the active ones. Inhibition was not observed (J. Li and B.P. Rosen, unpublished result). Although a negative result, it is consistent with intrasubunit interaction of A1 and A2 sites within each monomer. Finally, it remains to be determined whether both sites in the ArsA monomer are catalytic, either independently or cooperatively.

As mentioned above, ArsA ATPase activity is activated by arsenite or antimonite. Allosteric activation involves formation of soft metal-sulfur bonds between the metalloid and three cysteine thiolates. Sulfhydryl modifying reagents such as methyl methanethiosulfonate and N-ethylmaleimide were shown to inhibit ATPase, suggesting the involvement of cysteines in catalysis[60]. To investigate the role of individual cysteine residues in ArsA function, each cysteine was altered to a serine residue. ArsA has four cysteines, Cys26, Cys113, Cys172 and Cys422 (Fig. 6A). The C26S protein has essentially the same properties as wild type, indicating that Cys26 is not required for function. Cells expressing the other three mutant genes became sensitive to arsenite or antimonite. The purified C113S, C172S and C422S enzymes each exhibited approximately the same affinity for ATP as wild type. However, the affinity for arsenite or antimonite was reduced in the three altered enzymes. These results suggest that Cys113, Cys172 and Cys422 are each involved in metalloregulation of catalysis, leading to the hypothesis that ArsA contains a novel metalloid structure with three sulfur ligands coordinating to As(III) or Sb(III) (Fig. 6B)[61]. As soft metals As(III) and Sb(III) can inhibit the activity of enzymes by binding to two or three thiol groups in proteins. Usually metalloid binding involves interaction with vicinal thiols, but in ArsA the three cysteines are spatially distant from each other in the primary sequence. To be able to form the distinctive structures shown in Fig. 6B, Cys113, Cys172 and Cys422 must be with 3–4 Å of each other in the tertiary structure of ArsA. To determine the distance between the essential cysteine residues in ArsA, wild type enzyme and mutant ArsAs with one to three of essential cysteine substitutions were treated with the bifunctional alkylating agent dibromobimane, which reacts with sulfhydryl pairs within 3–6 Å to form a fluorescent adduct. ArsAs with two of the three essential cysteines formed fluorescent adducts. However, ArsAs with one of such residues did not form fluorescent adducts. These results demonstrate that Cys113, Cys172 and Cys422 are more than 3 Å but less than 6 Å from each other in the native enzyme, a distance consistent with formation of the three coordinate complex[61].

How does As(III) or Sb(III) binding at the effector binding site activates catalysis? A 12-residue sequence (DTAPTGHTIRLL) has been found to be conserved in proteins and open reading frames from a variety of proteins found in prokaryotes, archaea and eukaryotes[74] (see Fig. 9). The high degree of sequence conservation of this DTAP motif implies the function conservation. In ArsA there are two DTAP motifs, one in the A1 and the other in the A2 domain. Intrinsic tryptophan fluorescence was used as a spectroscopic probe of conformational changes in ArsA during catalysis[75]. ArsA has four tryptophan residues, but only the fluorescence of Trp159 (Fig. 6A), located at the C-terminal side of the DTAP motif, responded to addition of ligands such as ATP or metalloid. Altered ArsAs were constructed by site directed mutagensis in which a single tryptophan residue was introduced at either residue 141, the N-terminal side of the DTAP domain or at residue 159, the C-terminal side of the domain, with all other tryptophan residues changed to tyrosines[74]. In the absence of ligands, Trp141 is in a relatively nonpolar environment, and Trp159 is in a relatively hydrophilic environment. During ATP hydrolysis the carboxyl terminal end of the DTAP domain moves into a less polar environment; as product is formed the amino terminal end enters a more hydrophilic environment. During ATP hydrolysis there is accumulation of an intermediate conformation of the enzyme; addition of the metalloid activator converted the intermediate into a conformation resembling the initial state, consistent with acceleration of the reaction. These results suggest that the conserved domain experiences a rotational movement during the catalytic cycle, with transmission of binding information from the allosteric site to the catalytic site. A model for allosteric activation is that the two halves of the protein must be in contact with each other to be active

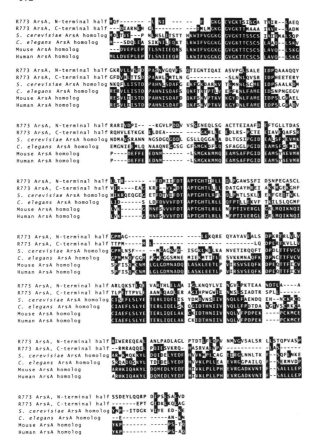

Figure 9. Multiple alignment of the amino acid sequences of ArsA homologues. The alignment was made using DNasis (Hitachi).

(Fig. 6C)[66]. In the absence of the metalloid activator the two A1 and A2 domains are free to move independently of each other. Without contact between the two nucleotide binding domains the enzyme catalyzes only basal level hydrolysis of ATP. When As(III) or Sb(III) interact with Cys113 and Cys172 in the A1 half and Cys422 in the A2 half, those domains are pulled together. The two nucleotide binding domains are then in contact with each other, producing an acceleration of catalysis. The release of energy from ATP hydrolysis in the ArsA subunit is transduced into the ArsB subunit of the pump, driving the transport reaction.

ArsB: The Arsenite Carrier. ArsAB complex is an obligatorily ATP-coupled pump, with ArsA serving as the energy-transducing subunit and ArsB the membrane carrier for arsenite[22, 53]. ArsB is postulated to bind arsenite or antimonite anion - a different molecule than the one bound at the allosteric site of ArsA - and to use the energy from hydrolysis to pump those toxic metalloid oxyanions out of the cells. From hydropathic analysis, the 45 kDa ArsB is a polytopic membrane protein[46]. From analysis of gene fusions of *arsB* with several types of reporter genes and from protease sensitivity from either side of the inner membrane, the topology of ArsB was determined[76]. The 429 residue ArsB has 12 transmembrane segments, most likely α-helices, with both the N- and C-termini located in the cytosol. Interestingly, this is more similar to the structure of secondary transporters than primary pumps[77]. The interaction between ArsA and ArsB is tight; ArsA can only be dissociated in the presence of high concentrations of urea or KCl[55]. When ArsB is expressed in the absence of ArsA, everted membrane vesicles containing ArsB can be isolated. Purified ArsA can be added to these everted vesicles and binds in a saturable manner. The affinity of ArsB for ArsA was increased by the presence of metalloid[53]. As discussed above, metalloid binding at the allosteric site of ArsA produces a conformational change and increases the concentration of dimer in solution. This suggests that the form of ArsA that binds to ArsB is the homodimer, and an increase in the concentration of homodimer facilitates interaction of the two subunits.

Dual Modes of Energy Coupling of ArsB. As discussed above, *ars* operons consist of either three (*arsRBC*) or five (*arsRDABC*) genes (Fig. 5). The *ars* operons from two staphylococcal plasmids and *E. coli* chromosome do not have an *arsA* gene, yet cells expressing them still extrude arsenite. Moreover, when the *arsA* gene was deleted from the R773 *ars* operon, cells expressing only *arsB* also conferred an intermediate level of resistance and still extruded $^{73}AsO_2^-$ [78]. How do cells expressing only *arsB* in the absence of *arsA* pump out arsenite? One possibility was that there is a chromosomal *arsA* gene. However, from genomic sequencing projects it is clear that neither *E. coli* nor *B. subtilis* chromosome has a homologous gene, and no chromosomal staphylococcal *arsA* homologue has been found.

These considerations led to an examination of the *in vivo* and *in vitro* energetics of arsenite transport. From the results of *in vivo*[78] and *in vitro*[22] studies it was demonstrated that the ArsAB complex is an obligatorily ATP-coupled pump. The *arsAB* genes were expressed in a Δunc *E. coli* strain lacking the H^+-translocating-ATPase (F_1F_0). The F_1F_0 catalyzes the equilibrium between ATP and the electrochemical proton gradient, so a mutant lacking this enzyme can be used to distinguish between chemical and electrochemical energy as the driving force for a transport reaction[79]. Following depletion of endogenous energy reserves, the mutant cells are able to produce only chemical energy if glucose is given in the presence of an inhibitor of respiration such as cyanide. In contrast, the cells will generate only electrochemical energy if given a respiratory substrate such as succinate. When the mutant cells were expressing both *arsA* and *arsB,* arsenite extrusion was coupled only to chemical energy, and electrochemical energy would not suffice[78]. However, when the cells expressed only *arsB*, opposite results were obtained; electrochemical energy was necessary and sufficient, and chemical energy was neither. From these *in vivo* results it appeared that the ArsA-ArsB complex was an obligatory pump, while ArsB alone could function as a secondary carrier coupled to the membrane potential (Fig. 7).

To demonstrate the energetics more conclusively, arsenite accumulation was measured in everted membrane vesicles prepared from the same types of cells[22, 80]. In everted membrane vesicles, which have an orientation inside-out relative to that of cells, accumulation of arsenite is the equivalent of extrusion from cells. In vesicles prepared from the *Dunc* strain expressing both *arsA* and *arsB* only ATP would drive transport of $^{73}AsO_2^-$. ATP could not be replaced with other nucleoside triphosphates or nonhydrolyzable ATP analog, ATPγS. ATP-dependent transport by the ArsA-ArsB complex was insensitive to uncouplers. Thus the R773 ArsA-ArsB complex is clearly an obligatorily ATP-coupled pump. In addition, transport in vesicles prepared from Δunc strains could not be driven by oxidation of lactate or NADH, demonstrating that electrochemical energy was neither necessary nor sufficient for the Ars pump. Like other transport ATPases, arsenite primary pump has an absolute requirement for a divalent cation, Mg^{2+} or Mn^{2+}. Neither vanadate, an inhibitor of P-type ATPases, nor azide, an inhibitor of F-type ATPases, inhibited arsenite accumulation[49, 81]. In contrast, in the absence of ArsA, ArsB functions as a secondary arsenite carrier[80]. ArsB-containing everted vesicles accumulated $^{73}AsO_2^-$ dependent on formation of an electrochemical gradient, positive interior. No transport was observed with ATP alone. Accumulation was uncoupler sensitive but insensitive to weak bases that would dissipate only the chemical gradient of protons. These results clearly demonstrate that ArsB by itself catalyzes arsenite transport coupled to the membrane potential, perhaps as an electrophoretic uniporter.

Why should there be two different ways for ArsB to function? ArsB may have evolved to produce a moderate level of resistance to metalloids. However, pumps are thermodynamically more efficient than carriers. Assuming that a single anion is transported, ArsB alone is theoretically capable of producing a 1000-fold gradient of arsenite such that the concentration of arsenite inside of a resistant cell would be 10^{-3} less than the medium concentration. On the other hand, the ArsA-ArsB pump theoretically could generate a 10^6-fold gradient if hydrolysis of one ATP were coupled to extrusion of one anion. Thus cells that express the pump would be expected to be more resistant than those with only ArsB. The ArsA-ArsB complex may have evolved later in response to exposure to higher environmental metalloid concentrations. This dual mode of energy coupling is novel but not unique. The F_1F_0 functions as an obligatory ATP-coupled proton pump, but the F_0 alone transports protons driven by the membrane potential. It may be that other pumps evolved from the association of carriers with ATPase subunits[82].

To fully understand the mechanisms of drug and metal resistances it is necessary to know the chemical nature of the interactions between drug or metal and resistance proteins. The chemical form recognized by regulatory elements may not be the same form recognized by the resistance enzymes. For example, two different metalloid chemistries are used by the gene products encoded by the R773 *ars* operon. For both transcriptional and allosteric regulation soft metal chemistry occurs between As(III) or Sb(III) and cysteine thiolates in ArsR, ArsD and ArsA[5, 83]. In contrast, the chemical form of the metalloid transported by the GlpF polyol carrier is conceivably an uncharged hydroxylated antimonite oligomer[41]. The substrate of the ArsB carrier appears to be the oxyanionic of arsenite or antimonite. First, the driving force for transport by ArsB alone is the membrane potential; the most parsimonious interpretation of that result is that ArsB is an anion-tranlocating uniporter. Second, the substrate of the transporter is free arsenite, with no thiols required[22, 80]. Third, ArsB does not use soft metal-thiol chemistry. There is only a single cysteine residue in the primary sequence of ArsB. Mutation of the codon for this single cysteine of ArsB to a number of other residues demonstrated that this cysteine is not essential for metalloid resistance or transport[84]. An effective transport system must be able to bind substrate on one side of the membrane and release it on the other. High affinity binding of As(III) as a soft metal to sulfur thiolates in the carrier would interfere with release, while low affinity oxyanion binding by ArsB is more conducive to a translocation mechanism.

EVOLUTION OF METALLOID RESISTANCES

All organisms - prokaryotes, archaea, eukaryotes - have evolved mechanisms for resistance to drugs and toxic metals. These are most likely ancient adaptations to environmental stresses. All organisms are exposed continually to toxic metals present naturally in the environment. In addition, bacteria constantly war against each other, synthesizing and extruding antibiotics for which the producing organism has evolved resistance mechanisms, and we have tailored these antibiotics to our own use. While it is not possible to determine experimentally when these resistances first arose, the first living cells arose in oceans rich in dissolved metals long before the biosynthesis of the first antibiotic. Indeed, bacterial resistance to arsenic was more common than antibiotic resistances before the modern era of clinical use of antibiotics[3], although it is not clear whether this was the result of exposure to natural sources of arsenic or to industrial production. As described above, arsenic resistance is found not only in prokaryotes but also in fungi, parasites and mammals. Are these resistances evolutionarily related or the products of parallel evolution?

ArsA Homologues

Our present knowledge about arsenical resistance genes in eukaryotes is limited primarily to DNA sequence analysis. A number of homologues have been identified by sequence comparison (Fig. 8). It appears that genes for three types of proteins diverged from a common ancestor. One branch led to bacterial cell division proteins such as MinD[85]. A second branch led to enzymes involved in nitrogen fixation such as dinitrogen reductase (NifH)[86]. The third branch are those closely related to ArsA. The ArsA family can be subdivided into representatives from the three kingdoms. The bacterial ArsAs arose from a gene duplication and fusion of the common ancestor (A), producing a gene product with A1 and A2 domains, although there are bacterial genes of unknown function that are single A[87]. Archaea have both. Methanogenic archaea have an A structure[88], while halobacteria have an A1-A2 organization (Ng,W.L., Ciufo,S.A., Smith,T.M., Bumgarner,R.E., Loretz,C., direct submission of *Halobacterium sp.* plasmid pNRC100). All eukaryotes known to date are single A domain proteins. A human homologue of the bacterial *arsA* (*harsA*) has been isolated recently [89]. The full-length *harsA* cDNA has 996 bp and encodes a 332 residue protein. Sequence analysis suggested that it is a member of the ArsA ATPase family with no transmembrane domain. If this is indeed the catalytic component of an arsenite pump, there must be a gene for a yet-unidentified membrane protein.

Biochemical analysis showed that hArsA has a low level of ATPase activity that is not metalloid activated. A mouse *arsA* gene (*marsA*) was identified from the expressed sequence tag (EST) database (H. Bhattacharjee and B.P. Rosen, direct submission of *Mus musculus* sequence, accesssion number AF039405). Complete sequencing of the *marsA* cDNA clone showed that the mArsA is 97.5% homologous with hArsA. The genomic sequencing of the small nematode, *Caenorhabditis elegans*[90] has revealed the presence of a hypothetical *C. elegans* ArsA homologue. This open reading frame encodes a 342 residue protein and shares 49% homology with the amino acid sequence of hArsA. An *arsA* has been identified in the genome of *Plasmodium falciparum* (D. Lawson, direct submission of *Plasmodium falciparum* sequence, accession number AL010250). This 379 residue protein exhibits 40% identity with hArsA. An *arsA* gene has also been located in chromosome IV of yeast, *Saccharomyces cerevisiae*[91]. The predicted protein has 354 amino acid residues and shows 47.9% identity and 68.4% similarity with *C. elegans* ArsA. The yeast ArsA also has about 29% identity and 49% similarity with either the A1 or A2 domains of the *E. coli* R773 plasmid encoded ArsA protein.

A multiple amino acid sequence alignment of ArsA homologues is shown in Fig. 9. A common feature is the presence of Walker A motif, or P loop (GKGGVGKT), formed by the glycine rich segment, which is thought to directly interact with the phosphate moiety of ATP or GTP[58]. As discussed above, *E. coli* ArsA has two such motifs, one in the N-terminal and the other in C-terminal half of the protein, both necessary for ArsA activity. The eukaryotic ArsA homologues have a single ATP binding domain. Another common feature of nucleotide binding proteins is the Walker B motif. In ArsA homologues the Walker B motif is predicted to form a hydrophobic ß-strand that terminates at an Asp residue in the conserved DTAP domain. The conserved aspartate is probably responsible for interaction with Mg^{2+} and is therefore important for catalysis[92, 93]. Another potential Mg^{2+} ligand is the conserved aspartate residue in the sequence DPA (corresponding to Asp45 in the A1 domain and Asp364 in the A2 domain of the R773 ArsA, T.Q. Zhou and B.P. Rosen, unpublished). There are other conserved residues within these ArsA homologous, but their functions are unknown.

It is assumed that there would be an allosteric metalloid binding site if these ArsA homologues are indeed the catalytic components of arsenite pumps. Although the ATP and Mg^{2+} binding sites are well conserved, the location of the putative metalloid binding site in the homologues is not as clear. In the R773 ArsA Cys113, Cys172 and Cys422 are involved in interaction with As(III) or Sb(III) (Fig. 6) These critical residues are however not conserved in eukaryotic ArsA homologues. Interestingly, Cys26, which is not involved in either catalysis or metalloactivation in *E. coli* ArsA, is conserved in the eukaryotic homologues. However, the eukaryotic homologues have conserved CXC and CXXC motifs, which can be high affinity metalloid binding sites. ArsR, the *trans*-acting repressor of bacterial *ars* operons, has a similar CXC motif that has been shown to be responsible for metal binding[94, 95]. The ArsA homologues from Archaea are more closely related to the bacterial ArsA (Fig. 8), but show interesting sequence similarities to both the prokaryotic and eukaryotic proteins. The *Halobacterium salinarum* ArsA has the A1-A2 duplication and has a cysteine triad corresponding to the R773 ArsA. In contrast the ArsAs of *Methanococcus jannaschii* and *Methanobacterium thermoautotrophicum* have the single A domain structure of the eukaryotic ArsA and lack the cysteine triad of the bacterial enzyme. Instead they have the CXXC sequence found in the eukaryotic homologues but not conserved CXC sequence. It is possible that Archaea acquired an *arsA* gene by horizontal transfer from either bacteria or a eukaryote. Arguing against this view is the fact that the methanogenic and halophilic ArsAs are more closely related to each other than to either the bacterial or eukaryotic members of the ArsA family. The fact that one branch of the Archaea has a bacterial-like ArsA and another branch has a eukaryotic-like ArsA suggests that the divergence of the two ArsA branches took place before the split between the kingdoms. However, until the function of other ArsA homologues are determined, the role of these proteins in arsenic resistance remains speculative.

ArsB Homologues

There appear to be two families of ArsB-like proteins, and it is not clear whether they arose from a common ancestor (Fig. 10). One family includes the R773 ArsB and other bacterial homologues that have 12 membrane spanning segments. A second family includes sequences from a diverse collection of organisms: a eukaryote (*Saccharomyces cerevisiae*)[39], two archaea (*Archaeoglobus fulgidus,* accession number AE001071,[96]) and *Methanobacterium thermoautotrophicum,* accession number 2621995,[97]), a prokaryote (*Synechocystis sp.,* accession number 2496798)[98], and a gene in the novel 48 kb skin element of *Bacillus subtilis*[99]. Unlike the ArsA homologues, these two groups of membrane proteins almost certainly have similar functions. ACR3 has been shown to confer arsenical resistance in *Saccharomyces cerevisiae*[38], and the skin element protein *yqcl* confers arsenic resistance in *B. subtilis*. Interestingly, ACR3 does not appear to confer resistance to antimonials, which differentiates it from the bacterial metalloid resistances. ACR3 is 37% identical to the skin element protein, which, in turn, is 60% identical to the *Archaeoglobus*

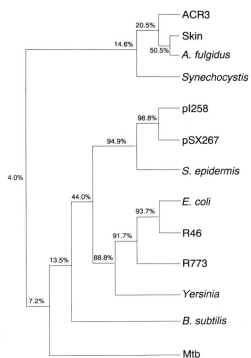

Figure 10. Phylogenetic relationship of the ArsB homologues and arsenic carrier proteins of prokaryotes, archaea and eukaryotes. The dendogram was made using DNasis (Hitachi). The calculated matching percentages are indicated at each branch point.

fulgidus protein. Thus there must have been a common ancestor before the divergence of these three kingdoms.

ACR3 and its homologues are most likely membrane proteins, but their topology is not clear; 10 membrane spanning regions have been suggested[38]. The hydropathy plots of ACR3 and the skin element protein are basically superimposible, but between members of this group and the bacterial ArsBs the hydropathy profiles cannot be superimposed. Usually similarities in structure are retained during evolution even after sequence similarities are lost. Thus it may be that the two groups evolved independently. Are the ArsA and ArsB homologues both involved in arsenic resistance? At this time there are no data pertaining to this question. On one hand, it is clear that the bacterial ArsB does not require ArsA, even though the complex functions more efficiently. On the other hand, many organisms in all kingdoms have ArsA homologues, and arsenic resistance is found in all representatives of every kingdom. We would postulate that, in at least some eukaryotes and archaea, arsenic detoxification systems would have an ArsA-ArsB structure.

ACKNOWLEDGMENTS

These studies were support in part by United States Public Health Service Grants GM52216 and GM55425.

REFERENCES

1. S. Dey, and B.P. Rosen Mechanisms of drug transport in prokaryotes and eukaryotes, in Drug Transport in Antimicrobial and Anticancer Chemotherapy, N.H. Georgopapadakou, Editor. Dekker. (1995).

2. B.P. Rosen. Resistance mechanisms to arsenicals and antimonials. J Basic Clin Physiol Pharmacol. 6:251 (1995).

3. V.M. Hughes, and N. Datta. Conjugative plasmids in bacteria of the pre-antibiotic era. Nature. 302:725 (1983).

4. B.P. Rosen, S. Dey, and D. Dou Anion-translocating ATPases, in Biomembranes, Vol. 5, ATPase. Jai Press, Inc.: London. (1996).

5. B.P. Rosen. Bacterial resistance to heavy metals. J. Biol. Inorg. Chem. 1:273 (1996).

6. C.J. Bacchi. Resistance to clinical drugs in african trypanosomes. Parasitology Today. 9:190 (1993).

7. W.E. Gultridge, and G.H. Cooms, Biochemistry of parasitic protozoa. 1st ed: McMillan, London. (1977).

8. A.H. Fairlamb, and A. Cerami. Metabolism and functions of trypanothione in the Kinetoplastida. Annual Review of Microbiology. 46:695 (1992).

9. A.H. Fairlamb, K. Smith, and K.J. Hunter. The interaction of arsenical drugs with dihydrolipoamide and dihydrolipoamide dehydrogenase from arsenical resistant and sensitive strains of Trypanosoma brucei brucei. Molec & Biochem Parasitol. 53:223 (1992).

10. D.J. Steenkamp, and H.S. Spies. Identification of a major low-molecular-mass thiol of the trypanosomatid Crithidia fasciculata as ovothiol A. Facile isolation and structural analysis of the bimane derivative. Eur J Biochem. 223:43 (1994).

11. H.S. Spies, and D.J. Steenkamp. Thiols of intracellular pathogens. Identification of ovothiol A in Leishmania donovani and structural analysis of a novel thiol from Mycobacterium bovis. Eur J Biochem. 224:203 (1994).

12. A.H. Fairlamb, N.S. Carter, M. Cunningham, and K. Smith. Characterisation of melarsen-resistant Trypanosoma brucei brucei with respect to cross-resistance to other drugs and trypanothione metabolism. Mol Biochem Parasitol. 53:213 (1992).

13. T.O. Frommel, and A.E. Balber. Flow cytofluorimetric analysis of drug accumulation by multidrug- resistant Trypanosoma brucei brucei and T. b. rhodesiense. Mol Biochem Parasitol. 26:183 (1987).

14. N.S. Carter, and A.H. Fairlamb. Arsenical-resistant trypanosomes lack an unusual adenosine transporter. Nature. 361:173 (1993).

15. S.L. Croft, K.D. Neame, and C.A. Homewood. Accumulation of [125Sb]sodium stibogluconate by Leishmania mexicana amazonensis and Leishmania donovani in vitro. Comp Biochem Physiol C. 68C:95 (1981).

16. H.L. Callahan, and S.M. Beverley. Heavy metal resistance: a new role for P-glycoproteins in Leishmania. J Biol Chem. 266:18427 (1991).

17. M. Ouellette, D. Legare, and B. Papadopoulou. Microbial multidrug-resistance ABC transporters. Trends in Microbiology. 2:407 (1994).

18. K. Grondin, B. Papadopoulou, and M. Ouellette. Homologous recombination between direct repeat sequences yields P- glycoprotein containing amplicons in arsenite resistant Leishmania. Nucleic Acids Res. 21:1895 (1993).

19. S. Dey, B. Papadopoulou, A. Haimeur, G. Roy, K. Grondin, D. Dou, B.P. Rosen, and M. Ouellette. High level arsenite resistance in Leishmania tarentolae is mediated by an active extrusion system. Mol Biochem Parasitol. 67:49 (1994).

20. B. Papadopoulou, G. Roy, S. Dey, B.P. Rosen, and M. Ouellette. Contribution of the Leishmania P-glycoprotein-related gene ltpgpA to oxyanion resistance. J Biol Chem. 269;11980 (1994).

21. B. Papadopoulou, G. Roy, S. Dey, B.P. Rosen, M. Olivier, and M. Ouellette. Gene disruption of the P-glycoprotein related gene pgpa of Leishmania tarentolae. Biochem Biophys Res Commun. 224:772 (1996).

22. S. Dey, D. Dou, and B.P. Rosen. ATP-dependent arsenite transport in everted membrane vesicles of Escherichia coli. J Biol Chem. 269:25442 (1994).

23. S. Dey, M. Ouellette, J. Lightbody, B. Papadopoulou, and B.P. Rosen. An ATP-dependent As(III)-glutathione transport system in membrane vesicles of Leishmania tarentolae. Proc Natl Acad Sci U S A. 93:2192 (1996).

24. R. Mukhopadhyay, S. Dey, N. Xu, D. Gage, J. Lightbody, M. Ouellette, and B.P. Rosen. Trypanothione overproduction and resistance to antimonials and arsenicals in Leishmania. Proc Natl Acad Sci U S A. 93:10383 (1996).

25. M. Ouellette, B. Papadopoulou, A. Haimer, K. Grondin, E. Leblanc, D. Legare, and G. Roy Transport of antimonials and antifolates in drug resistant Leishmania, in Drug transport in antimicrobial and anticancer chemotherapy, N.H. Georgopadakou, Editor. Dekker: New York. (1995).

26. K. Grondin, A. Haimeur, R. Mukhopadhyay, B.P. Rosen, and M. Ouellette. Co-amplification of the gamma-glutamylcysteine synthetase gene gsh1 and of the ABC transporter gene pgpA in arsenite-resistant Leishmania tarentolae. Embo J. 16:3057 (1997).

27. D. Legare, B. Papadopoulou, G. Roy, R. Mukhopadhyay, A. Haimeur, S. Dey, K. Grondin, C. Brochu, B.P. Rosen, and M. Ouellette. Efflux systems and increased trypanothione levels in arsenite-resistant Leishmania. Exp Parasitol. 87:275 (1997).

28. Z. Wang, and T.G. Rossman. Stable and inducible arsenite resistance in Chinese hamster cells. Toxicol Appl Pharmacol. 118:80 (1993).

29. Z. Wang, S. Dey, B.P. Rosen, and T.G. Rossman. Efflux-mediated resistance to arsenicals in arsenic-resistant and - hypersensitive Chinese hamster cells. Toxicol Appl Pharmacol. 137:112 (1996).

30. J.F. Lo, H.F. Wang, M.F. Tam, and T.C. Lee. Glutathione S-transferase pi in an arsenic-resistant Chinese hamster ovary cell line. Biochem J. 288:977 (1992).

31. H.F. Wang, and T.C. Lee. Glutathione S-transferase pi facilitates the excretion of arsenic from arsenic-resistant Chinese hamster ovary cells. Biochem Biophys Res Commun. 192:1093 (1993).

32. M. Delnomdedieu, M.M. Basti, J.D. Otvos, and D.J. Thomas. Transfer of arsenite from glutathione to dithiols: a model of interaction. Chem Res Toxicol. 6:598 (1993).

33. M. Delnomdedieu, M.M. Basti, J.D. Otvos, and D.J. Thomas. Reduction and binding of arsenate and dimethylarsinate by glutathione: a magnetic resonance study. Chem Biol Interact. 90:139 (1994).

34. A. Gyurasics, F. Varga, and Z. Gregus. Glutathione-dependent biliary excretion of arsenic. Biochem Pharmacol. 42:465 (1991).

35. T. Ishikawa. The ATP-dependent glutathione S-conjugate export pump. Trends Biochem Sci. 17:463 (1992).

36. S.P. Cole, K.E. Sparks, K. Fraser, D.W. Loe, C.E. Grant, G.M. Wilson, and R.G. Deeley. Pharmacological characterization of multidrug resistant MRP-transfected human tumor cells. Cancer Res. 54:5902 (1994).

37. G.J. Zaman, J. Lankelma, O. van Tellingen, J. Beijnen, H. Dekker, C. Paulusma, R.P. Oude Elferink, F. Baas, and P. Borst. Role of glutathione in the export of compounds from cells by the multidrug-resistance-associated protein. Proc Natl Acad Sci U S A. 92:7690 (1995).

38. R. Wysocki, P. Bobrowicz, and S. Ulaszewski. The Saccharomyces cerevisiae ACR3 gene encodes a putative membrane protein involved in arsenite transport. J Biol Chem. 272:30061 (1997).

39. P. Bobrowicz, R. Wysocki, G. Owsianik, A. Goffeau, and S. Ulaszewski. Isolation of three contiguous genes, ACR1, ACR2 and ACR3, involved in resistance to arsenic compounds in the yeast Saccharomyces cerevisiae. Yeast. 13:819 (1997).

40. A. Carlin, W. Shi, S. Dey, and B.P. Rosen. The ars operon of Escherichia coli confers arsenical and antimonial resistance. J Bacteriol. 177:981 (1995).

41. O.I. Sanders, C. Rensing, M. Kuroda, B. Mitra, and B.P. Rosen. Antimonite is accumulated by the glycerol facilitator GlpF in Escherichia coli. J Bacteriol. 179:3365 (1997).

42. S. Silver, and L.T. Phung. Bacterial heavy metal resistance: new surprises. Annu Rev Microbiol. 50:753 (1996).

43. G. Ji, and S. Silver. Regulation and expression of the arsenic resistance operon from Staphylococcus aureus plasmid pI258. J Bacteriol. 174:3684 (1992).

44. R. Rosenstein, A. Peschel, B. Wieland, and F. Gotz. Expression and regulation of the antimonite, arsenite, and arsenate resistance operon of Staphylococcus xylosus plasmid pSX267. J Bacteriol. 174:3676 (1992).

45. H.J. Sofia, V. Burland, D.L. Daniels, G. Plunkett, 3rd, and F.R. Blattner. Analysis of the Escherichia coli genome. V. DNA sequence of the region from 76.0 to 81.5 minutes. Nucleic Acids Res. 22:2576 (1994).

46. C.M. Chen, T.K. Misra, S. Silver, and B.P. Rosen. Nucleotide sequence of the structural genes for an anion pump. The plasmid-encoded arsenical resistance operon. J Biol Chem. 261:15030 (1986).

47. D.F. Bruhn, J. Li, S. Silver, F. Roberto, and B.P. Rosen. The arsenical resistance operon of IncN plasmid R46. FEMS Microbiol Lett. 139:149 (1996).

48. K. Suzuki, N. Wakao, T. Kimura, K. Sakka, and K. Ohmiya. Expression and Regulation of the Arsenic Resistance Operon of Acidiphillium multivorum AIU301 Plasmid pKW301 in Escherichia coli. Applied and Environmental Microbiology. 64:411 (1998).

49. H.L. Mobley, and B.P. Rosen. Energetics of plasmid-mediated arsenate resistance in Escherichia coli. Proc Natl Acad Sci U S A. 79:6119 (1982).

50. S. Silver, and D. Keach. Energy-dependent arsenate efflux: the mechanism of plasmid-mediated resistance. Proc Natl Acad Sci U S A. 79:6114 (1982).

51. J. Wu, and B.P. Rosen. The ArsR protein is a trans-acting regulatory protein. Mol Microbiol. 5:1331 (1991).

52. J. Wu, and B.P. Rosen. The arsD gene encodes a second trans-acting regulatory protein of the plasmid-encoded arsenical resistance operon. Mol Microbiol. 8:615 (1993).

53. S. Dey, D. Dou, L.S. Tisa, and B.P. Rosen. Interaction of the catalytic and the membrane subunits of an oxyanion- translocating ATPase. Arch Biochem Biophys. 311:418 (1994).

54. C.M. Hsu, and B.P. Rosen. Characterization of the catalytic subunit of an anion pump. J Biol Chem. 264:17349 (1989).

55. L.S. Tisa, and B.P. Rosen. Molecular characterization of an anion pump. The ArsB protein is the membrane anchor for the ArsA protein. J Biol Chem. 265:190 (1990).

56. K.L. Oden, T.B. Gladysheva, and B.P. Rosen. Arsenate reduction mediated by the plasmid-encoded ArsC protein is coupled to glutathione. Mol Microbiol. 12:301 (1994).

57. T.B. Gladysheva, K.L. Oden, and B.P. Rosen. Properties of the arsenate reductase of plasmid R773. Biochemistry. 33:7288 (1994).

58. J.E. Walker, M. Saraste, M.J. Runswick, and N.J. Gay. Distantly related sequences in the alpha- and beta-subunits of ATP synthase, myosin, kinases and other ATP-requiring enzymes and a common nucleotide binding fold. Embo J. 1:945 (1982).

59. B.P. Rosen, U. Weigel, C. Karkaria, and P. Gangola. Molecular characterization of an anion pump. The arsA gene product is an arsenite(antimonate)-stimulated ATPase. J Biol Chem. 263:3067 (1988).

60. H. Bhattacharjee, J. Li, M.Y. Ksenzenko, and B.P. Rosen. Role of cysteinyl residues in metalloactivation of the oxyanion- translocating ArsA ATPase. J Biol Chem. 270:11245 (1995).

61. H. Bhattacharjee, and B.P. Rosen. Spatial proximity of Cys113, Cys172, and Cys422 in the metalloactivation domain of the ArsA ATPase. J Biol Chem. 271:24465 (1996).

62. S. Lutsenko, and J.H. Kaplan. Organization of P-type ATPases: significance of structural diversity. Biochemistry. 34:15607 (1995).

63. C.E. Karkaria, and B.P. Rosen. Trinitrophenyl-ATP binding to the ArsA protein: the catalytic subunit of an anion pump. Arch Biochem Biophys. 288:107 (1991).

64. C.E. Karkaria, C.M. Chen, and B.P. Rosen. Mutagenesis of a nucleotide-binding site of an anion-translocating ATPase. J Biol Chem. 265:7832 (1990).

65. P. Kaur, and B.P. Rosen. Mutagenesis of the C-terminal nucleotide-binding site of an anion- translocating ATPase. J Biol Chem. 267:19272 (1992).

66. J. Li, S. Liu, and B.P. Rosen. Interaction of ATP binding sites in the ArsA ATPase, the catalytic subunit of the Ars pump. J Biol Chem. 271:25247 (1996).

67. P. Kaur, and B.P. Rosen. Identification of the site of [α-32P]ATP adduct formation in the ArsA protein. Biochemistry. 33:6456 (1994).

68. S. Ramaswamy, and P. Kaur. Nucleotide binding to the C-terminal nucleotide binding domain of ArsA: Studies with an ATP analogue, 5' -p-fluorosulfonylbenzoyladenosine. Journal of Biological Chemistry. in press: (1998).

69. P. Kaur, and B.P. Rosen. Complementation between nucleotide binding domains in an anion- translocating ATPase. J Bacteriol. 175:351 (1993).

70. P. Kaur, and B.P. Rosen. In vitro assembly of an anion-stimulated ATPase from peptide fragments. J Biol Chem. 269:9698 (1994).

71. J. Li, and B.P. Rosen. Steric limitations in the interaction of the ATP binding domains of the ArsA ATPase. J Biol Chem. in press: (1998).

72. C. Hsu, P. Kaur, C.E. Karkaria, R.F. Steiner, and B.P. Rosen. Substrate-induced dimerization of the ArsA protein, the catalytic component of an anion-translocating ATPase. J Biol Chem. 266:2327 (1991).

73. J.P. Abrahams, A.G. Leslie, R. Lutter, and J.E. Walker. Structure at 2.8 Å resolution of F1-ATPase from bovine heart mitochondria. Nature. 370:621 (1994).

74. T. Zhou, and B.P. Rosen. Tryptophan fluorescence reports nucleotide-induced conformational changes in a domain of the ArsA ATPase. J Biol Chem. 272:19731 (1997).

75. T. Zhou, S. Liu, and B.P. Rosen. Interaction of substrate and effector binding sites in the ArsA ATPase. Biochemistry. 34:13622 (1995).

76. J. Wu, L.S. Tisa, and B.P. Rosen. Membrane topology of the ArsB protein, the membrane subunit of an anion- translocating ATPase. J Biol Chem. 267:12570 (1992).

77. P.C. Maloney. Bacterial transporters. Curr Opin Cell Biol. 6:571 (1994).

78. S. Dey, and B.P. Rosen. Dual mode of energy coupling by the oxyanion-translocating ArsB protein. J Bacteriol. 177:385 (1995).

79. E.A. Berger, and L.A. Heppel. Different mechanisms of energy coupling for the shock-sensitive and shock-resistant amino acid permeases of Escherichia coli. J Biol Chem. 249:7747 (1974).

80. M. Kuroda, S. Dey, O.I. Sanders, and B.P. Rosen. Alternate energy coupling of ArsB, the membrane subunit of the Ars anion-translocating ATPase. J Biol Chem. 272:326 (1997).

81. B.P. Rosen, and M.G. Borbolla. A plasmid-encoded arsenite pump produces arsenite resistance in Escherichia coli. Biochem Biophys Res Commun. 124:760 (1984).

82. B.P. Rosen, S. Dey, D. Dou, G. Ji, P. Kaur, M. Ksenzenko, S. Silver, and J. Wu. Evolution of an ion-translocating ATPase. Ann N Y Acad Sci. 671:257 (1992).

83. B.P. Rosen, Bhattacharjee, H. and Shi, W.P. Mechanisms of metalloactivation of an anion-translocating AT-Pase. J. Bioenerget. Biomemb. 27:85 (1995).

84. Y. Chen, S. Dey, and B.P. Rosen. Soft metal thiol chemistry is not involved in the transport of arsenite by the Ars pump. J Bacteriol. 178:911 (1996).

85. P.A. de Boer, R.E. Crossley, A.R. Hand, and L.I. Rothfield. The MinD protein is a membrane ATPase required for the correct placement of the Escherichia coli division site. Embo J. 10:4371 (1991).

86. S.T. Murphy, D.M. Jackman, and M.E. Mulligan. Cloning and nucleotide sequence of the gene for dinitrogenase reductase (nifH) from the heterocyst-forming cyanobacterium Anabaena sp. L31. Biochim Biophys Acta. 1171:337 (1993).

87. S. Chung, G. Frank, H. Zuber, and D.A. Bryant. Genes encoding two chlorosome components from the green sulfur bacteria Chlorobium vibrioforme strain 8327D and Chlorobium tepidum. Photosynthesis Research. 41:261 (1994).

88. C.J. Bult, O. White, G.J. Olsen, L. Zhou, R.D. Fleischmann, G.G. Sutton, J.A. Blake, L.M. FitzGerald, R.A. Clayton, J.D. Gocayne, A.R. Kerlavage, B.A. Dougherty, J.F. Tomb, M.D. Adams, C.I. Reich, R. Overbeek, E.F. Kirkness, K.G. Weinstock, J.M. Merrick, A. Glodek, et al. Complete genome sequence of the methanogenic archaeon, Methanococcus jannaschii. Science. 273:1058 (1996).

89. B. Kurdi-Haidar, S. Aebi, D. Heath, R.E. Enns, P. Naredi, D.K. Hom, and S.B. Howell. Isolation of the ATP-binding human homolog of the arsA component of the bacterial arsenite transporter. Genomics. 36:486 (1996).

90. J. Sulston, Z. Du, K. Thomas, R. Wilson, L. Hillier, R. Staden, N. Halloran, P. Green, J. Thierry-Mieg, L. Qiu, and et al. The C. elegans genome sequencing project: a beginning. Nature. 356:37 (1992).

91. J. Boskovic, A. Soler-Mira, J.M. Garcia-Cantalejo, J.P. Ballesta, A. Jimenez, and M. Remacha. The sequence of a 16,691 bp segment of Saccharomyces cerevisiae chromosome IV identifies the DUN1, PMT1, PMT5, SRP14 and DPR1 genes, and five new open reading frames. Yeast. 12:1377 (1996).

92. H.G. Yan, and M.D. Tsai. Mechanism of adenylate kinase. Demonstration of a functional relationship between aspartate 93 and Mg2+ by site-directed mutagenesis and proton, phosphorus-31, and magnesium-25 NMR. Biochemistry. 30:5539 (1991).

93. R.M. Story, and T.A. Steitz. Structure of the recA protein-ADP complex. Nature. 355:374 (1992).

94. W. Shi, J. Wu, and B.P. Rosen. Identification of a putative metal binding site in a new family of metalloregulatory proteins. J Biol Chem. 269:19826 (1994).

95. W. Shi, J. Dong, R.A. Scott, M.Y. Ksenzenko, and B.P. Rosen. The role of arsenic-thiol interactions in metalloregulation of the ars operon. J Biol Chem. 271:2427 (1996).

96. H.P. Klenk, R.A. Clayton, J.F. Tomb, O. White, K.E. Nelson, K.A. Ketchum, R.J. Dodson, M. Gwinn, E.K. Hickey, J.D. Peterson, D.L. Richardson, A.R. Kerlavage, D.E. Graham, N.C. Kyrpides, R.D. Fleischmann, J. Quackenbush, N.H. Lee, G.G. Sutton, S. Gill, E.F. Kirkness, et al. The complete genome sequence of the hyperthermophilic, sulphate- reducing archaeon Archaeoglobus fulgidus. Nature. 390:364 (1997).

97. D.R. Smith, L.A. Doucette-Stamm, C. Deloughery, H. Lee, J. Dubois, T. Aldredge, R. Bashirzadeh, D. Blakely, R. Cook, K. Gilbert, D. Harrison, L. Hoang, P. Keagle, W. Lumm, B. Pothier, D. Qiu, R. Spadafora, R. Vicaire, Y. Wang, J. Wierzbowski, et al. Complete genome sequence of Methanobacterium thermoautotrophicum deltaH: functional analysis and comparative genomics. J Bacteriol. 179:7135 (1997).

98. T. Kaneko, S. Sato, H. Kotani, A. Tanaka, E. Asamizu, Y. Nakamura, N. Miyajima, M. Hirosawa, M. Sugiura, S. Sasamoto, T. Kimura, T. Hosouchi, A. Matsuno, A. Muraki, N. Nakazaki, K. Naruo, S. Okumura, S. Shimpo, C. Takeuchi, T. Wada, et al. Sequence analysis of the genome of the unicellular cyanobacterium Synechocystis sp. strain PCC6803. II. Sequence determination of the entire genome and assignment of potential protein-coding regions. DNA Res. 3:109 (1996).

99. K. Takemaru, M. Mizuno, T. Sato, M. Takeuchi, and Y. Kobayashi. Complete nucleotide sequence of a skin element excised by DNA rearrangement during sporulation in Bacillus subtilis. Microbiology. 141:323 (1995).

10

THE IMPACT OF BACTERIAL GENOMICS ON ANTIBACTERIAL DISCOVERY

David J. C. Knowles[1] and Frank King[2]

[1]Ladywell House
York Road, Boroughbridge
York YO51 9EB, UK
[2]New Frontiers Science Park (North)
SmithKline Beecham Pharmaceuticals
Harlow, Essex CM19 5AW, UK

INTRODUCTION

The period between 1945 and 1970 has been described as the 'golden age' of antibiotic discovery. Large scale screening programmes for new antibiotics within the pharmaceutical industry resulted in the discovery of virtually all the current, structurally diverse, antibiotic classes with clinical utility. Indeed, based on the perceived potential for these drugs, by the end of the 1960's it was widely believed that bacterial infection would soon be conquered. This apparent success in infection control caused a number of pharmaceutical companies to reduce their antibacterial research effort in favour of alternative therapeutic areas. Some even exited the field entirely.

Those companies that continued antibacterial research have faced technological and commercial barriers to the discovery of new drugs and it is a fact that no new classes of antibiotic (defined as acting on a new bacterial molecular target) have been commercialised in the last 25 years (Bax, 1997). The traditional, semi-empiric approaches of chemical modification of known antibiotic classes and the search for new structures *via* natural product screening programmes have yielded progressively fewer development candidates. More often than not, the compounds identified could not be progressed on commercial grounds because their advantages over existing, increasingly generic, antibiotics were largely incremental and not sufficient to justify the development costs.

Against this background, antimicrobial drug resistance, arising through genetic transfer and mutation, has become a mounting and threatening public health problem (Cohen, 1992; Neu, 1992; Tomasz, 1994; Tenover & Hughes, 1996; Kunin, 1997). For example, strains of bacteria now exist which remain susceptible to only a single clinically

Resolving the Antibiotic Paradox, edited by Rosen and Mobashery.
Kluwer Academic / Plenum Publishers, New York, 1998.

available antibiotic, vancomycin. Furthermore, vancomycin resistance in enterococci has been described as the 'Physician's worst nightmare' (Travis, 1994), since its spread to staphylococci and pneumococci would place many common diseases beyond the reach of effective therapy. The recent reports of vancomycin-resistant *Staphylococcus aureus* from Japan (Hiramatsu *et al.,* 1997a&b) are therefore of real concern and strengthen the need for new antibacterial drugs which are not subject to current resistance mechanisms.

Thankfully, this worsening medical situation is occurring during something of a renaissance of both biological and chemical sciences, being driven principally by revolutions in genomics and medicinal chemistry respectively. As a consequence, the pharmaceutical and biotechnology industries, which have made major investments in the development and application of a vast array of associated technologies, now have the means to break the apparent deadlock in the discovery of radically new anti-infective agents. To do this, two principle technical hurdles, at the very beginning of the discovery process, need to be overcome. These relate to the paucity of new molecular targets and to the limited chemical diversity available for screening

This chapter describes the impact of these scientific revolutions on the discovery of new classes of anti-infectives.

Microbial Genomic Sequencing

A systematic approach to the identification of new therapeutic molecular targets is now afforded by the recent progress made in bacterial genome sequencing. Bacterial genomes are comparatively small (between 0.6 and 6Mb) and since a high proportion of their DNA sequence encodes gene products, it is now cost-effective to sequence entire genomic libraries to facilitate the search for new molecular targets for classes of anti-infective therapies.

In 1994, SmithKline Beecham began a bacterial genome sequencing initiative involving two key Gram positive pathogens, *Staphyolococcus aureus* and *Streptococcus pneumoniae*. The first complete bacterial genome sequence (*Haemophilus influenzae*) was published in 1995 (Fleischmann et al., 1995). Since then, the number of microbial

Table 1. Microbial genomes: Complete sequences in the public domain

Organism	Size (Mb)	Reference
Eubacteria		
Aquifex aeolicus	1.50	Deckert et al. (1998)
Bacillus subtilis	4.20	Kunst et al. (1997)
Borrelia burgdorferi	1.44	Fraser et al. (1997)
Escherichia coli K-12	4.60	Blattner et al. (1997)
Haemophilus influenzae Rd	1.83	Fleischmann et al. (1995)
Helicobacter pylori	1.66	Tomb et al. (1997)
Mycoplasma genitalium	0.58	Fraser et al. (1995)
Mycoplasma pneumoniae	0.81	Himmelreich et al. (1996)
Synechocystis sp.	3.57	Kaneko et al. (1996)
Archaea		
Archaeoglobus fulgidus	2.18	Klenk et al. (1997)
Methanobacterium thermoautotrophicum	1.75	Smith et al. (1997)
Methanococcus jannaschii	1.66	Bult et al.(1996)
Eukaryotes		
Saccharomyces cerevisiae	13	Goffeau et al. (1997)

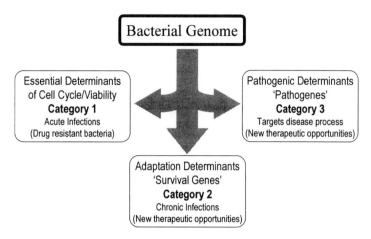

Figure 1. Potential for genomics in anti-infective discovery.

genomes sequenced has expanded explosively. There are now thirteen completed and published microbial genomes (Table 1) and at least nine more are expected to be completed in 1998.

There are also proprietary genome sequence databases, containing annotated sequence data from many pathogenic bacteria available to subscribers. Additionally, there are considered to be at least another 43 microbial genomes in the process of being sequenced (Ash, 1997; see also the TIGR website http://www.tigr.org/tigr_home/tdb/mdb/mdb.html) The rapidity by which progress is being made in this area is such that it is anticipated that 100 bacterial genomes will have been sequenced by the year 2000 (Metting and Romine, 1997).

IDENTIFICATION OF MOLECULAR TARGETS FROM GENOMIC SEQUENCE

Completed bacterial genome sequences, correctly assembled and annotated, obviously contain all therapeutic molecular targets associated with the pathogens themselves. The challenge is to identify them.

Fundamentally, these molecular targets can be classified into three different categories (Fig. 1).

Essential Determinants of Cell Cycle and Viability

All antibiotics used medically today either inhibit bacterial growth or are otherwise lethal to susceptible bacteria. Their principle molecular targets represent essential determinants of cell growth and viability *in vitro* and the identification of new targets is required to circumvent many existing antibiotic resistance determinants.

Even from a purely numerical standpoint, the impact that bacterial genomics is set to make in this context is substantial. An organism such as *Staphylococcus aureus* with a genome size of 2.8Mb, contains ~2000 genes, approximately 10% of which (200) may be essential for bacterial growth *in vitro*. The proportion of such genes common to a range of different pathogens is not yet known but if new antibiotics are successfully developed that interact with the gene products of only 5% of the 200 such potential molecular targets, this would represent 10 new antibiotic classes. This alone would more than double the number of antibiotic classes currently available for medical use.

A rapid means of identifying such new molecular targets is by homlogy to genes known to be essential in other organisms. Often however, the extent of homology may be sufficient only to indicate putative biochemical function without giving any information regarding the physiological role of the gene product. For example, there are 80 ABC transporters in *Escherichia coli* K-12 (Blattner et al., 1997), many of which are not well characterised. Perhaps of greater importance to drug discovery is the fact that when the full *E.coli* sequence was published, 38% of the protein coding regions annotated (over 1600 genes) had no attributed function (Blattner et al., 1997). Clearly, the systematic disruption of such genes represents an additional and necessary approach to obtain the full list of potential essential targets.

Prioritisation of this list of targets for screen development is still largely pragmatic. Attributes used frequently include the likely cellular location of the expressed gene product, its similarity to known human genes and any detailed information regarding its biochemical mechanism. Molecular targets external to the plasma membrane avoid issues of cell penetration and lack of extensive homology to known human genes can provide a degree of comfort with regard to the likelyhood of developing bacterio-selective agents. Information on function can clearly help guide the discovery of inhibitors (see below).

Adaptation and Pathogenicity Determinants

Genomic sequence information from pathogenic microorganisms also offers the exciting prospect of expanding the horizons for anti-infective therapy beyond the confines of agents that are merely bactericidal or bacteriostatic. The identification of molecular targets associated with bacterial adaptation/survival in infection and indeed those associated directly with the disease process (pathogenesis) provide an additional focus for anti-infective therapy. Compounds acting on such targets may significantly improve the prospects of treating severely immunocompromised patients or those suffering from chronic infections, for whom current treatment is frequently suboptimal.

These molecular targets represent gene products which may not be essential to micro-organisms growing *in vitro* but which are essential for bacteria to survive in infection foci and cause disease. The reason for differentiating these two target categories is that different search strategies can sometimes be adopted. Some adaptation determinants may be identified *in vitro* more readily than pathogenic determinants, for example by subjecting bacteria to various culture conditions and environmental stresses. The identification of suitable pathogenic determinants as molecular targets generally requires animal infection models that closely mimic the human disease and/or a detailed knowledge of aspects of the disease process that can be modelled *in vitro*.

The laboratory techniques developed to identify such determinants generally answer one of two basic questions; (1) what bacterial genes are expressed during infection? and (2) what bacterial genes are essential to infection?

All such genes, including some which currently have no known function, constitute potential drug targets and although some of the experimental approaches are not totally reliant on genomic sequence information, such knowledge considerably speeds the identification process. Access to large amounts of genomic sequence provides full length sequences of the genes of interest and an understanding of local gene architecture (to identify potential polarity effects related to highlighted genes). In addition, the need to clone genes for subsequent expression and/or genetic disruption studies is substantially reduced, if not removed altogether.

The use of bacterial gene expression data in the identification of drug targets relies on the premise that if a particular gene is expressed/upregulated in disease, it at least represents a possible drug target. The corollary is false (that if expression of a particular gene is not detected it is unlikely to be a good target) since it is probable that certain key genes are weakly expressed and fall below the detection level of some of the techniques mentioned below.

In its first manifestation, IVET (In Vivo Expression Technologies) constituted a positive selection strategy whereby populations of *Samonella typhimurium purA* mutants (purine auxotrophs containing a promotorless purA gene hooked up to random *S. typhimurium* DNA fragments) were inoculated into mice (Mahan et al., 1993a). Only those bacteria in which the random genome fragment contained a promoter which resulted in the expression of PurA during infection were able to multiply *in vivo*. The technique carried a subtle refinement in that the promotorless purA gene was transcriptionally fused to a lacZ reporter gene. Bacteria isolated from the animal formed blue colonies if the gene was 'on' *in vitro* but white if 'off' *in vitro*. Attention could therefore be focused on DNA fragments that switched *purA* 'on' *in vivo* and 'off' *in vitro* and the genomic fragment. A potential limitation of positive selection in this context is that the unidentified promoter would need to be 'on' throughout most of the infection in order to be well represented in the pool of isolated bacteria.

A subsequent IVET approach, based on enrichment rather than positive selection, was later developed that circumvented this issue (Mahan et al., 1993b). A promoter-less resolvase was used in conjunction with an antibiotic resistance gene flanked by two resolvase cleavage sites. If a fragment of DNA inserted upstream of the resolvase contained a promoter which switched it on, even transiently, the resistance determinant would be clipped out and the bacterium became antibiotic-sensitive. Comparison of the genomic fragments associated with reversion to antibiotic sensitivity with the originating genome reveals genes of potential relevance to infection. Other variations of this IVET approach have also been reported (Mahan et al., 1995).

Signature tagged mutagenesis (STM) takes this concept a stage further by identifying genes which are not only expressed, but which are essential, to infection in laboratory animals (Hensel et al., 1995; Shea et al., 1996; Mei et al., 1997). Pools of independently tagged, unknown mutants are inoculated into animals. After the infection has become established, bacterial mutants with disrupted genes essential for infection, will not be represented amongst those subsequently recovered from the animal. Comparison of the 'input' mutant pools with the 'output' pools by hybridisation using the molecular tags as probes, reveals such mutants by their absence. Again, access to genomic information shortens the time to identify the nature of such negatively selected genes, which by definition, have been shown to be essential for infection.

Various non-genetic approaches have also been used to identify potentially therapeutically relevant genes in a number of important pathogens. These include subtractive hybridisation techniques and global transcript analysis. Examples of the use of subtractive hybridisation can be found in *Listeria monocytogenes* (Utt et al., 1995), *Haemophilus influenzae* (Utt and Quinn, 1994) and *Mycobacterium tuberculosis* (Kikuta-Oshima et al., 1994). However, it is likely that global transcript analysis will become much more widely used in the next few years.

There have already been a number of approaches based on global transcript analysis. Chuang et al. (1993) used reverse transcriptase to prepare cDNA from *Escherichia coli* re-

covered from infected gnotobiotic mice, followed by dot-blot hybridisation to an ordered
E. coli genomic library. A multiplex PCR-based approach, using primers based on open
reading frames identified from SmithKline Beecham's genomics database, has been used
to good effect to highlight genes expressed during infection (M. Burhnam et al., unpublished, see Knowles, 1997). Recent reports of using micro-array, chip-based technologies
to examine mRNA expression in bacteria and fungi (de Saizieu et al., 1998; Wodicka et
al., 1997) may provide a rapid and highly sensitive 'snapshot' of microbial gene expression under a variety of different conditions. This may ultimately lead to the identification
of regulatory genetic networks associated with disease (de Saizieu et al., 1998), particularly if coupled with data relating to global gene expression at the protein level by 2D gel
electrophoresis (Schmid et al., 1997; Bernhardt et al., 1997). From this information, it is
anticipated that further candidates for gene disruption experiments can be selected.

The application of the molecular techniques referred to above will undoubtedly lead
to the identification of a wide range of new drug targets for subsequent screening of in-
hibitors/mediators. In cases where the biochemical function of a target gene product can
be deduced directly from the gene sequence (e.g. a novel protease), a suitable biochemical
screen can be readily configured. In other cases, cell-based screens, exploiting a characteristic phenotype bestowed by the disrupted gene, may be more appropriate.

Although in many instances, natural product libraries will no doubt continue to provide an excellent starting place for lead generation (Demain, 1998), the major response to
the impact of genomics in drug discovery has been in the area of medicinal chemistry.
Furthermore, advances in screening technologies mean that the prospect of screening tens,
and even hundreds, of thousands of compounds in just one day is becoming a reality (Rogers, 1997). It is against this background that medicinal chemists are facing their greatest
challenge yet.

THE CHALLENGES TO MEDICINAL CHEMISTRY

Historically, the number of different kinds of targets successfully addressed by traditional medicinal chemistry has been relatively limited. The genomics-based approaches
discussed above are likely to identify a rich and diverse collection of proteins, some of
which will act by totally novel mechanisms. These will require novel types of molecules
to intervene in the required manner. This poses a problem since the current compound
banks of pharmaceutical companies contain a historical bias towards previously examined
receptor and enzyme targets. Thus the probability of finding molecules among these libraries, that interact with totally novel systems is likely to be low. We have already seen
early signs of this phenomenon. For example, the Abbott screening of bacterial topoisomerase I produced few leads, none of which were believed to be suitable for designing
drugs (Lerner et al., 1996).

A separate generic issue is that potency of a molecule for its target is just one of the
attributes necessary for successful development of a new antibiotic. The majority of targets identified via genomics are likely to be intracellular targets, thus the molecules will
need to penetrate the bacterial cell wall. If a broad spectrum (Gram negative and Gram
positive) agent is required, then two totally different penetration issues will be encountered and some balance of properties will be required to optimise its antibacterial potential
(Nikaido and Vaara, 1985). The molecular properties required for bacterial cell wall penetration are poorly understood. In addition, antibacterial activity alone does not produce a
drug, as evidenced from the exceptionally high failure rate of antibacterials in develop-

ment (>95%) for metabolism and pharmacokinetic reasons (Halliday et al., 1992). Thus the properties required for bacterial cell penetration are not necessarily the properties required for good oral absorption, or aqueous solubility for a parenteral product, or for maintenance of blood levels and appropriate distribution kinetics.

The magnitude of these challenges cannot be understated, so how is the medicinal chemist tackling these challenges?

COMBINATORIAL CHEMISTRY

Lead Identification

An obvious pre-requisite of any pharmaceutical is possession of appropriate activity at the target and the initial attempt to find this will be invariably by high throughput screening. Success or failure will depend upon the size, quality and diversity of the compound "bank". This problem was first encountered in the late 80's and early 90's by the biotechnology industry. Many such companies had access to good, validated biological targets, but did not have large banks of compounds for screening. The need to produce a large number of compounds as quickly as possible gave rise to the birth of combinatorial chemistry in which relatively few reactions can generate large numbers of compounds. This same issue is now faced throughout the pharmaceutical industry in companies working on new, genomics-derived, molecular targets. In many cases, appropriate classes of chemicals interacting with such molecular targets are poorly represented within existing compound banks. If the target is totally novel, with low homology to any known target and no known mediators (exactly the kinds of targets that may come from genomics), the problem is even worse!

The "split and mix" procedure on solid phase leads to each bead containing a single chemical entity and very large libraries are possible. This was amply illustrated by Lam and co-workers. (Lam et al., 1991) in the generation of a pentapeptide library "in a few days" using 19 naturally-encoded amino acids to afford 19^5 (~2.5M) peptides on beads where each bead carries only one peptide. The production of these libraries was coupled with novel screening methodologies, in this case biopanning with a monoclonal antibody against beta-endorphin identified high affinity peptide ligands. The whole library was screened "in an afternoon" and the active peptides identified by microsequencing from a single bead. However, for such large libraries with less amenable acceptor molecules, the identification of the active component is an issue, although an iterative method for the identification of sub-nM hexapeptide antagonists for the opioid receptors from a >52 million member library has been described (Dooley et al., 1993). This challenge of identifying the active component from the library has also been addressed in several highly innovative ways, for example parallel tagging of the beads (Nestler et al., 1994) or by affinity capillary electophoresis coupled with mass spectrometric identification of the ligand (Chu et al., 1995).

Such large libraries have been effective for identifying lead molecules, but successful screening of bead-bound libraries is limited to soluble targets with highly accessible binding sites. An alternative procedure is to cleave the library, then screen the mixture with an immobilized target, but again this is limited to functionally relevant targets that can be immobilised. Under more standard screening procedures, deconvolution can become a nightmare and cross-compound interference such as positive, mutual enhancement of activity, can lead to hits on screening which disappear on deconvolution. A way to avoid this is by screening much smaller sub-libraries (~20–100 compounds), perfectly possible with the "split and mix" procedure which simplifies deconvolution and reduces the risk of false positives.

As each bead contains only one compound, the above risks and the problems of deconvolution can be eliminated by bead arraying and partial cleavage of the compound. With the advent of ultra-high throughput screening, the screening of hundreds of thousands of compounds becomes a reality. Thus the individual beads in these libraries can be separated, cleaved and tested as individual compounds. By using the larger beads, it is possible to produce sufficient compound on a single bead for multiple screens whilst retaining material on the bead for additional cleavage and identification, either spectroscopically (e.g. by NMR, Keifer, 1997) or by cleaving the parallel tag. Statistically, for libraries with n components, a selection of n beads only samples 65% of compounds. To sample a satisfactory number of components, 3 fold oversampling is often used to get ~95% of compounds (~0.95n). However, where biological evaluation is rate limiting, alternative strategies need to be employed. Multiple beads can be cleaved and the compounds tested as mixtures, and with small numbers, deconvolution by retesting single beads is not an issue. An alternative approach, where the chemistry is possible, is to make the original library three times bigger, 3n components. A single arraying of that library, covering ~65% of compounds, would then test over twice as many compounds for the same number of screens (~1.95n).

In Vitro Lead Optimisation

There is a growing opinion that combinatorial libraries may only produce ~10% of drug candidates, so that in the majority of cases in vitro and/or in vivo optimisation of the combinatorial lead will be needed (Metcalf, 1998). The screening of library mixtures would not give structure activity relationship information (SAR) suitable for lead optimisation, although screening of diverse, well characterised sub-libraries may provide information on modifications leading to inactivity. For SAR the chemist needs individual data on validated, well characterised individual compounds. Bead arraying methodology is also not appropriate due to the generally lower compound validation standards, uncertainty over the concentration of compound being tested and to the inability to test all of the compounds prepared, even with 3-fold oversampling. Therefore to overcome the limitations of traditional iterative chemistry, rapid parallel synthesis methodologies are being used. Various scenarios are possible and will be discussed below.

If the lead has come from a solid-phase synthesized library, then the same synthetic methodology can be applied to the rapid synthesis of individual compounds. There have been considerable advances in the versatility of synthesis machines capable of automated solid phase synthesis under ever refined conditions of high and low temperatures and inert atmospheres. There has also been a rapid increase in the number of reactions possible on solid phase (Hermkens et al., 1996; Hermkens et al., 1997) and an ever increasing selection of linkers to the resin. Most linker groups require residual functionality which, if not an essential component of the pharmacophore of the active series, can severely limit analogue design. However, "traceless" linkers have been designed, for example the arylsilane linker developed within SmithKline Beecham laboratories (Chenera et al., 1995), which can be either protodesilylated, or removed with an alternative electrophile to add diversity at the point of attachment. An alternative solid phase approach is to use the IRORI SMART technology in which the resin is contained within a MicroKan or MicroTube including a radio-marker that is used to follow and identify the reaction history (Nicolaou et al., 1997).

Alternatively, if the lead has come from compound bank screening, solid phase synthesis may not be immediately applicable. Depending upon the complexity of the chemistry, rapid solution phase synthesis may be possible, again with the help of automated synthesisers capable of solution-phase techniques (Storer, 1996). Most currently available machines are limited in their solution phase capability but there are some very exciting parallel synthesis automated machines on the horizon which overcome many of the limitations of current machines in terms of reaction condition versatility and liquid handling techniques.

However, if none of these techniques is applicable to the lead molecule, the medicinal chemist may have to resort to initial traditional iterative synthesis with the aim of simplifying the chemistry so that automation now becomes a possibility. For example, the lead molecule may have an ethylene link, but the amide may retain activity but, say, 10 fold lower potency. Amide synthesis is exquisitely applicable to rapid parallel synthesis, with acids and amines very readily available, so the SAR optimisation could be automated on the less active series, and the lessons learnt from that applied to the more active, but more intractable series. The assumption is that the SAR's of the two series are roughly parallel, and care must be taken to ensure that this assumption is reasonably valid. This approach is a risk and a judgement decision must be made of a case-by-case basis depending upon the likelihood of success. However, with the pressure on for quick results, the plethora of targets, and hopefully the increased number of lead compounds available, the possibility of a rapid synthesis approach is becoming a key selection criterion for progression of a research effort.

STRUCTURE-BASED DESIGN

Although the power of combinatorial chemistry to generate ever increasingly diverse masses of compounds is fulfilling a need, the potential of structure-based design should not be forgotten. The ready availability of recombinant proteins, either in their natural form or with specific site directed mutagenesis, makes knowledge-based design an ever more attractive alternative. This approach has a number of advantages including giving much more knowledge about the target and how it interacts with the natural and unnatural mediators. This information is invaluable in in vitro lead optimisation where structural information of ligand-target complexes supplements the traditional "black-box SAR" and is essential for de novo design.

The further potential for structure-based design has recently been elegantly exemplified by the "SAR by NMR" technique where two simple molecules which interact at two adjacent sites on the target are identified from NMR (Shuker et al., 1996). This is conceptually equivalent to the independent identification of two elements of a pharmacophore. The appropriate linking of these elements can have a marked co-operative effect to the affinity, thus from separate mM binding affinity components, sub-μM leads can be identified.

IN VIVO LEAD OPTIMISATION

Whilst relatively large quantities of compounds are required for whole animal pharmacokinetic and/or pharmacodynamic studies, compounds will need to be prepared individually. These animal studies are normally rate-limiting to progress, although combinatorial pharmacokinetic methods are being investigated (Halm, 1996). Therefore where these in vivo methods are required, rapid, parallel synthesis of compounds is unlikely to reduce the cycle times. However, more and more we are using in vitro techniques earlier in Discovery to help with the in vivo lead optimisation process. A consciousness of physicochemical parameters, such as those based on the "Lipinski rule of 5" (Lipinski et al., 1997) in the design of libraries and individual compounds should improve the chances of adequate in vivo activity. In vitro techniques increasingly used for predicting in vivo bioavailability include ever more sophisticated partition measurements across both artificial and natural membranes (Navia and Chaturvedi, 1996; Chan and Stewart, 1996) and both cytochrome P450 and liver microsome/hepatocyte degradation experiments. These have dramatically increased the understanding of the problems associated with bioavailability and persistence, but follow-up in vivo studies are still required for validation. In addition, cyclic or polycyclic compounds may need to be targeted to overcome bioavailability issues such as metabolism (King et al., 1993a), or to improve selectivity (King et al., 1993b) or to reduce the number of acidic protons for improved distribution (Bromidge et al., 1997). For such individualistic compounds, standard iterative processes using chemistry not currently amenable to automation may be required.

CONCLUSION

The impact of bacterial genomics on antibacterial discovery is potentially immense. After nearly 30 years without the discovery of a major new class of antibiotic, bacterial genomics represents a gateway into a new (and possibly final!) 'golden era' in antibiotic discovery. This optimism is based on the following.

First, microbial genome sequence data, together with appropriate computational (bioinformatics) and laboratory (functional genomics) approaches, provides a rational basis upon which to select molecular targets for anti-infective therapy. Furthermore, not only is there the exciting prospect of developing new antibiotic classes to combat the rising tide of bacterial resistance, but also there is the possibility of discovering new types of therapies that act by modulation of pathogen adaptation/survival strategies within their mammalian hosts. It may even be that every possible target will have been identified within a few years.

Secondly, the challenges that such new types of drug target impose on the drug discovery process are likely to be met initially by new combinatorial chemistry strategies and associated developments in ultra-high throughput screening.

Together, these will result in the discovery and optimisation of new pharmacophores and lead series. This will shift the pressure point in antibiotic discovery towards the later stages of the process in which drug candidates with appropriate pharmacodynamic properties are the goal. Here, equivalent improvements will need to be made to ensure rapid progress is maintained so that a commercial return on the increased research and development investment is achieved (Drews, 1997).

REFERENCES

Ash, C., 1997, Year of the genome, *Trends Microbiol.* 5:135.
Bax, R., 1997, Antibiotic resistance: a view from the pharmaceutical industry, *Clin. Infect. Dis.* 24:S151.

Bernhardt, J., Volker, U., Volker, A., Antelmann, H., Schmid, R., Mach, H., and Hecker, M., 1997, Specific and general stress proteins in *Bacillus subtilis* – a two-dimensional protein electrophoresis study, *Microbiology* 143:999.

Blattner, F.R., Plunkett, G. 3rd., Bloch, C.A., Perna, N.T., Burland, V., Riley, M., Collado-Vides, J., Glasner, J.D., Rode, C.K., Mayhew, G.F., Gregor, J., Davis, N.W., Kirkpatrick, H.A., Goeden, M.A., Rose, D.J., Mau, B., and Shao, Y., 1997, The complete genome sequence of *Escherichia coli* K12, Science 277:1453.

Bromidge, S.M., Duckworth, M., Forbes, I.T., Ham, P., King, F.D., Thewlis, K.M., Blaney, F.E., Naylor, C.B., Blackburn, T.P., Kennett, G.A., Wood, M.D., and Clarke, S.E., 1997, 6-Chloro-5-methyl-1-[[2-[(2-methyl-3-pyridyl)oxy]-5-pyridyl]carbamoyl]-indoline (SB-242084): The first selective and brain penetrant 5-HT2C receptor antagonist, *J Med. Chem.* 40:3494.

Bult, C.J., White, O., Olsen, G.J., Zhou, L., Fleischmann, R.D., Sutton, G.G., Blake, J.A., Fitzgerald, L.M., Clayton, R.A., Gocayne, J.D., Kerlavage, A.R., Dougherty, B.A., Tomb, J.F., Adams, M.D., Reich, C.I., Overbeek, R., Kirkness, E.F., Weinstock, K.G., Merrick, J.M., Glodek, A., Scott, J.L., Geoghagen, N.S.M., and Venter, J.C., 1996, Complete genome sequence of the methanogenic archaeon, *Methanococcus jannaschii*, Science 273:1058

Chan, O.H., and Stewart, B.H., 1996, Physicochemical and drug-delivery considerations for oral drug bioavailability, *Drug Discovery Today* 1:461.

Chenera, B., Finkelstein, J.A., and Veber, D.F., 1995, Protodetachable aryl silane polymer linkages for use in solid phase organic synthesis, *J. Amer. Chem. Soc.* 117:11999.

Chu, Y.-H., Kirby, D.P., and Larger, B.L., 1995, Free solution identification of candidate peptides from combinatorial libraries by affinity capillary electrophoresis/mass spectrometry, *J. Amer. Chem. Soc.* 117:5419.

Chuang, S.E., Daniels, D.L., and Blattner, F.R., 1993, Global regulation of gene expression in *Escherichia coli*, *J. Bacteriol.* 175:2026

Cohen, M.L., 1992, Epidemiology of drug resistance: implications for a post-antimicrobial era, *Science* 257,1050.

Deckert, G., Warren, P.V., Gaasterland, T., Young, W.G., Lenox, A.L., Graham, D.E., Overbeek, R., Sneed, M.A., Keller, M., Aujay, M., Huber, R., Feldman, R.A., Short, J.M., Olsen, G.J, and Swanson, R.V., 1998, The complete genome sequence of the hyperthermophilic bacterium Aquifex aeolicus, Nature 392:353.

de Saizieu, A., Certa, U., Warrington, J., Gray, C., Keck, W., and Mous, J., 1998, Bacterial transcript imaging by hybridization of total RNA to oligonucleotide arrays, *Nature Biotechnology* 16:45.

Demain, A., 1998, Microbial natural products: alive and well in 1998, *Nature Biotechnology* 16:3.

Dooley, C.T., Chung, N.N., Schiller, P.W., and Houghten, R.A., 1993, Acetalins: Opioid receptor antagonists determined through the use of synthetic peptide combinatorial libraries, *Proc. Natl. Acad. Sci.* 90:10811.

Drews, J., 1997, Strategic choices facing the pharmaceutical industry: a case for innovation, *Drug Discovery Today*, 2:72.

Fleischmann, R.D., et al. (40 authors), 1995, Whole genome random sequencing and assembly of *Haemophilus influenzae* Rd., *Science* 269:496.

Fraser, C.M., et al. (29 authors), 1995, The minimal gene complement of *Mycoplasma genitalium*, *Science* 270:397.

Fraser, C.M., et al. (38 authors), 1997, Genomic sequence of a Lyme disease spirochaete, *Borrelia burgdorferi*, *Nature* 390: 580.

Goffeau, A., et al. (633 authors), 1997, The yeast genome directory, *Nature* 387 (Suppl.) 5.

Halliday, R.G., Walker, S.R., Lumley, C.H., 1992, R and D philosophy and management in the world's leading pharmaceutical companies, J. Pharm. Med. 2:139.

Halm, K., 1996, N-in-One dosing in the dog: LC/MS as a tool for higher throughput in vivo pharmacokinetic screening of 'drug discovery' compound mixtures, Drug Discovery Technology Conference, International Business Communications, August 1996, Boston, USA.

Hensel, M. Shea, J.E., Gleeson, C., Jones, M.D., Dalton, E., and Holden, D.W., 1995, Simultaneous identification of bacterial virulence genes by negative selection, *Science* 269:400.

Hermkens, P.H.H., Ottenheijm, H.C.J., and Rees, D.C., 1996, Solid-phase organic reactions: a review of the recent literature, *Tetrahedron*, 52:4527.

Hermkens, P.H.H., Ottenheijm, H.C.J., and Rees, D.C., 1997, Solid-phase organic reactions - II. A review of the literature November 1995-November 1996, *Tetrahedron*, 53:5643.

Himmelreich, R., Hilbert, H., Plagens, H., Pirkl, E., Li, B.C., and Herrmann, R., 1996, Complete sequence analysis of the genome of the bacterium *Mycoplasma pneumoniae, Nuc. Acid Res.* 24:4420.

Hiramatsu, K., Aritaka, N., Hanaki, H., Kawasaki, S., Hosoda, Y., Hori, S., Fukuchi, Y., Kobayashi, I., 1973a, Dissemination in Japanese hospitals of strains of *Staphylococcus aureus* heterogenously resistant to vancomycin, *Lancet* 350:1670.

Hiramatsu, K., Hanaki, H., Ino, T., Yabuta, K., Oguri, T., and Tenover, F.C., 1997b, Methicillin-resistant *Staphylococcus aureus* clinical strain with reduced vancomycin susceptibility, *J. Antimicrob. Chemother.* 40:135.

Kaneko, T., Sato,S., Kotani, H., Tanaka, A., Asamizu,E., Nakamura, Y., Miyajima, N., Hirosawa, M., Sugiura, M., Sasamoto, S., Kimura, T., Hosouchi, T., Matsuno,A., Muraki, A., Nakazaki, N., Naruo, K., Okumura, S., Shimpo, S., Takeuchi, C., Wada, T., Watanabe, A., Yamada, M., Yasuda, M., and Tabata, S., 1996, Sequence analysis of the genome of the unicellular cyanobacterium *Synechocystis sp.* Strain PCC6803. II. Sequence determination of the entire genome and assignment of potential protein-coding regions, *DNA Res.* 3:109.

Keifer, P.A., 1997, High-resolution NMR techniques for solid-phase synthesis and combinatorial chemistry, *Drug Discovery Today*, 2:468.

Kikuta-Oshima, L.C., King, C.H., Shinnick,T.M., and Quinn, F.D., 1994, Methods for the identification of virulence genes expressed in *Mycobacterium tuberculosis* strain H37 Rv, *Ann. NewYork Acad. Sci.* 730:263.

King, F.D., Brown, A.M., Gaster, L.M., Kaumann, A.J., Medhurst, A.D., Parker, S.G., Parsons, A.A., Patch, T.L., and Raval, P., 1993a, (±) 3-Amino-6-carboxamido-1,2,3,4-tetrahydrocarbazole: A conformationally restricted analogue of 5-carboxamidotryptamine with selectivity for the serotonin 5-HT1D receptor, *J. Med. Chem.* 36:1918.

King, F.D., Hadley, M.S., Joiner, K.T., Martin, R.T., Sanger, G.J., Smith, D.M., Smith, G.E., Smith, P., Turner, D.H., and Watts, E.A., 1993b, Substituted benzamides with conformationally restricted side chains. 5. Azabicyclo[x.y.z] derivatives as 5-HT4 receptor agonists and gastric motility stimulants, *J. Med. Chem.* 36:683.

Klenk, H.P., et al. (51 authors), 1997, The complete genome sequence of the hyperthermophilic, sulphate-reducing archaeon *Archaeoglobus fulgidis*, *Nature* 390:364.

Knowles, D.J.C., 1997, New strategies for antibacterial design, *Trends Microbiol.* 5:379.

Kunin, C.M., 1997, Antibiotic armageddon, *Clin. Infect. Dis.* 25:240.

Kunst, F., et al. (151 authors), 1997, The complete genome sequence of the gram-positive bacterium *Bacillus subtilis*, *Nature* 390:249.

Lam, K.S., Salmon, S.E., Hersh, E.M., Hruby, V.J., Kazmierski, W.M., and Knapp, R.J., 1991, A new type of synthetic peptide library for identifying ligand-binding activity, *Nature* 354:82.

Lerner, C.G., Chiang Saiki, A.Y., MacKinnon, A.C.,and Xuei, X., 1996, High throughput screen for inhibitors of bacterial DNA topoisomerase 1 using the scintillation proximity assay, *J. Biomol. Screening* 1:135.

Lipinski, C.A., Lombardo, F., Dominy, B.W., and Feeney, P.J., 1997, Experimental and computational approaches to estimate solubility and permeability in drug discovery and development settings., *Adv. Drug Del Revs.* 23:3.

Mahan, M.J., Slauch, J.M., and Mekalanos, .J.J., 1993a, Selection of bacterial virulence genes that are specifically induced in host tissues, *Science* 259:686.

Mahan, M.J., Slauch, J.M., Hanna, P.C., Camilli, A., Tobias, J.W., Waldor, M.K., and Mekalanos, J.J., 1993b, Selection for bacterial genes that are specifically induced in host tissues: the hunt for virulence factors, *Infect. Agents Dis.* 2:263.

Mahan, M.J., Tobias, J.W., Slauch, J.M., Hanna, P.C., Collier, R.J., and Mekalanos, J.J., 1995, Antibiotic-based selection for bacterial genes that are specifically induced during infection of a host, *Proc. Natl. Acad. Sci. USA.* 92:669.

Mei, J.M., Nourbakhsh, F., Ford, C.W., and Holden,D.W., 1997, Identification of *Staphylococcus aureus* virulence genes in a murine model of bacteraemia using signature-tagged mutagenesis, *Mol. Microbiol.* 26: 399.

Metcalf, B.W., 1998, The impact of genomics on medicinal chemistry, *J. Pure Appl. Chem.* (in press)

Metting, F.B., and Romine, M.F., 1997, Microbial genomics: the floodgates open, *Trends Microbiol.* 5:91.

Navia, M.A., and Chaturvedi,P.R., 1996, Design principles for orally bioavailable drugs, *Drug Discovery Today* 1, 179

Nestler, H.P., Bartlett, P.A., and Still, W.C., 1994, A general method for molecular tagging of encoded combinatorial chemistry libraries, *J. Org. Chem.*, 1994, 59:4723.

Neu, H.C., 1992, The crisis in antibiotic resistance, *Science* 257:1064.

Nicolaou, K.C., Vourloumis, D., Li, T., Pastor, J., Winssinger, N., He, Y., Ninkovic, S., Sarabia, F., Vallberg, H., Roschangar, F., King, N.P., Ray, M., Finlay, V., Giannakakou, P., Verdier-Pinard, P., and Hamel,E., 1997, Designed epothilones: combinatorial synthesis, tubulin assembly properties, and cytotoxic action against taxol-resistant tumor cells, *Angew. Chem. Int Ed. Engl.* 36:2097.

Nikaido, H., and Vaara, M., 1985, Molecular basis of bacterial outer membrane permeability, *Microbiol. Rev.* 49:1

Rogers, M.V., 1997, Light on high-throughput screening: flourescence-based assay technologies, *Drug Discovery Today* 2:156.

Schmid, R., Bernhardt, J., Antelmann, H., Volker, A., Mach, H., Volker, U., and Hecker, M., 1997, Identification of vegetative proteins for a two-dimensional protein index of *Bacillus subtilis*, *Microbiology* 143:991.

Shea, J.E., Hensel,M., Gleeson, C., and Holden, D.W., 1996, Identification of a virulence locus encoding a second type III secretion locus system in *Salmonella typhimurium*, *Proc. Natl. Acad. Sci. USA.* 93:2593.

Shuker, S.B., Hajduk, P.J., Meadows, R.P., and Fesik, S.W., 1996, Discovering high-affinity ligands for proteins: SAR by NMR, *Science* 274:1531.

Smith, D.R., et al. (37 authors), 1997, Complete genome sequence of *Methanobacterium thermoautotropicum* deltaH: functional analysis and comparative genomics, *J. Bacteriology* 179:7135.

Storer, R., 1996, Solution-phase synthesis in combinatorial chemistry: Applications in drug discovery, *Drug Discovery Today* 1:248.

Tenover, F.C., and Hughes, J.M., 1996, The challenges of emerging infectious diseases. Development and spread of multiply-resistant bacterial pathogens, *J. Am. Med. Assoc.* 275:300.

Tomasz, A., 1994, Multiple antibiotic-resistant pathogenic bacteria. A report on the Rockefeller University Workshop, *N. Engl. J. Med.* 330:1247.

Tomb, J.F., et al. (42 authors), 1997, The complete genome sequence of the gastric pathogen *Helicobacter pylori*, *Nature* 388:539.

Travis, J., 1994, Reviving the antibiotic miracle?, *Science* 264:360.

Utt, E.A., and Quinn, F.D., 1994, mRNA subtractive hybridisation for the isolation and identification of tissue culture-induced determinants from *Haemophilus influenzae* biogroup aegyptus, the causative agent of Brazilian purpuric fever, *Ann. New York Acad. Sci.* 730:269.

Utt, E.A., Brousal, J.P., Kikuta-Oshima, L.C., and Quinn, F.D., 1995, The identification of bacterial gene expression differences using mRNA-based isothermal subtractive hybridization, *Can. J. Microbiol.* 41:152.

Wodicka L., Dong, H., Mittman, M., Ho M-H., and Lockhart D., 1997, Genome-wide expression monitoring in *Saccharomyces cerevisiae*, *Nature Biotechnology* 15:1359.

11

PEPTIDOGLYCAN BIOSYNTHESIS

Unexploited Antibacterial Targets within a Familiar Pathway

Kenny K. Wong and David L. Pompliano

Department of Biochemistry
Merck Research Laboratories
Rahway, New Jersey 07065

INTRODUCTION

No other single medical advance has had greater salutary effect on public health than the discovery of antibiotics. Truly the miracle drugs of the 20th century, antibiotics such as penicillin, streptomycin and erythromycin, enabled physicians to cure ancient bacterial scourges like tuberculosis (TB) and syphillis, and to prevent complications brought on by bacterial infections (Russel and Chopra, 1990). In 1969, confident that the microbial threat had been neutralized by antibiotic therapy, the US Surgeon General declared that it was time to "close the book on infectious disease" (Fisher, 1994). With the hindsight of 30 years, the Surgeon General's comment appears to be a bit premature. The current crisis of antibiotic resistance is now serious news, covered sensationally in newspapers and with statistical coldness in the scientific and medical literature. Resistance exists to virtually every known antibiotic. Very scary are the organisms, like methicillin resistant *Staphyloccocus aureus* (MRSA), that are resistant to everything except vancomycin, and that leave infected patients with few treatment options. Bacteria that were formerly of little threat are now potential killers, because antibiotics that were taken for granted are no longer effective.

Our predicament is the result of an unwitting experiment in bacterial evolution conducted over the past 50 years. Victims of their own success, antibiotics were used with abandon, becoming an evolutionary force that selected for and enhanced the survival of bacterial strains that could resist them. Ironically, the hospital setting breeds the most aggressive resistant bacteria (Goetz and Yu, 1997), because intense use of antibiotics in crowded and less-than-sterile conditions provide an extremely rigorous evolutionary training ground. Physicians contribute to the problem--often prescribing antibiotics in greater quantity and higher potency than is required. This practice often has been unavoidable since treatment of putative infections had to commence before culture results were back (so called empiric therapy). Broad spectrum agents--the "big guns"--are preferred under

Resolving the Antibiotic Paradox, edited by Rosen and Mobashery.
Kluwer Academic / Plenum Publishers, New York, 1998.

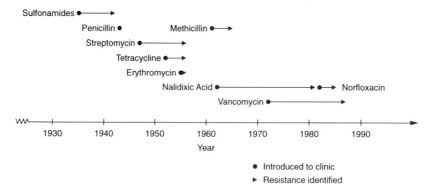

Figure 1. A timeline indicating the date when an antibiotic was introduced clinically (closed circles) and when resistance was first identified (arrow head).

these conditions to insure that all possible organisms were covered. Part of the blame also belongs to patients who demand antibiotics for maladies other than bacterial infections. When these same patients really do have a bacterial infection, they do not finish their course of antibiotic therapy, selecting for bacteria with better tolerance to the drug.

That resistance to a new agent will develop is inevitable, but it is striking how quickly it happens. Fig. 1 shows the time between introduction of a new class of antibiotic into the clinic and the first report of a resistant isolate (Davies, 1997). Regardless of the structural class of the antibiotic or its biochemical target, new agents have only a few years of unfettered clinical use before resistance arises. Although resistance doesn't vitiate the usefulness of the drug, it does sound an alarm and may preclude using the drug in empiric therapy (because one cannot be sure of the drug's spectrum).

While the adaptability that allows bacteria to escape a drug insult is formidable, it is the readiness and ease with which bacteria can exchange genetic material that is responsible for the rapid spread of resistance. Bacteria can pass plasmids and fragments of DNA between species and even between genera (Amabile-Cuevas and Chicurel, 1992). Considering the evolutionary distance between different species of bacteria, these transactions are remarkable. Thus a heritable resistance determinant need only be selected for once, by nearly any bacterial species, and then it can be propagated genetically. Apart from the obvious advantage of sharing resistance determinants that confer survival, this transmission of DNA also enhances the chances of evolving a defense mechanism by submitting a larger population of organisms, each of which has diverse genetic capabilities, to the test of survival.

The development and spread of vancomycin resistance is an especially worrisome example. Vancomycin, the last new class of antibiotic introduced (in 1972), works not by inhibiting an enzyme, but by binding to and sequestering the substrate necessary for the final step in cell wall biosynthesis. The resistance mechanism that evolved is complex, involving several gene products whose combined effect is to produce an altered cell wall (Walsh et al., 1996). In 1980, the incidence of MRSA in hospitals was less than 5% of the total Staphylococcal isolates, and, at that time, vancomycin was used in less than 0.1% of the patients. However, the frequency of MRSA began to rise noticeably in 1982 and has continued unabated. Since MRSA is resistant to every drug except vancomycin, the use of vancomycin shot up so that, by 1990, >10% of patients receiving antibiotics were receiving vancomycin. This 100-fold increase in the use of vancomycin selected for resistant Enterococcal strains (in 1986). The incidences of vancomycin-resistant Enterococci (VRE) and of MRSA are now increasing at the same rate (Swartz, 1994). Thus, there is a fatalistic aspect to antibacterial therapy, where the growing ineffectiveness of one drug drives the increased use of a more potent alternative drug. The predestined result is resistance to both agents.

Against this backdrop of bacterial evolutionary prowess, the task is to develop new agents that will not only be active against existing resistant bacteria, but will also forestall the emergence of a new mechanism of resistance (Chopra et al., 1996; Chu et al., 1996; Desnottes, 1996; Knowles, 1997; Setti et al., 1997).

ANTIBACTERIAL DRUG DISCOVERY: TARGET SELECTION

The goal is to *kill* bacteria. Elimination of all invading bacteria from the host is required to cure the infection. Killing organisms (as opposed to preventing their further growth, as protein synthesis inhibitors do) removes the host's reliance upon its immune system to clear the infection. This is especially important given the growing population of older and immunocompromised patients. There is evidence that bacteria can hypermutate during stasis, essentially trying out new genotypes to see which is best for survival (Riesenfeld et al., 1997; Hall, 1990). A swiftly acting cidal agent would reduce the incidence of resistance by this mechanism. Empiric therapy currently demands broad spectrum agents, although genomics and new technologies may permit rapid determination of the infecting organism, and thus allow administration of highly refined, narrow spectrum agents that selectively act on the invading pathogen. Therefore, a cidal agent that acts against many species of bacteria is the aim. Such a compound should have a novel structure, so that it would be inert to the action of existing resistance mechanisms. Finally it should itself be recalcitrant to resistance development, perhaps by inhibiting more than one molecular target simultaneously.

Although a cidal agent would be ideal, a strategy to disarm bacteria is also viable. For example, preventing further growth of the bacteria should give the host immune system time to mount an effective defense against the infection. The success of protein synthesis inhibitors, such as tetracycline and the macrolides, suggests that this works well for immunocompetent patients. Another possibility is to inactivate the resistance mechanism of a known antibiotic, restoring the drug to original efficacy. For example, inhibiting ß-lactamases with clavulanic acid has extended the useful life of penicillins. Lastly, enhancing the uptake of an antibiotic or preventing its export would return potency to existing antibiotics. Inhibition of drug efflux pumps is just one potential approach.

Having defined the desired properties of the next-generation antibacterials, how do we go about finding the small molecule that will eventually be a new drug? Given that resistant organisms are the threat, and given that they have mechanisms in place to render ineffectual all known classes of antibiotic, incremental improvement of a known chemical class, although the historical approach of choice, will not lead to a longlasting solution. Therefore, the focus must be on *novel structural classes of chemicals*, compounds for which no mode of resistance currently exists. Whether such molecules are inhibitors of familiar biochemical targets, a non-β-lactam penicillin-binding-protein (PBP) inhibitor for instance, or disruptors of unexploited targets is less crucial. Consequently, choice of a cellular target against which to screen compounds can be quite broad.

In theory, four criteria are necessary to qualify as a good antibacterial target. First, the function of the molecular entity must be essential to the survival of the organism. Conditional lethal alleles of the target (in an otherwise wild type background) can validate this requirement. Paradoxically, this criterion for the selection of targets is restrictive because it demands that the disruption of a single target gene will lead to death. By this measure, the PBPs--the targets of the ß-lactam antibiotics--would not surface as a good molecular targets. At least two PBPs must be inactivated to kill *E. coli* (Kato et al., 1985) or *S. aureus* (Beise et al., 1988). ß-Lactams kill bacteria because they bind to many of the PBPs simultaneously. This example should point out the value of identifying protein families whose concerted action is required for survival (Silver and Bostian, 1990). A molecule that inhibits the entire class will be a cidal agent. Histidine protein kinases may fall into this target category.

Second, the target should be unique to bacteria so that inhibitors will not harm the organisms they are intended to help. Eucaryotic orthologs of the target imply commonalities of structure that could make finding molecules that bind differentially to the bacterial and eucaryotic orthologs difficult. Mammalian toxicity is a potential problem for non-selective compounds. Third, the structure (and function) of the target protein should be highly conserved across bacterial species, so that inhibitors discovered against one ortholog can be presumed to be active against its congeners. Such inhibitors will be broad spectrum agents.

Finally, resistance to inhibitors of the target should not be easily acquired. Predicting this quality is difficult. An inhibitor of the target that has antibacterial activity must be available so that the frequency of resistance development can be measured empirically (by looking for survivors in the presence of drug). However, if the target is a member of a larger structurally-related protein family, finding a molecule that inhibits more than one of these targets, a multimodal inhibitor, might be possible (Silver and Bostian, 1993). Assuming that all of the inhibited targets are essential, the frequency of target-mediated resistance would be negligible, since mutations conferring resistance would have to occur in at least two different target genes during a single generation.

With all due respect to bacterial genomics discoveries, there are already plenty of good targets. In general, they are in pathways of macromolecular synthesis: DNA, RNA, protein and cell wall biosynthesis. Most of them have been validated both genetically (by conditional lethal mutants), pharmacologically (through use in the clinic) and evolutionarily (because they are the targets of natural products). For example, DNA replication is the site of action of the quinolones. mRNA synthesis is inhibited by rifampin. Protein synthesis is stopped by tetracyclines and macrolides. Cell wall metabolism is blocked by penicillins, cephalosporins and vancomycin. By and large, these compounds were identified originally as agents that possessed antibacterial activity; their biochemical targets were elucidated much later. Focusing on whole cell activity, rather than on specific inhibition of biochemical activity, obviates the difficult chemical task of converting an inhibitor of an isolated enzyme into a compound that has antibacterial activity. More often than not, the lack of antibacterial activity of such an inhibitor is due to its inability to penetrate to its site of action.

Since diffusion and transport of putative small molecule inhibitors from the extracellular milieu into the cytoplasm is poorly understood, a major *practical* consideration is the cellular location of the target. Intracellular targets are difficult because they hide behind the barrier of the cell membrane. Impermeability of the bacterial cell wall and membrane to polar molecules has been the downfall of many very potent enzyme inhibitors. For example the phosphinate inhibitors of D-Ala-D-Ala ligase (Parsons et al., 1988) could not be modified synthetically to achieve significant antibacterial activity. This permeability factor cannot be overemphasized, especially when screening a biochemical target. Finding inhibitors of the isolated intracellular enzyme is comparatively easy. But, even with a dedicated medicinal chemistry effort, there is no synthetic chemical recipe for transforming an enzyme inhibitor that cannot permeate the bacterium into a drug that can; this process is completely empirical.

The question now becomes how to best find an antibacterial drug. There are two choices: (1) in vitro assays using isolated components of the cellular machinery or (2) whole cell assays. Having pointed out the main disadvantage of the biochemical approach (i.e. that an in vitro assay cannot predict whole cell activity), it seems only fair to highlight the advantages. First, biochemical assay conditions are well-defined and reproducible. The sensitivity of the enzyme to inhibitors can be altered in a predictable manner by adjusting concentrations of substrates. In fact, for multisubstrate enzymes, conditions can be set to favor competitive inhibitors of only one of the substrates. Moreover, biochemical assays, compared to whole cell assays, are generally much easier to establish and more amenable to high throughput screening methods. Third, isolated target proteins can be the subject of structural studies (by NMR or X-ray crystallography) to aid in the design of inhibitors. The conclusion is that a biochemical approach will generate lead compounds. Since these compounds will probably have at best weak antibacterial activity, a chemistry program will be required to turn them into drugs.

The greatest strength of the cell based approach is that it offers an immediate test of biological activity. Caution is warranted, however, because many compounds with antibacterial activity do not have modes of action that are specific to bacterial cells. To avoid generally cytotoxic agents (such as detergents, DNA intercalators and ionophores), a whole cell assay must be reasonably specific for the intended bacterial protein target. For example, by constructing two strains, one of which underexpresses and the other of which overexpresses a defined target protein, inhibitors of the target may be found by comparing the responses of the underexpressing strain to the overexpressing strain. Still, the mode of action of a putative inhibitor is not certain and may not be specific to the desired target. Tying the antibacterial activity of a such a compound to the inhibition of a particular cellular target can be difficult. Also, metabolic control mechanisms of whole cells may cloak weakly active molecules, thereby dismissing a molecule that might warrant optimization by synthetic chemistry. Another drawback is the incompatibility of whole cells with the liquids (like DMSO) used to dissolve the test compounds.

There are two special cases where the choice of screening methodology is clear. First, when improving the potency or spectrum of a known class of antibiotic, the whole cell approach is superior. Here since the biochemical mode of action is likely already known, the only issue is antibacterial activity. Second, a biochemical screen is better for extracellular (or membrane-bound) targets where the worries of permeability are moot. In this case, biological activity will tend to track with potency of inhibition. Inhibition of the target is not complicated with the vagaries of whole cell metabolism. One example is finding inhibitors of PBPs in Gram-positive bacteria.

Thus our philosophy can be distilled down to a few points. Irrespective of their cellular location, single enzyme targets are suspect because of the ease of evolving resistance by single point mutation, either in the structural gene, in the promoter or in genes involved in transport or permeability. Targeting multiple enzymes that are structurally related or that recognize common substrate motifs, and offer the possibility of finding a small molecule that binds to more than one family member, is much preferred. Unless there is a synthetic chemistry effort committed to converting good enzyme inhibitors into permeative antibiotics, screening intracellular protein targets--particularly lone enzymes--promises to be frustrating. Extracellular targets are always attractive, especially for biochemical screens, because penetration of the cellular boundary is not required. Finally, experience suggests that it is easier to find the cellular target of an antibacterial compound than it is to engineer permeability into an enzyme inhibitor. Thus, whole cell assays are best for finding a lead compound that has a modicum of antibacterial activity, but biochemical assays are necessary to determine the mode of action of these leads. In fact, a cryptic hit identified by whole cell screening methods can be assayed against a bank of purified bacterial enzyme targets to help identify its molecular target. Biochemical and structural studies may also help direct the path of synthetic chemistry, by well-defined structure-activity relationships, to produce more potent analogues. In the end, the advantages of biochemical and whole cell assays are complementary; both methodologies must be pursued in parallel.

While target selection and assay methodology are key, the most important factor when searching for new drugs is the variety or diversity of chemicals available to screen. The chemical collections of most large pharmaceutical companies have been panned for possible antibacterials. The lowlying fruit from the antibiotic tree has probably already been picked. What is needed are new sources of compounds. Combinatorial chemistry has been heralded as the cavalry in this regard, but the technology for generating chemical diversity is not quite ready. Fortunately, nature is not yet tapped out of novel compounds. Bizarre organisms are being isolated from all sorts of odd niches, bringing with them their own chemical defense mechanisms (Pace, 1997). These naturally occurring organisms, together with recombinant organisms generated using combinatorial genetics (Hutchinson, 1995; Khosla, 1996) and having new chimeric metabolic pathways, promise to deliver a wealth of new compounds.

BACTERIAL PEPTIDOGLYCAN BIOSYNTHESIS: GOOD TARGETS ABOUND

An intact cell wall is critical for the survival of the bacteria. The bacterial cell wall or peptidoglycan consists of a single polymeric molecule, the murein sacculus, that girdles the plasma membrane and cytoplasm of the cell (for reviews, see Ghuysen & Hakenbeck, 1994; Bugg & Walsh, 1992). Assembled by crosslinking glycan chains with short, unusual peptide bridges, the completed structure is strong enough to maintain cell integrity against an osmotic pressure differential of over four atmospheres, but also flexible enough to allow the cell to move, grow and divide. In Gram-negative bacteria, the murein sacculus may only be only a few layers thick and is surrounded by an additional lipid bilayer, the lipopolysaccharide. In Gram-positive bacteria, the cell wall is thick, often more than 20 layers (25 nm) deep (Beveridge, 1981), and no outer membrane exists. Eucaryotes do not contain a peptidoglycan cell wall.

The biosynthesis of this structure starts in the cytoplasm (Stage I) with the condensation of phosphoenolpyruvate (PEP) and UDP-N-acetylglucosamine (UDP-GlcNAc) catalyzed by MurA (Fig 2). This reaction, followed by a stereospecific reduction catalyzed by MurB, results in the placement of a lactyl group on the 3-OH of the glucosamine moiety. Next a series of ATP-dependent amino acid ligases (MurC, MurD, MurE, and MurF) catalyze the stepwise synthesis of the pentapeptide sidechain using the newly synthesized lactyl carboxylate as the first acceptor site. Attachment of the sugar pentapeptide to a lipid carrier in the plasma membrane (Stage II) and addition of another glucosamine unit to the 4-OH of the muramic acid moiety completes the synthesis of the monomeric building block. The finished precursor is moved across the membrane into the periplasm where it is stitched enzymatically by the penicillin-binding proteins into the fabric of the growing cell wall (Stage III).

The assembly of the peptidoglycan is the target of many antibiotics. That over 40 agents in clinical use target the penicillin binding proteins (PBP's) attest to the usefulness of drugs

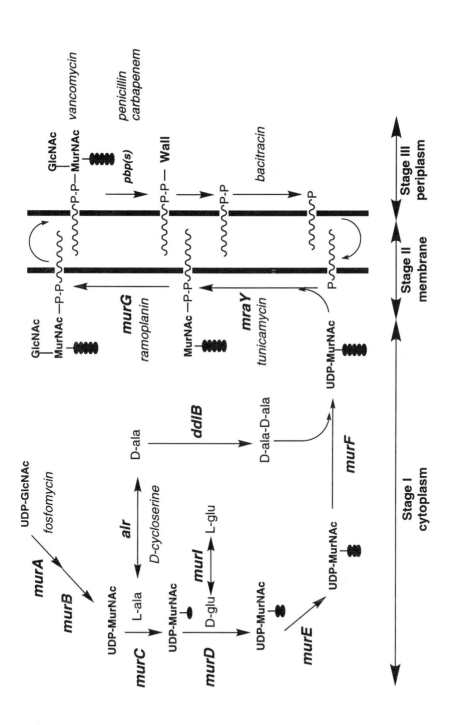

Figure 2. Pathway of bacterial peptidoglycan biosynthesis. Genes encoding the enzymes are indicated in italics. Inhibitors of individual enzymes are in bold italics.

that block the later stages of cell wall biosynthesis. But PBP's are only a small subset of the enzymes involved in the murein biosynthetic pathway. Earlier steps in the pathway, especially those catalyzed by Stage I enzymes, offer a plethora of attractive antibacterial targets. The genes encoding these intracellular enzymes have only recently been identified in both Gram-negative and Gram-positive bacteria. The difficulty associated with isolating pure Mur enzymes, never mind their substrates, has hindered research efforts in this area. However, advancements in cloning and protein expression have allowed the large-scale production of active recombinant proteins for enzymological and structural studies. The stage is now set for understanding the structure and function of these enzymes, hopefully culminating in the design or discovery of antibiotics that act in this segment of the pathway.

The chemical complexity of the precursor's pentapeptide side chain supports the idea that novel inhibitors specific for cytoplasmic peptidoglycan synthesis should be possible to find (or make). The pentapeptide sidechain is not synthesized ribosomally and so it may contain more diverse chemical functionality than a typical peptide, both structurally and stereochemically. Two of the enzymes catalyze the addition of D-amino acids (MurD and MurF) and MurE mediates the formation of an isopeptide bond between the γ-carboxylate of D-glutamate and the amino group of L-lysine. Presumably these structures render the exposed peptidoglycan resistant to the action of proteases, but they also imply that the active sites of the biosynthetic enzymes must have unusual structures in order to handle the somewhat uncommon substrates. It is into these unusual active sites that novel inhibitors are expected to bind.

As a target for antibiotic discovery, it is difficult to find fault with the peptidoglycan biosynthetic pathway. All of the murein biosynthetic genes are essential; conditional lethal mutations are lytic (Lugentburg and van Schijndel-van Dam, 1972; Lugentburg and van Schijndel-van Dam, 1973; Lugentburg et al., 1972). Thus, chemical disruption of the proteins they encode should be lethal. The enzymes within this pathway are ubiquitous in eubacteria, prophesying broad spectrum antibiotic effects of inhibitors. Since the murein sacculus is uniquely bacterial, drugs directed against the pathway of its synthesis will likely be safe in eucaryotes. Indeed, no yeast or mammalian homologs of these enzymes have been found. In this review, we will first summarize the enzymology of the cytoplasmic (Stage I) enzymes, then detail our in vitro approach to screening for inhibitors of these enzymes, and finally discuss the advantages and limitations of our approach with respect to the time-tested method of whole cell screening.

UDP-N-ACETYLGLUCOSEAMINE ENOLPYRUVYLTRANSFERASE (MURA)

MurA (EC 2.5.1.7), formerly named MurZ, catalyzes an addition/elimination reaction to form UDP-GlcNAc-enolpyruvate (UDP-GlcNAc-EP) and inorganic phosphate from UDP-GlcNAc and PEP, the first committed step of the peptidoglycan biosynthetic pathway. The enzyme from *Escherichia coli* has been most extensively studied, but the enzymes from *Enterobacter colocae* and *Staphylococcus epidermidis* have also been examined (Zemel & Anwar, 1975; Wickus & Strominger, 1973). Steady-state and pre-steady-state kinetic analyses of the reaction catalyzed by MurA implies that two distinct enzyme-bound tetrahedral intermediates are formed on the reaction coordinate to product (Fig. 2). The first is a phospholactoyl-tetrahedral adduct and the second is a tightly-bound phospholactoyl-UDP-GlcNAc adduct (Wanke & Amrhein, 1993; Brown et al., 1995). The stereochemical course of the reaction has been shown to be either an

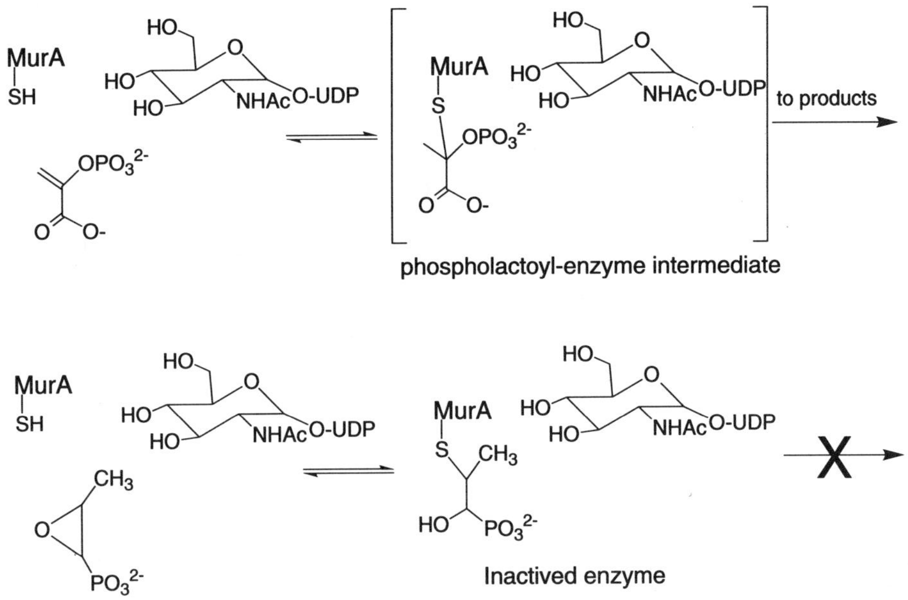

Figure 3. Mechanism of action of fosfomycin (bottom). Fosfomycin is a PEP mimic which inactivates MurA via covalent modification. This reaction is proposed to be similar to the formation of the phospholactoyl-enzyme intermediate between MurA and PEP during normal catalysis (top).

anti/syn or syn/anti addition-elimination reaction (Lees & Walsh, 1995; Kim et al., 1996), similar to the enzyme enolpyruvyl shikimate phosphate (EPSP) synthase. Studies with the pseudo-substrate, (Z)-3-fluorophosphoenolpyruvate further substantiated the two-intermediate mechanism; however, quantitation of the rate constants of the steady-state and presteady-state data suggests a branched mechanism (Kim et al., 1995).

During the early 1970's, researchers at Merck identified a natural product antibiotic, fosfomycin, from whole-cell screening (Gadebusch et al., 1992) that caused spheroplasting of bacteria in isotonic media, a sign that this agent disrupted cell wall biosynthesis. Subsequent studies on the mechanism of action of fosfomycin revealed that the molecular target was MurA. Fosfomycin inhibition is depended on the presence of UDP-GlcNAc and mediated through the modification of an enzymic cysteine residue (Kahan et al., 1974). Development of fosfomycin, first in Europe and more recently in the US, led to the marketing of Monurol™ (fosfomycin tromethamine)

Monurol™ is currently being used as a one-dose oral antibiotic for uncomplicated urinary tract infection (de Jong et al., 1991; Moroni, 1987). Both the pharmacokinetics and the safety profile of Monurol™ are very good. It is rapidly absorbed into the blood and displays no serum binding capability. It has a half life of ~6 hours and is excreted unmetabolized. Although fosfomycin exhibits broad spectrum bactericidal activity, the high rate of resistance to fosfomycin limits its use to acute cystitis only. Administration of fosfomycin synergized β-lactams against *Staphylococci* and *Pseudomonas,* suggesting that fosfomycin could be more broadly utilized (Chin, et al., 1986). Resistance to fosfomycin is due to either decreasing drug uptake (Kahan et al., 1974) or destroying fosfomycin via a novel plasmid-encoded glutathione transferase (Suarez & Mendoza, 1991; Bernat et al., 1997). A third mechanism of resistance depends upon mutation of MurA to a form that is not reactive to fosfomycin (Venkateswaren & Wu, 1973). Mechanistic studies on recombinant MurA identified Cys115 as the site of modification by fosfomycin (Marquardt et al., 1994). Interestingly, site-directed mutagenesis of the Cys115 to Asp resulted in an active enzyme that escaped inactivation (Kim et al., 1996). That the enzyme from *Mycobacterium tuberculosis* uses an Asp in place of the conserved Cys115 may explain why fosfomycin is ineffective against this organism.

The crystal structure of the enzyme was recently reported (Schonbrunn et al., 1996) The enzyme is a two-domain protein containing an unusual "inside out" α/β barrel. The structure is similar to the crystal structure of EPSP synthase and confirms the stereochemical similarities (Stalling et al., 1991). Despite their common structural features and stereochemistry, the chemical mechanisms of these two enzymes are actually quite different. In the case of EPSP synthase, only one intermediate (phospholactoyl-shikimate-3-phosphate) is formed during the course of the catalytic turnover. However, in the case of MurA, the enzyme proceeds through two intermediates. Fosfomycin specifically inhibits the formation of the first of these intermediates, the enzyme-lactoyl adduct that results from the condensation of Cys115 with PEP (Fig. 3). Noteworthy is that an inhibitor for EPSP synthase, glyphosate, blocks the formation of the substrate-tetrahedral intermediate (Steinrucken and Amrheim, 1984; Anderson et al., 1988; Anderson and Johnson, 1990), but that fosfomycin and glyphosate exhibit no cross-reactivity. Physiologically, the enzymes from *E. coli*, *E. cloacae*, and *B. cereus* (rod-shaped bacteria) were feedback inhibited by UDP-MurNAc-tripeptide and UDP-MurNAc-pentapeptide (Venkateswaran et al., 1973; Zemel and Anwar, 1975). However, the enzyme in Gram-positive cocci does not exhibit feedback inhibition. This suggests that the Stage I enzymes may be controlled differently between rods and cocci. A detailed comparison of MurA from these two classes of bacteria is warranted to further examine this hypothesis.

UDP-N-ACETYLGLUCOSAMINE ENOLPYRUVATE REDUCTASE (MurB)

The second enzyme of the pathway is a flavoprotein reductase that catalyzes the conversion of the 3-enoylpyruvyl moiety to a lactoyl group, which acts as a "primer" for amino acids to be appended by the ligases. The *E. coli* enzyme has been the subject of detailed mechanistic studies. MurB proceeds through a ping-ping Bi-Bi kinetic mechanism. A reduced enzyme intermediate is formed during catalysis (Dhalla et al., 1995). Steady-state kinetic analyses demonstrate the enzyme is prone to both substrate and product inhibition. The physiological relevance of this potentially regulatory phenomenon remains to be determined.

The three dimensional structure of MurB has been determined using X-ray crystallography, both in the free and substrate bound forms (Benson et al., 1995; Benson et al., 1996). Comparison of these structures revealed a large domain movement from a tight conformation to a loose conformation upon substrate binding. This loosening of the enzyme global structure actually closes the substrate channel after the binding of UDP-GlcNAc-EP. Since a NADPH complex of MurB was not crystallized, the site of the NADPH binding could not be deduced from the data. Closer analysis suggested that there is a single binding site for UDP-GlcNAc-EP and NADPH. Support for this hypothesis came from comparative NMR analysis of the chemical shifts of the MurB unliganded enzyme, the enzyme-NADP+ and enzyme-UDP-GlcNAc-EP complexes (Farmer et al., 1996). Similar chemical shift perturbations were observed in the enzyme-NADP+ and enzyme-UDP-GlcNAc-EP complexes leading to the conclusion that NADPH binds to the same site as UDP-GlcNAc-EP does. Thus, MurB follows a single site ping-pong Bi-Bi ki-

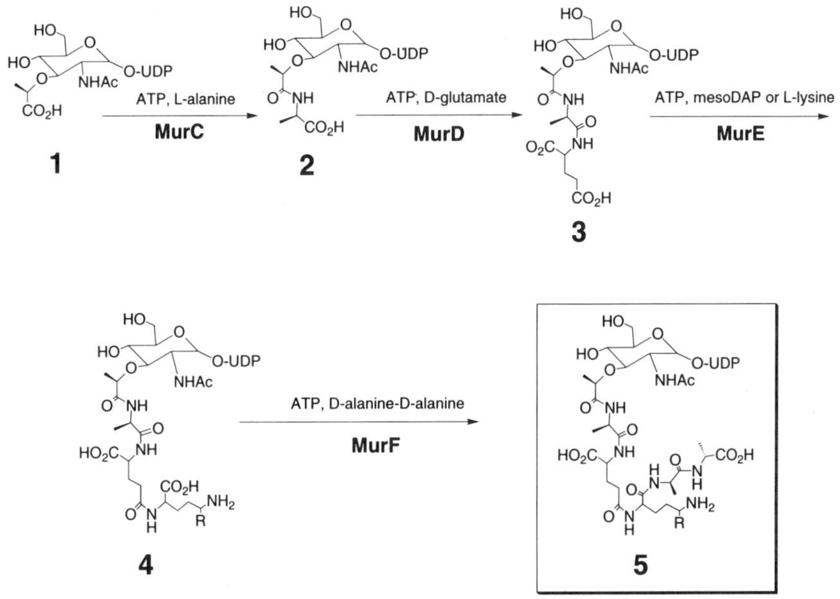

Figure 4. Reaction catalyzed by the Mur amino acid ligases. All reactions require Mg-ATP. L-alanine is ligated by MurC, D-glutamate by MurD, L-lysine or mesoDAP by MurE and D-alanine-D-alanine by MurF, to form **5**, the basic building block for the cell wall.

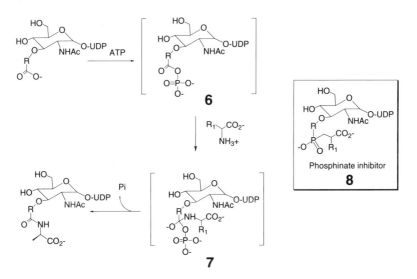

R = lactoyl, lactoyl-L-ala, lactoyl-L-ala-D-glu,or lactoyl-L-ala-D-glu-γ-mDAP

Figure 5. General mechanism of the Mur amino acid ligases. The acceptor carboxylate is first activated by phosphorylation to form **6**. Then the in-coming amino acid reacts to form the tetrahedal intermediate, **7**. The collapse of this intermediate releases inorganic phosphate and the amide product.

netic mechanism and this kinetic mechanism explains why the enzyme is inhibited by both substrates and products. The domain changes upon binding to substrate may also be the cause for the changes in the visible spectrum of the enzyme-bound flavin (Axley et al., 1997). Both substrates cause a red shift of the flavin chromophore. This shift will allow the determination of binding constants for both substrates and for potential inhibitors. Finally, the stereochemical course of the reduction has been carefully mapped (Lees et al., 1996). The pro-R hydride of NADPH is transferred to the si face of the flavin. Upon binding of UDP-GlcNAc-EP to the reduced enzyme, the hydride is then transferred to the C-3 methylene of the enoylpyruvate moiety. This stereochemistry of hydride transfer between NADPH and the enzyme-bound flavin is unusual, and only one other enzyme, methylenetetrahydrofolate reductase, displays this stereochemistry.

THE MUR ATP-DEPENDENT AMINO ACID LIGASES (MurC, MurD, MurE, AND MurF)

The reactions catalyzed by the next four enzymes of the pathway are related in that they all catalyze an ADP-forming addition of D- or L- amino acids (Fig.4). UDP-MurNAc-pentapeptide (5) is a biologically unique structure where three out of the five constituent amino acids are of D-configuration. The high D-amino acid content and the γ-glutamyl isopeptide linkage catalyzed by MurE protects bacteria from foreign proteolytic assault on the cell wall. The general mechanism of this class of ligases involves an acyl phosphate intermediate 6, (Fig. 5) produced from the phosphorylation of the acceptor carboxylate by ATP (Falk et al., 1996). This phosphorylation activates the carbonyl group for attack by the incoming amino acid. The highly conserved sequence of the pentapeptide moiety is thought to be due to the exquisite specificity of each of the four amino acid ligases for their respective amino acid. Insights into the close relationship among these ligases were first identified by Ikeda and coworkers (1990). They identified two domains, a glycine rich region and a region of high hydrophobicity. Subsequently, detailed re-examination of the *mur* genes by

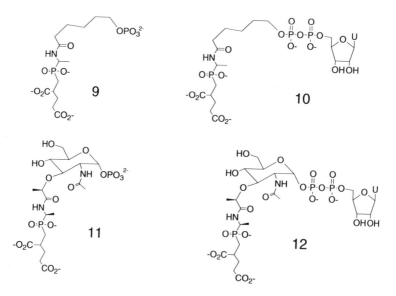

Figure 6. Potent phosphinate inhibitors of MurD.

Eveland et al. (1997) identified two additional regions of homologies between the nucleotide binding domain (Region I) and the hydrophobic domain (Region IV). The additional regions of homologies were later confirmed by two other groups (Betrand et al., 1997; Bouhuss et al., 1997). Region two is the most interesting region since it contains five highly conserved ionic residues. Since the reaction involves charged intermediates, these conserved residues are good candidates for being active site amino acids. Indeed site-directed mutagenesis of His188 and E158 (in Region II) are deleterious to the catalytic activity of *E coli* MurF (Eveland et al., 1997). This is also the case for H199G and H199A (Region II) mutants of *E. coli* MurC (Reddy et al., unpublished results). Further support of the notion that the conserved residues of Region II are indeed active site residues comes from the recently reported crystal structure of *E. coli* MurD (Betrand et al., 1997). H188 is situated within hydrogen binding distance of the carboxylate of UDP-MurNAc-L-alanine, while E158 is one of two metal ligands for Mg-ATP. Taken together, these data imply a role for H188 in catalysis. Further mechanistic studies are required to substantiate this hypothesis. Additional evidence of the high degree of relationship among these ligases comes from steady-state kinetic analysis. MurF proceeds through a sequential Ter-Ter kinetic mechanism (Anderson et al., 1996) as does MurC (Emanuele et al., 1996). Thus these data suggest that MurD and MurE also proceeds through the same kinetic mechanism. The mechanistic and structural similarities of the Mur ligases bode well for the design of an inhibitor, a multimodal inhibitor, that binds to more than one of the Mur ligases.

The first D-amino acid ligase of the pathway is MurD which catalyzes the addition of D-glutamate to UDP-MurNAc-L-alanine. Recently several potent inhibitors of this enzyme have been synthesized. Using the chemical mechanism of the ligase reaction as a guide, Tanner et al. (1996) synthesized a series of acyclic phosphinate, **9** and **10** inhibitors (Fig. 6) designed to mimic the tetrahedral transition state, **7** (Fig. 5). Many structural elements of the substrate were required for potent inhibition (for **10**, IC_{50} = 600 nM). More recently, even more potent inhibitors were synthesized where the N-acetylmuramyl moiety was incorporated (Gegnas et al., 1998). Examination of their inhibition characteristics with *E. coli* MurD revealed excellent inhibition with IC_{50} values reaching the sub-nanomolar range for **11** and **12**. Unfortunately, these compounds were not antibacterial, probably due to a lack of cellular penetration. This approach has also been attempted to inhibit MurE and MurF (Le Roux et al., 1992; Miller et al., 1998), but the compounds synthesized did not contain the UDP-MurNAc moiety. As a result, the potency of inhibition of their target enzymes were unimpressive. These data indicates that there is significant binding energy associated with the interactions of the UDP-MurNAc portion of the substrate with all of the Mur ligases.

THE ANCILLARY ENZYMES

Although not part of the main pathway, glutamate racemase (MurI), alanine racemase (Alr) and D-alanyl-D-alanine ligase (DdlA and DdlB) catalyze the reactions necessary to produce D-amino acids for the incorporation into the pentapeptide moiety. Glutamate racemase (MurI) provides the intracellular pool of D-glutamate for the second amino acid position of the pentapeptide. Unlike alanine racemase, glutamate racemase from *Bacillus subtilus* contains no known co-factor. With a mechanism similar to proline racemase (Cardinale & Abeles, 1968, Rudnick & Abeles, 1975), MurI interconverts the D and L forms of glutamate using a two-cysteine mechanism (Gallo et al., 1993; Gallo and Knowles 1993; Tanner et al, 1993). The activity of the enzyme from *E. coli* is allosterically regulated by the substrate of MurD (Ho et al., 1995). Intriguing is that this type of regulation does not appear to operate in Gram-positive bacteria.

Alanine racemase is a pyridoxal-phosphate-containing enzyme that converts naturally occurring L-alanine into D-alanine. D-Alanyl-D-alanine ligase joins two D-alanine molecules, forming the dipeptide substrate for MurF. Several natural product inhibitors have been reported for these enzymes (Lynch and Neuhaus, 1966; Reitz et al., 1967; Neuhaus & Hammes, 1981). During the 1980's, several groups synthesized a number of inhibitor classes of alanine racemase and D-alanyl-D-alanine ligase (Walsh, 1989). The mechanism-based halo-alanine class of inhibitors of alanine racemase involve an enzyme-catalyzed dehalogenation step. The formation of an aminoacrylate intermediate results in the covalent modification of the pyridoxal cofactor. Alanine phosphonate and alanine boronate are slow binding inhibitors of alanine racemase (Duncan et al., 1989). For D-alanyl-D-alanine ligase, synthetic efforts by the Merck group resulted in the preparation of (aminoalkyl)phosphinates (Parsons et al., 1988) which were excellent slow binding inhibitors of the enzyme (Duncan and Walsh, 1988). The phosphinate inhibitor is phosphorylated by ATP during partial turnover of the enzyme, resulting in a molecule that forms a very tight complex. None of these inhibitors are used in the clinic.

MINING THE MUR PATHWAY FOR NOVEL ANTIBIOTICS

Based on genetic and pharmacological studies, the Stage I enzymes of peptidoglycan biosynthesis are valid targets for antibiotic development. As already detailed above, much is known about the structure and mechanism of the cytoplasmic enzymes. Given a multitude of excellent targets, how do we choose which one to pursue? If the targets are all equally good (from a theoretical point of view), it is impossible to know, *a priori,* which of them will be susceptible to permeative small molecule inhibitors. Ideally, we would like to let the leads tell us which are the best targets. Our strategy therefore has been *not* to make a choice, but to screen all six (MurA-MurF) of the validated cytoplasmic targets. If carried out in the conventional manner, this approach calls for many individual enzyme assays, each of which must be optimized and validated. Every assay will require large quantities of substrates and enzymes, especially if the target is to be run though a high volume screening facility. Finally each enzyme must actually be screened, and this could take from only a few weeks to six months or more, depending on the size of the sample collection and the complexity of the assay. To gain some of the advantages of whole cell screening, while retaining the control over assay conditions that in vitro methods allow, we developed a Mur pathway assay that consists of all of the enzymes in the biosynthetic sequence.

The advantages of such a system are obvious. Screening throughput is increased directly by increasing the number of targets (assayed against the same number of test samples). At the same time, assaying six enzymes simultaneously reduces the number of times the sample collection must be screened. High throughput screening has introduced concern that sample collections are being depleted faster than they can be restocked. One-pot screening of many enzymes certainly will conserve limited samples. But the savings in resources goes beyond this. By assaying the enzymes together as a metabolic sequence, in which the product of one enzyme is the substrate for the next enzyme in the pathway, the effort of preparing substrate for each individual enzyme is obviated. Only the first substrate, in our case, UDP-GlcNAc, need be prepared. The co-substrates of the pathway (PEP, ATP, NADH, amino acids) are all common biochemicals. In fact, the in situ synthesis of substrates for downstream enzymes is what makes screening for enzymes that have rare substrates (i.e. not commercially available) possible. An added feature from a theoretical point of view is that pathway metabolites have common structural features that must be recognized by different enzymes. Thus inhibitors that recognize these shared motifs will likely bind to more than one enzyme in the pathway. The cumulative effect of weakly inhibiting several enzymes might reduce flux through the pathway more effectively than an inhibitor of a single enzyme. Such mulimodal inhibitors can only be selected in a pathway context.

To reconstruct the Mur pathway in vitro, purified Mur enzymes are required. Since the DNA sequences from *E. coli* encoding the cytoplasmic enzymes were known, it was straightforward to clone each of them into an expression vector of our own design (Pryor and Leiting, 1997). Maximal soluble expression is gained by making a dual fusion protein that includes maltose binding protein (MBP; Maina et al., 1988) and hexahistidyl (His6) tag (Gentz et al., 1988). Although MBP fusions tend to be highly soluble proteins, unlike glutathione-S-transferase protein fusions that have a propensity to form inclusion bodies, MBP fusions did not purify cleanly on the amylose affinity column. Therefore the His6 tag was included in the vector to aid in purification (Pryor and Leiting, 1997). There is a thrombin proteolytic site located between the affinity tags and the protein of interest. Thus a one-step purification using the nickel affinity column, followed by cleavage with thrombin, yields 200–500 mg/L of pure soluble protein. This procedure was used to express and purify all of the Mur pathway enzymes.

Equally important for soluble expression of the target proteins is the correct growth conditions. Most bacterial proteins can be produced in soluble form by adjusting the growth media and the temperature (Pryor and Leiting, 1997). Surprisingly, minimal media actually increased the yield of soluble protein, most likely because rich media contains peptides and small proteins that induce various scavenger pathways. These scavenger pathways use proteases to break down the peptides in the media to amino acids for use in protein biosynthesis. However, these proteases can also degrade the target protein. Lower growth temperature (even 4 °C) also increases the fraction of soluble protein expressed.

With the enzymes in hand, the next concern is the substrates. To kinetically characterize each of the Mur enzymes, an ample supply of each of substrate must be available. A glance at the structures of the murein intermediates explains why there has been a lack of detailed kinetic studies of the pathway enzymes: the substrates are complex nucleoside-containing molecules that are neither commercially available nor easy to synthesize chemically. As was just described, however, the enzymes catalyzing their biosynthesis are available in large quantities and can be used as chemical reagents to make the intermediates. Using commercially available UDP-GlcNAc as starting material and adding the appropriate co-substrates and Mur pathway enzymes, hundreds of milligrams of any one of the UDP-containing substrates in the pathway can be produced enzymatically. Note that UDP-GlcNAc itself also can be synthesized enzymatically (Leiting et al., 1998). These reactions are high-yielding because they are all thermodynamically favored (with most of them coupled to the hydrolysis of ATP). The pathway intermediates are purified readily by reverse phase HPLC or anion exchange FPLC (Jin et al., 1996; Reddy et al., unpublished results). Some of the substrates can also be purified from bacteria treated with a metabolic inhibitor. For example, cells grown in the presence of cycloserine accumulate UDP-MurNAc-tripeptide, the MurF substrate (Nakatani et al., 1968; Anderson et al., 1996). Likewise, using vancomycin will cause a buildup of the UDP-MurNAc-pentapeptide. Presently there are no known cell-active inhibitors of MurB, MurC, MurD or MurE, so this method does not apply to earlier metabolites of the pathway. From enzymatic synthesis, we can prepare all of the pathway intermediates for enzymological studies, or for use as reference standards.

Monitoring the progress of the pathway assay has taken several forms. For rapid screening, only the rate of formation of the final product of the pathway is measured. Using radiolabelled D-alanyl-D-alanine as the reporter, radiolabeled product UDP-MurNAc-pentapeptide is separated from the substrate D-alanyl-D-alanine and quantified. Since all the Stage I intermediates can be separated by HPLC, using radiolabelled UDP-GlcNAc as the reporter provides a complete picture of the time-dependent change in concentrations of all seven metabolites. Radiolabelled UDP-GlcNAc and D-alanyl-D-alanine are commercially available, but they are quite expensive. However, a cheaper synthesis of UDP-GlcN[^{14}C]Ac via enzymatic means is available (Leiting et al., 1998).

The last issue to be considered is the kinetic behavior of the pathway. The goal is to discover inhibitors of the pathway enzymes, not to recreate a test tube version of the in vivo Mur pathway. The relative concentrations of the enzymes in the screening assay are going to be different than those that exist in vivo. For the screen, concentrations of the enzymes and substrates must be optimized so that an inhibitor of any one of the enzymes in the pathway is equally likely to be detected. In order for this to occur, the flux of substrate through each enzyme should be nearly the same. Under such conditions, inhibition of any one of the enzymes will result in the diminution of the final product, UDP-MurNAc-pentapeptide. However, if the fluxes through each enzyme step are not equal, inhibitors of some enzymes might be missed. By analogy with kinetic isotope effects, if one enzyme in a metabolic sequence is rate limiting, inhibitors of that enzyme will be found preferentially, just as the rate-limiting elementary step of an enzyme-catalyzed reaction is most sensitive to an isotope effect. Likewise a pathway enzyme following one that is rate-limiting will be less sensitive to inhibition; the effects of an inhibitor on a non-rate-determining step will be masked by the sluggishness of the rate-limiting step.

There are two ways to set the conditions of the pathway assay correctly. The first is an empirical method. With arbitrary concentrations for all enzymes and the concentrations of the substrates set at their value of Km, the rate of product UDP-MurNAc-peptide is determined. The enzyme concentration of the first enzyme is reduced incrementally, keeping the other enzyme concentrations fixed, until the rate of product formation begins to decrease linearly with the decrease in the varied enzyme concentration. This concentration of the first enzyme is then fixed. The same experiment is performed for subsequent enzymes in the pathway until all the concentration for all enzymes are adjusted to values where the flux of the pathway is equally determined by each of the constituent enzymes.

The necessary relative enzyme concentrations in the pathway assay can also be predicted using the combination of kinetic parameters for each individual enzyme with a numeric model of the coupled sequential enzyme systems. The kinetic parameters for each individual enzyme, if unknown, can be determined through conventional enzymological methods in conjunction with a non-linear modeling of the kinetic data to extract the relevant rate constants for each enzyme. The experimentally determined kinetic parameters can then be used in a computer simulation of the sequential enzyme system. Software was devised to fit kinetic constants to experimental data and to simulate the time course of multiple enzyme systems. This approach utilizes the Runge-Kutta algorithm to solve general chemical and enzyme kinetic rate equations as non-linear, coupled differential equations. The approach also allows for the simulation of multiple enzyme systems under various initial conditions in which no closed form solutions either analytic or approximated are available. Thus, enzyme and chemical reaction pathways may be simulated and rate constants derived from experimental data without resorting to approximations based

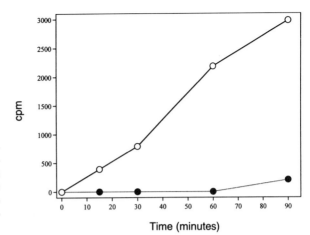

Figure 7. Mur pathway in action. Analysis of UDP-MurNAc-pentapeptide formation using [³H]-D-alanyl-D-alanine in the absence (open circles) and in the presence (filled circles) of 4 µM **11** demonstrates inhibition of the pathway by specifically inhibiting MurD.

on initial conditions or a particular kinetic model. Additionally, the time course of all components of multiple enzyme systems may be simulated under any initial concentration conditions.

The empirical approach offers the advantage of a solution without knowing a priori the kinetic parameters for each of the enzymes within the pathway. Since the kinetic characterization of unfamiliar enzymes takes time and consumes an exorbitant amount of substrates, this trial and error method is the quickest way to a solution. However, if the kinetic parameters are known, the mathematical model should allow the conditions to be established easily, and the effects of perturbations (inhibitors, substrate concentration changes, etc.) can be anticipated. Since few of the kinetic parameters of the Stage I enzymes of the peptidoglycan biosynthetic pathway were known when we began, we determined the concentrations of the components of the pathway assay empirically. However, kinetic characterization of all the constituent enzymes is underway so as to feed the mathematical model.

Screening of the six Stage I enzymes is now possible in a single pathway assay. Shown in Figure 7 is a progress curve for the formation of radiolabeled UDP-MurNAc-pentapeptide using [³H]D-alanyl-D-alanine as the reporter substrate. Note the pre-steady state lag in product formation while the intermediates accumulate to their steady-state concentrations. The addition of a potent MurD inhibitor dramatically attenuated the rate of product formation. If a compound inhibits the pathway, individual Stage I enzyme assays are in place to identify which of the enzymes is the target.

Used in high throughput mode, the Stage I pathway screen is an efficient method to screen a large number of validated antibacterial targets. It is a perfect complement to whole cell assays specific for cell wall biosynthesis (Gadebusch et al., 1992) in the search for the next generation of antibacterial drugs. Furthermore, this approach can be generally applied to any therapeutically relevant metabolic pathway. It is hoped that this review will spawn new ideas that will accelerate the rate of drug discovery, not only in antibiotic research, but in many other therapeutic areas.

ACKNOWLEDGMENTS

We are indebted to all of our colleagues involved in peptidoglycan biosynthesis research at Merck. We also thank John O'Connell for sharing his preliminary pathway modeling studies, Matt S. Anderson and Lynn L. Silver for reviewing the manuscript, and John W. Kozarich for his unflagging support of our work.

REFERENCES

Amabile-Cuevas, C.F., and Chicurel, M.E., 1992, Bacterial plasmids and gene flux. *Cell* 70:189.

Anderson K.S., Sikorski J.A., and Johnson K.A., 1988, Evaluation of 5-enolpyruvoylshikimate-3-phosphate synthase substrate and inhibitor binding by stopped-flow and equilibrium fluorescence measurements, *Biochemistry* 27:1604.

Anderson, K.S., and Johnson, K.A., 1990, Kineic and Structural analysis of enzyme intermediates: Lessons from EPSP synthase, *Chem. Rev.* 90:1131.

Anderson, M.S., Eveland, S.S., Onishi, H.R., and Pompliano, D.L., 1996, Kinetic mechanism of the *Escherichia coli* UDPMurNAc-tripeptide D-alanyl-D-anlanine-adding enzyme: use of a glutathione S-transferase fusion, *Biochemistry* 35:16264.

Axley, M.J., Fairman, R., Yanchunas, Jr, J., Villafranca, J.J., and Robertson, J.G., 1997, Spectroscopic properties of *Escherichia coli* UDP-N-acetylpyruylglucosamine reductase, *Biochemistry* 36, 812.

Beise, F., Labischinski, H., and Giesbrecht, P., 1988, Role of penicillin-binding proteins of *Staphylococcus aureus* in the induction of bacteriolysis, in: *Antibiotic Inhibition of Bacterial Cell Surface Assembly and Function*, Actor, P., Daneo-Moore, L. Higgins, M.L., Salton, M.R.J., and Schockman, G.D., eds., American Society for Microbiology, Washington, DC.

Benson, T.E., Filman, D.J., Walsh, C.T., and Hogle, J.M., 1995, An enzyme-substrate complex involved in bacterial cell wall biosynthesis, *Nature Struc. Biol.* 2:644.

Benson, T.E., Walsh, C.T. and Hogle, J.M., 1996, The structure of the substrate-free form of MurB, an essential enzyme for the synthesis of bacterial cell walls, *Structure* 4:47.

Bernat, B.A., Laughlin, L.T., and Armstrong, R.N., 1997, Fosfomycin resistance protein (FosA) is a manganese metalloglutathione transferase related to glyoxalase I and the extradiol dioxygenases, *Biochemistry* 36, 3050.

Bertrand, J.A., Auger, G., Fanchon, E., Martin, L., Blanot, D., van Heijenoort, J., and Dideberg, O., 1997, Crystal structure of UDP-N-acetylmuramoyl-L-alanine:D-glutamate ligase from *Escherichia coli*, *EMBO J.* 16:3416.

Beveridge, T.J., 1981, Ultrastructure, chemistry and function of the bacterial cell wall, *Int. Rev. Cytol.*, 72:229.

Bouhss, A., Mengin-Lecreulx, D., Blanot, D., van Heijenoort, J., and Parquet, C., 1997, Invariant amino acids in the Mur peptide synthetases of bacterial peptidoglycan synthesis and their modiication by site-directed mutagenesis in the UDP-MurNAc:L-alanine ligase from *Escherichia coli*, *Biochemistry* 36:11556.

Brown, E.D., Vivas, E.I., Walsh, C.T., and Kolter, R., 1995, MurA(MurZ), the enzyme that catalyzes the first committed step in peptidoglycan biosynthesis is essential in *Escherichia coli*, *J. Bacteriol.* 177:4194.

Bugg, T., and Walsh, C.T., 1992, Intracellular steps of bacterial cell wall peptidoglycan biosynthesis: enzymology, antibiotic, and antibiotic resistance, *Nat. Prod. Rep.* 9:199.

Cardinale, G.J., and Abeles, R.H., 1968, Purification and mechanism of action of proline racemase, *Biochemistry* 7:3970.

Chin, N.X., Neu, N.M., and Neu, H.C., 1986, Synergy of fosfomycin with beta-lactam antibiotics against staphylococci and aerobic gram-negative bacilli, *Drugs Exp. Clin. Res.*, 12, 943.

Chopra, I., Hodgson, J., Metcalf, B., and Poste, G., 1996, New approaches to the control of infections caused by antibiotic-resistant bacteria, *J. Am. Med. Assoc.* 275:401.

Chu, D.T.W., Plattner, J.J., and Katz, L., 1996, New directions in antibacterial research, *J. Med. Chem.* 39:3853.

Davies, J.E., 1997, Origins, acquisition, and dissemination of antibiotic resistance determinants, In: *Antibiotic Resistance: Origins, Evolution and Spread*, Chadwick, D.J. & Goode, J., eds., Ciba Foundation Symposium 207, John Wiley & Sons.

de Jong, Z., Pontonnier, F., and Plante, P., 1991, Single-dose fosfomycin trometamol (Monuril) versus multiple-dose norfloxacin: results of a multicenter study in females with uncomplicated lower urinary tract infections, *Urol. Int.*, 46, 344.

Desnottes, J-F., 1996, New targets and strategies for the development of antibacterial agents. *TIBTECH* 14:134.

Dhalla, A.M., Yanchunas, Jr., J., Ho, H.-T., Falk, P.J., Villafranca, J.J., and Robertson, J.G., 1995, Steady-sate kinetic mechanism of *Escherichia coli* UDP-N-acetylenolpyruvyl-glucosamine reductase, *Biochemistry*, 34:5390.

Duncan, K., and Walsh, C.T., 1988, ATP-dependent inactivation and slow binding inhibition of *Salmonella ty-phimurium* D-alanine:D-alanine ligase (ADP) by aminoalkyl)phosphinate and aminophosphonate analogues of D-alanine, *Biochemistry* 27:3709.

Duncan, K., Faraci, W.S., Matteson, D.S., and Walsh, C.T., 1989, (1-Aminoethyl)boronic acid: A novel inhibitor for Bacillus stearothermophilus alanine racemase and *Salmonella typhimurium* D-alanine:D-alanine ligase, *Biochemistry* 28:3541.

Emanuele, Jr., J.J., Jin, H., Jacobson, B.L., Chang, C.Y., Einspahr, H.M., and Villafranca, J.J., 1996, Kinetic and crystallographic studies of *Escherichia coli* UDP-N-acetylmuramate:L-alanine ligase, *Protein Sci.* 5:2566.

Eveland, S.S., Pompliano, D.L., and Anderson, M.S., 1997, Conditional lethal *Escherichia coli* murein mutants contain point defects that map to regions conserved among murein and folyl poly-γ-glutamate ligases:identification of a ligase superfamily, *Biochemistry* 36, 6223.

Falk, P.J., Ervin, K.M., Volk, K.S., and Ho, H.-T., 1996, Biochemical evidence for the formation of a covalent acyl-phosphate linkage between UDP-N-acetylmuramate and ATP in the *Escherichia coli* UDP-N-acetylmuramate:L-alanine ligase-catalyzed reaction, *Biochemistry* 35: 1417.

Farmer, II, B.T., Constantine, K.L., Goldfarb, V., Friedrichs, M.S., Wittekind, M., Yanchunas, Jr., J., Robertson, J.G., and Mueller, K., 1996, Localizing the NADP+ binding site on the MurB enzyme by NMR, *Nature Struc. Biol.* 3:995.

Fisher, J.A., 1994, *The Plague Makers*, Simon and Schuster, New York.

Gadebusch, H.H., Stapley, E.O., Zimmerman, S.B., 1992, The discovery of cell wall active antibacterial antibiotics, *Crit. Rev. Biotech.* 12:225.

Gallo, K.A. and Knowles, J.R., 1993, Purification, cloning, and cofactor independence of glutamate racemase from Lactobacillus, *Biochemistry* 32:3981.

Gallo, K.A., Tanner, M.E., and Knowles, J.R., 1993, Mechanism of the reaction catalyzed by glutamate racemase, *Biochemistry* 32:3991.

Gegnas, L.D., Waddell, S.T., Chabin, R.M., Reddy, S., Wong, K.K., 1998, Inhibitors of the bacterial cell wall biosynthesis enzyme MurD, *Bioorg. Med. Chem. Let.* in press.

Gentz, R., Certa, U., Takacs, B., Matile, H., Dobeli, H., Pink, R., Mackay, M., Bone, N., Scaife, J.G., 1988, Major surface antigen p190 of *Plasmodium falciparum*: detection of common epitopes present in a variety of Plasmodia isolates, *EMBO J.* 7:225–230.

Ghuysen, J.-M., and Hakenbeck, R., Eds., 1994, *Bacterial Cell Wall. New Comprehensive Biochemistry*, Vol. 27, Elsevier, Amsterdam.

Goetz, A., Yu, V.L., 1997, The intensive care unit: the hottest zone, *Curr. Opin. Infect. Dis.* 10:319.

Hall, B.G., 1990, Spontaneous point mutations that occur more often when advantageous than when neutral, *Genetics* 126, 5.

Ho, H.T., Flak, P.J., Ervin, K.M., Krishnan, B.S., Discotto, L.F., Dougherty, T.J., and Pucci, M.J., 1995, UDP-N-acetylmuramyl-L-alanine functions as an activator in the regulation of the *Escherichia coli* glutamate racemase activity, *Biochemistry* 34:2464.

Hutchinson, C.R., 1995, Drug synthesis by genetically engineered microorganisms. *Biotechnology* 12: 375.

Ikeda, M., Wachi, M., Jung, H.K., Ishino, F., and Matsuhashi, M., 1990, Homology among MurC, MurD, MurE and MurF proteins in *Escherichia coli* and that between *E. coli* MurG and a possible MurG protein in *Bacillus subtilis*, *J. Gen. Appl. Microbiolog.*, 36: 179.

Jin, H., Emanuele, Jr., J.J., Fairman, R., Robertson, J.G., Hail, M.E., Ho, H.-T., Falk, P.J., and Villafranca, J.J., 1996, Structural studies of *Escherichia coli* UDP-N-acetylmuramate:L-alanine ligase, *Biochemistry* 35:1423.

Kahan, F.M., Kahan, J.S., Cassidy, P.J., and Kropp, H., 1974, The mechanism of action of fosfomycin (phosphonomycin), *Ann. NY Acad. Sci.* 235:364.

Kato, J., Suzuki, H., and Hirota, Y., 1985. Dispensability of either penicillin-binding protein-1a or -1b involved in the essential process for cell elongation in *Escherichia coli*, *Mol. Gen. Genet.* 200:272.

Khosla, C., 1996, Combinatorial chemistry and biology: an opportunity for engineers, *Curr-Opin-Biotechnol.* 7: 219.

Kim., D.H., Lees, W.J., Haley, T.M., and Walsh, C.T., 1995, Kinetic characterization of the inactivation of UDP-GlcNAc-enoylpyruvyl transferase by (Z)-3-fluorophosphoenol-pyruvate: Evidence for two oxocarbenium ion intermediates in enolpyruvl transfer catalysis, *J. Am. Chem. Soc.* 117:1494.

Kim., D.H., Lees, W.J., Kempsell, K.E., Lane, W.S., Duncan, K., and Walsh, C.T., 1996, Characterization of a Cys115 to Asp substitution in the *Escherichia coli* cell wall biosynthetic enzyme UDP-GlcNac enolpyruvyl transferae (MurA) that confers resistence to inactivation by the antibiotic fosfomycin, *Biochemistry* 35:4923.

Knowles, D.J.C., 1997, New strategies for antibacterial drug design, *Trends Microbiol.* 5:379.

Le Roux, R., Auger, G., van Heijenoort, J., and Blanot, D., 1992, Synthesis of new peptide inhibitors of the meso-diaminopimelate-adding enzyme, *Eur. J. Med. Chem.* 27:899.

Lees, W.J., and Walsh., C.T., 1995, Analysis of the enol ether transfer catalyzed by UDP-GlcNac enolpyruvyl transferase using (E)- and (Z)-isomers of phosphoenolbutyrate: sterochemical, partitioning and isotope effect studies, *J. Am. Chem. Soc.* 117:7329.

Lees, W.J., Benson, T.E., Hogle, J.M., and Walsh, C.T., 1996, (E)-Enolbutyryl-UDP-N-acetylglucosamine as a mechanistic probe of UDP-N-acetylenolpyruvylglucosamine reductase (MurB), *Biochemistry* 35:1342.

Leiting, B., Pryor, K.-A.D., Eveland, S.S., and Anderson, M.S., 1998, One-day enzymatic synthesis and purification of UDP-N-[1–^{14}C]acetylglucosamine, *Anal. Biochem.*, 256:185.

Lugtenberg, E.J.J., de Haas-Menger, L., and Ruyters, W.H.M., 1972, Murein synthesis and identification of cell wall precursors of temperature-sensitive lysis mutants of *Escherichia coli*, *J. Bacteriol.* 109:326.

Lugtenberg, E.J.J., and van Schijndel-van Dam, A., 1972, Temperature-sensitive mutant of *Escherichia coli* K-12 with low activifies of the L-alanine adding enzyme and the D-alanyl-D-alanine adding enzyme, *J. Bacteriol.* 110:35.

Lugtenberg, E.J.J., and van Schijndel-van Dam, A., 1973, Temperature-sensitive mutant of *Escherichia coli* K-12 with an impaired D-alanine:D-alanine ligase. *J. Bacteriol.* 113:96.

Lynch, J.L., and Neuhaus, F.C., 1966, On the mechanism of action of the antibiotic O-carbamyl-d-serine in *Streptococcus faecalis*, *J. Bacteriol.* 91:449.

Maina, C.V., Riggs, P.D., Grandea, A.G., III, Slatko, B.E., Moran, L.S., Tagliamonte, J.A., McReynolds, L.A., and di Guan, C., 1988, An *Escherichia coli* vector to express and purify foreign proteins by fusion to and separation from maltose-binding protein, *Gene* 74:365.

Marquardt, J. Brown, E.D., Lane, W.S., Haley, T.M., Ichikawa, Y., Wong, C.-H., and Walsh, C.T., 1994, Kinetics, stoichiometry, and identification of the reactive thiolate in the inactivation of UDP-GlcNAc enoylpyruvoyl transferase by the antibiotic fosfomycin, *Biochemistry* 33:10646.

Miller, D.J., Hammond, S.M., Anderluzzi, D., and Bugg, T.D.H., 1998, Aminoalkylphosphinate inhibitors of D-ala-D-ala adding enzyme, *J. Chem. Soc., Perkin Trans.* 1:131.

Moroni, M., 1987, Monuril in lower uncomplicated urinary tract infection in adults, *Eur. Urol.*, 13 (Suppl 1), 101.

Nakatani, T., Araki, Y., Ito, E., 1968, Preparation and characterization of uridinediphosphate-N-acetylmuramyl-L-alanyl-D-glutamyl-meso-2,6-diaminopimelic acid, *Biochim Biophys Acta* 156:210.

Neuhaus, F.C., and Hammes, W.P., 1981, Inhibition of cell wall biosyntheisis by analogues of alanine, *Pharmacol. Ther.* 14:265.

Pace, N.R., 1997, A molecular view of microbial diversity and the biosphere, *Science* 276: 734

Parsons, W.H, Patchett, A.A., Bull, H.G., Schoen, W.R., Taub, D., Davidson, J., Combs, P.L., Springer, J.P., Gadebusch, H., Weissberger, B.,Valiant, M.E., Mellin, T.N., and Busch, R.D., 1988, Phosphinic acid inhibitors of D-alanyl-D-alanine ligase, *J. Med. Chem.* 31:1772.

Pryor, K.D., and Leiting, B., 1997, High-level expression of soluble protein in *Escherichia coli* using a His6-tag and maltose-binding-protein double-affinity fusion system, *Protein Expr Purif.* 10: 309.

Reitz, R.H., Salde, H.D., and Neuhaus, F.C., 1967, The biochemical mechanism of resistance by streptococci to the antibiotic D-cycloserine and O-carbamyl-D-serine, *Biochemistry* 6:2561.

Riesenfeld, C., Everett, M., Piddock, L.J., and Hall, B.G., 1997, Adaptive mutations produce resistance to ciprofloxacin, *Antimicrob. Agents. Chemother.* 41:2059.

Rudnick, G., and Abeles, R.H., 1975, Reaction mechanism and structure of the active site proline racemase, *Biochemistry* 14:4515.

Russel, A.D., and Chopra, I., 1990, *Understanding Antibacterial Action and Resistance*, Ellis Horwood, New York.

Schonbrunn, E., Sack, S., Eschenburg, S., Perralis, A., Krekel, F., Amrhein, N., and Mandelkow, E., 1996, Crystal structure of UDP-N-acetylglucoamine enolpyruvatetransferase, the target of the antibiotic fosfomycin, *Structure* 4:1065.

Setti, E.L., Quattrocchio, L., and Micetich, R.G., 1997, Current approaches to overcome bacterial resistance, *Drugs Fut.* 22:271.

Silver, L.L., and Bostian, K.A., 1990, Screening of natural products for antimicrobial agents, *Eur. J. Clin. Microbiol. Infect. Dis.* 9:455.

Silver, L.L., and Bostian, K.A., 1993, Discovery and development of new antibiotics: the problem of antibiotic resistance, *Antimicrob. Agents Chemother.* 37:377.

Stallings, W.C., Abdel-Meguid, S.S., Lim, L.W., Shieh, H.-S., Dayringer, H.E., Leimgruber, N.K., Stegman, R.A., Anderson, K.S., Sikorski, J.A., Padgetter, S.R., and Kishore, G.M., 1991, Structure and topological symmetry of the glyphosate target 5-enol-pyruvaylshikimate-3-phosphate synthase: A distinctive protein fold, *Proc. Natl. Acad. Sci. USA* 88:5046.

Steinrucken, H.C., and Amrhein, N., 1984, 5-Enolpyruvylshikimate-3-phosphate synthase of *Klebsiella pneumoniae* 2. Inhibition by glyphosate [N-(phosphonomethyl)glycine], *Eur. J. Biochem.* 143:351.

Suarez, J.E., and Mendoza, M.C., 1991, Plasmid-encoded fosfomycin resistance, *Antimicrob. Agents Chemother.* 35:791.

Swartz, M.N., 1994, Hospital-acquired infections: diseases with increasingly limited therapies, *Proc. Natl. Acad. Sci. USA* 91:2420.

Tanner, M.E., Vanganay, S., van Heijenoort, J., and Blanot, D., 1996, Phosphinate inhibitor of the D-glutamate acid-adding enzyme of peptidoglycan biosynthesis, *J. Org. Chem.* 61:1756.

Tanner, M.E., Gallo, K.A., and Knowles, J.R., 1993, Isotope effects and the identification of catalytic residues in the reaction catalyzed by glutamate racemase, *Biochemistry* 32:3998.

Venkateswaran, P.S., Lutenburg, E.J., and Wu, H.C., 1973, Inhibition of phosphoenoylpyruvate:uridine diphosphate N-acetylglucoseamine enoylpyruvyl transferase by uridine diphosphate N-acetylmuramyl peptides, *Biochimica et Biophysica Acta* 293:570.

Walsh, C.T., 1989, Enzymes in the D-alanine branch of bacterial cell wall peptidoglycan assembly, *J. Biol. Chem.* 264:2393.

Walsh, C.T. Fisher, S.L., Park, I.S., Prahalad, M., and Wu, Z., 1996, Bacterial resistance to vancomycin: five genes and one missing hydrogen bond tell the story, *Chem. Biol.* 3: 21.

Wanke, C. and Amrhein, N., 1993, Evidence that the reaction of the UDP-N-acetylglucoamine 1-carboxyvinyltransferase proceeds through the O-phosphothioketal of pyruvic acid bound to Cys115 of the enzyme, *Eur. J. Biochem.* 218:861.

Wickus, G.G., and Stromynger, J.L., 1973, Partial purification and properties of the pyruvate-uridine diphospho-N-acetylglucosamine transferase from *Staphylococcus epidermidis*, *J. Bacteriol.* 113:287.

Zemell, R.I., and Anwar, R.A., 1975, Pyruvate-uridine diphospho-N-acetylglucosamine transferase: purification to homogeneity and feedback inhibition, *J. Biol. Chem.* 250:3185.

DESIGN, SYNTHESIS, AND EVALUATION OF NOVEL OXAZOLIDINONE ANTIBACTERIAL AGENTS ACTIVE AGAINST MULTIDRUG-RESISTANT BACTERIA

Michael R. Barbachyn,[*] Steven J. Brickner, Robert C. Gadwood,
Stuart A. Garmon, Kevin C. Grega, Douglas K. Hutchinson,
Kiyotaka Munesada, Robert J. Reischer, Mikio Taniguchi,
Lisa M. Thomasco, Dana S. Toops, Hiromi Yamada, Charles W. Ford,
and Gary E. Zurenko

Pharmacia & Upjohn
Kalamazoo, Michigan 49007

INTRODUCTION

Throughout the human experience, diseases caused by pathogenic bacteria have exerted an enormous negative impact on society. Today, for example, approximately one third of the world's population is infected with *Mycobacterium tuberculosis* and tuberculosis remains the leading cause of death in the world from infectious disease (Bloom, 1994). The emergence of effective antibacterial agents, from penicillin to more contemporary drugs, was initially thought to mark an end to the burden of microbial disease. However, subsequent events have illustrated the resiliency of bacteria to environmental pressures, including the threat of antibacterial agents.

Some particularly problematic organisms include multidrug-resistant *M. tuberculosis* (Bloch et al., 1996), penicillin- and cephalosporin-resistant *Streptococcus pneumoniae* (Tomasz, 1997; McCracken, 1996; Spangler et al., 1996; Breiman et al., 1994), methicillin-resistant *Staphylococcus epidermidis* (MRSE) and *Staphylococcus aureus* (MRSA) (Ayliffe, 1997; Moreno et al., 1995; Voss et al., 1994; Tomasz, 1994), and vancomycin-resistant *Enterococcus faecalis* and *Enterococcus faecium* (VREF) (Leclercq, 1997; Leclercq and Courvalin, 1997; McDonald et al., 1997; Coque et al., 1996). Of par-

---

[*] Author to whom all correspondence should be addressed

Resolving the Antibiotic Paradox, edited by Rosen and Mobashery.
Kluwer Academic / Plenum Publishers, New York, 1998.

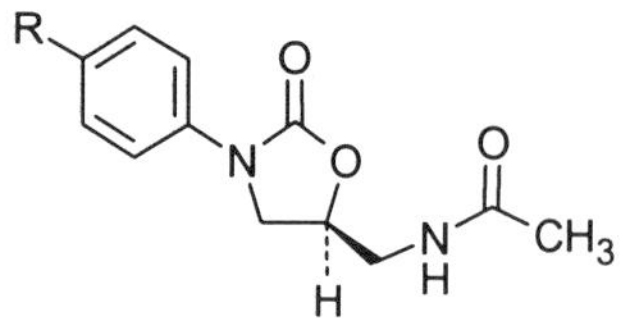

DuP 105: R = CH$_3$SO
DuP 721: R = CH$_3$CO

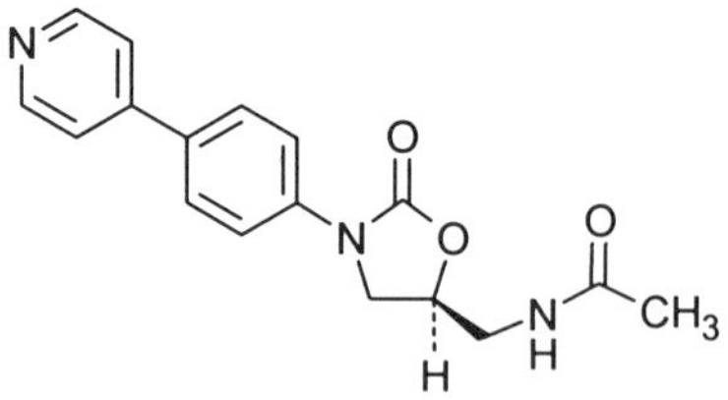

E3709

Figure 1. DuPont lead oxazolidinones

ticular concern is the strong possibility that the enterococci will transfer their vancomycin resistance determinants to the more virulent staphylococci via a plasmid mediated process, a scenario that has already been demonstrated in experimental studies (Noble et al., 1992). When this event occurs in the clinical setting there will be no effective treatment for infections caused by such organisms, in lieu of alternative efficacious therapies. In a disturbing recent development, the first vancomycin intermediate-resistant *S. aureus* (VISA) clinical strains have been isolated (Hiramatsu et al., 1997; Martin et al., 1997).

A number of solutions to the bacterial resistance problem have been suggested (Silver and Bostian, 1993). One example involves the structural modification of known drugs to overcome resistance liabilities. Combination therapies, for example the combination of a β-lactam antibiotic with a β-lactamase inhibitor, have also been utilized with some success. New therapeutic approaches such as the use of narrow spectrum agents with improved diagnostics are possible. However, the best solution to the bacterial resistance dilemma remains the identification of novel antibacterial agents employing a unique mechanism of action (Chopra et al., 1996; Chu et al., 1996).

OXAZOLIDINONES

DuPont Oxazolidinones

A new and promising group of antibacterial agents, collectively known as the oxazolidinones, have recently emerged (Brickner, 1996). The discovery and preliminary evolution of these compounds was reported by workers at DuPont in 1987 (Slee et al., 1987; Eustice and Slee, 1987). Two lead analogs, DuP 105 and DuP 721, were described at that time, but subsequently dropped from clinical development (Figure 1) (*Scrip*, 1987; *Pharmaprojects*, 1995; *Pharmcast-International*, 1995). In later animal studies at Phamacia and Upjohn, (±)-DuP 721 was found to exhibit significant toxicity in a chronic rat model (Piper, 1989). Further DuPont oxazolidinones with improved levels of antibacterial activity, exemplified by E3709, were subsequently described (Brumfitt and Hamilton-Miller, 1992; Carlson, Park and Gregory, 1990).

Some of the dogmas that emerged from the early DuPont structure-activity relationships (SAR) are highlighted below (Figure 2) (Park et al., 1992). As subsequent events will illustrate, several of these notions require revision.

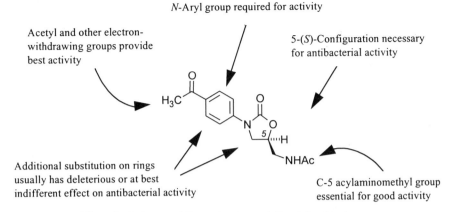

N-Aryl group required for activity

Acetyl and other electron-withdrawing groups provide best activity

5-(*S*)-Configuration necessary for antibacterial activity

Additional substitution on rings usually has deleterious or at best indifferent effect on antibacterial activity

C-5 acylaminomethyl group essential for good activity

Figure 2. Early oxazolidinone structure-activity relationship dogmas.

Pharmacia & Upjohn Oxazolidinones

Conceptually, we wondered whether the 4-pyridyl moiety of the DuPont lead, E3709, might be amenable to replacement by suitable saturated heterocyclic bioisosteres. In connection with this notion, and in an inverse sense, we were cognizant of the successful replacement of the piperazine ring system of, for example, ciprofloxacin, with a pyridine fragment, as seen in Win-57273, in the quinolone antibacterial agent area (Figure 3) (Reuman et al., 1989). Another important aspect of the existing quinolone SAR was the finding that strategically located fluorine atoms were found to not only increase potency, but also to confer enhanced oral pharmacokinetic performance to the compounds (Nix and Schentag, 1988; Chu and Fernandes, 1989). Contemporaneous to our plans to explore the piperazine surrogate, we speculated that the small but highly electron-withdrawing fluo-

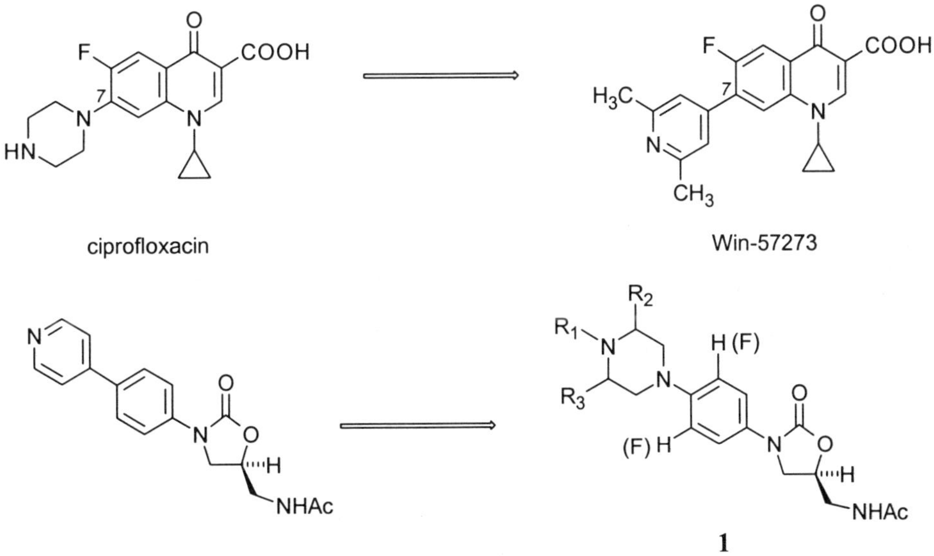

ciprofloxacin

Win-57273

1

Figure 3. Genesis of the fluorinated piperazinylphenyloxazolidinones.

Table 1. The effect of fluorine substitution on antibacterial activity

				MIC (μg/mL)[1]			ED_{50}
PNU-No.	R_1	R2	R_3	SA^2	EF3	SP4	(mg/kg)[5]
107399	CO_2Me	H	H	4	4	2	NT[6]
98257	CO_2Me	H	F	4	2	1	3.7 (1.6)
98170	CO_2Me	F	F	2	2	0.5	2.5 (1.3)
108946	$COCH_2OH$	H	H	4	2	1	NT
100592	$COCH_2OH$	H	F	4	1	<0.5	3.3 (5.0)
100675	$COCH_2OH$	F	F	2	1	0.25	1.6 (1.8)
143145	$COCH_2OH$	H	OMe	>16	>16	>16	NT
97665	CH_2CN	H	F	8	4	1	4.0 (2.2)
98172	CH_2CN	F	F	4	2	1	2.8 (2.7)
99200	$(CH_2)_2OMe$	H	F	16	16	2	7.9 (1.7)
99372	$(CH_2)_2OMe$	F	F	8	4	1	7.7 (2.0)
100762	$(CH_2)_2F$	H	F	16	8	2	8.6 (5.0)
100349	$(CH_2)_2F$	F	F	4	2	1	5.0 (2.8)

[1]MIC = minimum inhibitory concentration
[2]SA = *Staphylococcus aureus* UC9213
[3]EF = *Enterococcus faecalis* UC9217
[4]SP = *Streptococcus pneumoniae* UC9912
[5]ED_{50} = effective dose$_{50}$ - dose that protects 50% of the animals; oxazolidinones administered orally; subcutaneously administered vancomycin in parentheses
[6]NT = not tested

rine atom would be tolerated at the *meta* position(s) of the central phenyl ring and confer enhanced antibacterial activity and/or other desirable properties to the targeted oxazolidinones (see generic structure).

Eperezolid (PNU-100592): The First Clinical Oxazolidinone. A number of piperazinylphenyloxazolidinones of generic structure **1** were synthesized. Many of these analogs exhibited interesting levels of *in vitro* (MIC) and *in vivo* (ED_{50}) antibacterial activity. Of particular note was the gratifying finding that one or two fluorine atoms flanking the *para* piperazine appendage exerted a significant potentiating effect on the antibacterial activity (see Table 1), a finding consistent with observations in other oxazolidinone subclasses (Barbachyn, Toops, et al., 1996; Barbachyn, Hutchinson, Brickner et al., 1996). Ultimately, based on a consideration of other factors beyond the scope of this discussion, the most interesting

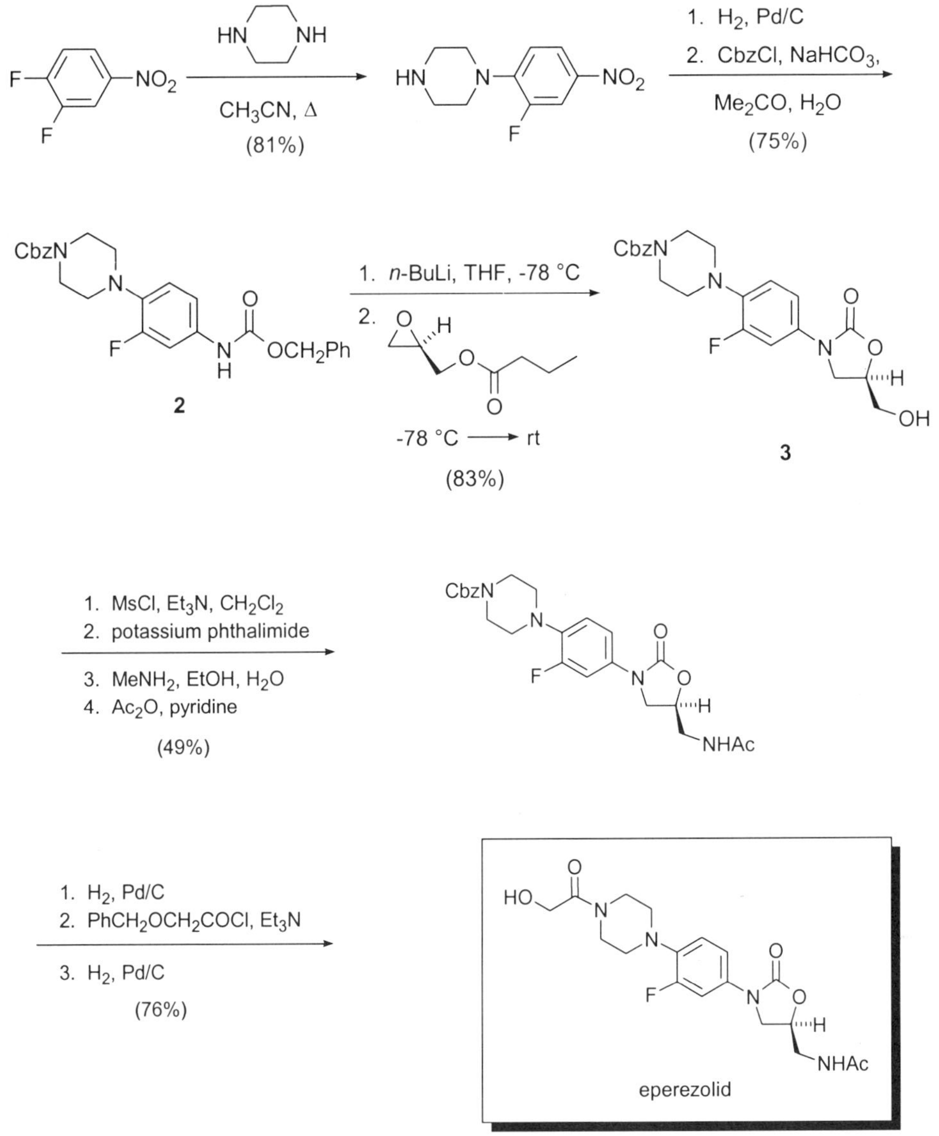

Scheme 1

compound to emerge from this preliminary series was eperezolid (PNU-100592) (Brickner, Hutchinson, Barbachyn et al., 1996. Orally or subcutaneously administered eperezolid displays vancomycin-like activity levels against clinically relevant gram-positive organisms in animal infection models and has successfully completed phase I clinical safety trials.

A synthesis of eperezolid in enantiomerically enriched form is outlined in Scheme 1. The key step in the sequence is the reaction of lithiated carbamate **2** with commercially available (R)-glycidyl butyrate to generate high yields of the advanced 5-(hydroxymethyl)oxazolidinone intermediate **3** (Brickner, Manninen et al., 1993). Further elaboration of **3** proceeded uneventfully to furnish eperezolid (Brickner, Hutchinson, Barbachyn et al., 1996).

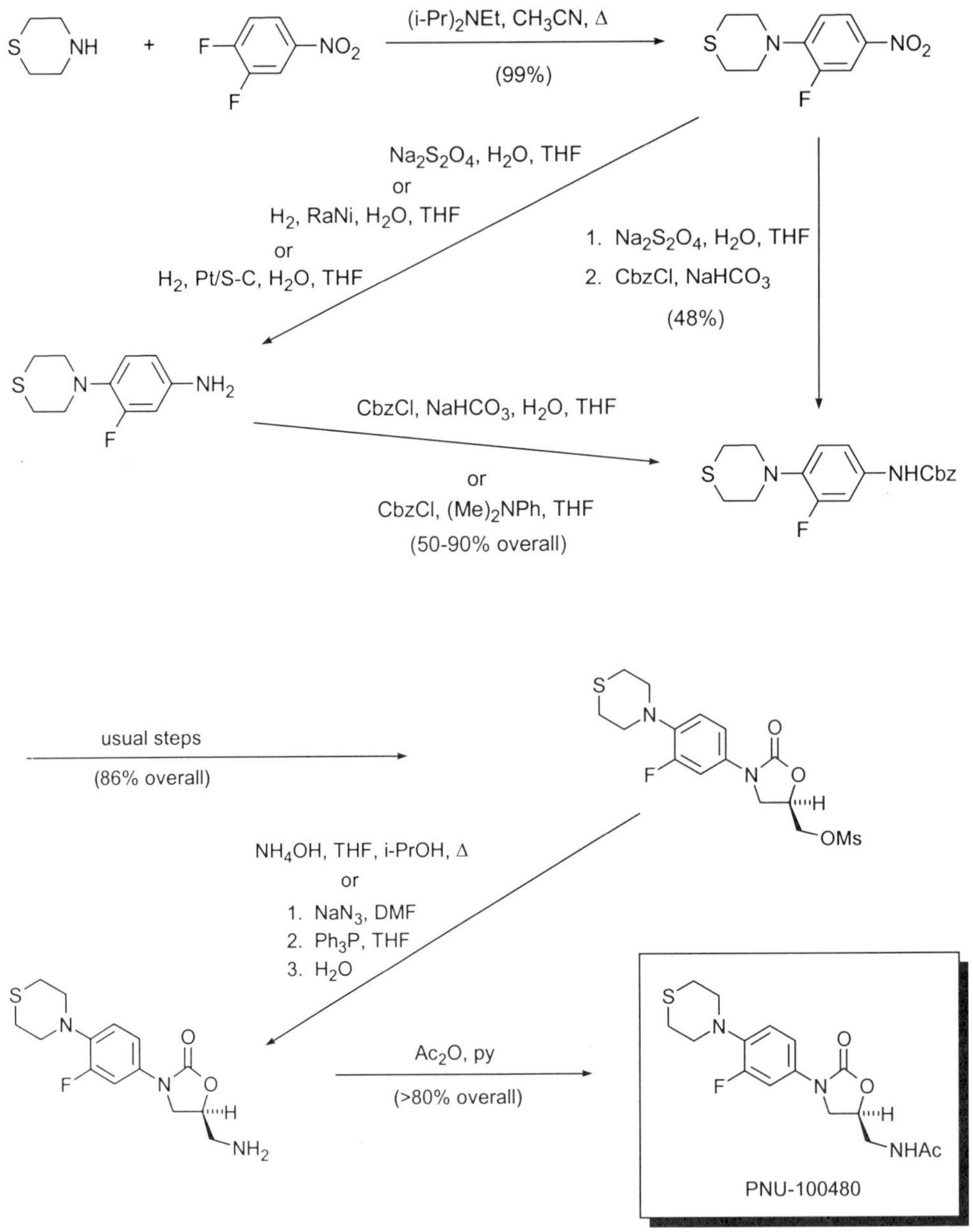

Scheme 2

PNU-100480: A Potent Antimycobacterial Agent. In an extension of the piperazinyl-phenyloxazolidinone subclass, we have also examined the preparation of morpholinyl- and thiomorpholinylphenyloxazolidinones. A preparation of the parent thiomorpholine analog, PNU-100480 (Barbachyn, Hutchinson, Brickner, Cynamon, Kilburn, Klemens et al., 1996), which closely parallels the synthesis of eperezolid, is depicted in Scheme 2. Not surprisingly, due to the presence of the sulfur residue, some alternative conditions

Table 2. *In vitro* activity of PNU-100480 against selected mycobacteria

Organism	MIC (μg/mL)[1]		
	PNU-100480	isoniazid	azithromycin
M. tuberculosis H37Rv	≤0.125	0.2	NT[2]
M. avium ATCC 49601	4	NT	4
M. avium 101	0.5	NT	4
M. simiae	2	NT	4
M. xenopi	2	NT	1
M. malmoense	2	NT	16
M. fortuitum	8	NT	>64

[1]MIC = minimum inhibitory concentration
[2]NT = not tested

were necessary for some of the synthetic transformations, especially the various reduction steps.

Interestingly, PNU-100480 exhibits potent *in vitro* and *in vivo* antimycobacterial activity (Barbachyn, Hutchinson, Brickner, Cynamon, Kilburn, Klemens et al., 1996; Klemens, Sharpe and Cynamon, 1995; Zamkoff, Cline, Klemens and Cynamon, 1995). Table 2 shows that the activity of PNU-100480 against several mycobacterial species is comparable or superior to that of currently used clinical agents such as isoniazid and azithromycin.

This activity extends to multiple clinical isolates of *M.tuberculosis*, including strains resistant to conventional antituberculosis drugs, and *M. avium* complex (see Table 3) (Barbachyn, Hutchinson, Brickner, Cynamon, Kilburn, Klemens et al., 1996). The latter organism is an opportunistic pathogen commonly associated with the acquired immune deficiency syndrome (AIDS).

Linezolid (PNU-100766): An Oxazolidinone in Advanced Clinical Studies. The most significant oxazolidinone prepared to date is PNU-100766 (linezolid) (Brickner, Hutchinson, Barbachyn et al., 1996). This morpholine derivative is readily prepared in seven steps from commercially available starting materials (scheme 3).

Linezolid exhibits *in* vitro activity (see Table 4) similar to that of vancomycin against *S. aureus*, including MRSA and VISA strains, penicillin- and cephalosporin-resistant *S. pneumoniae*, and *E. faecalis* and *E. faecium*, including VREF strains (Zurenko et

Table 3. *In vitro* activity of PNU-100480
against multiple clinical isolates

Organism	No. strains	MIC (μg/mL)	
		Range	90%
M. tuberculosis	10[1]	0.03-0.5	0.5
M. avium complex	20	0.5-4	4

[1]Panel of 5 "drug-sensitive" and 5 "drug-resistant" isolates (including resistance to one or more of: streptomycin, isoniazid, rifampin, ethionamide and ethambutol).

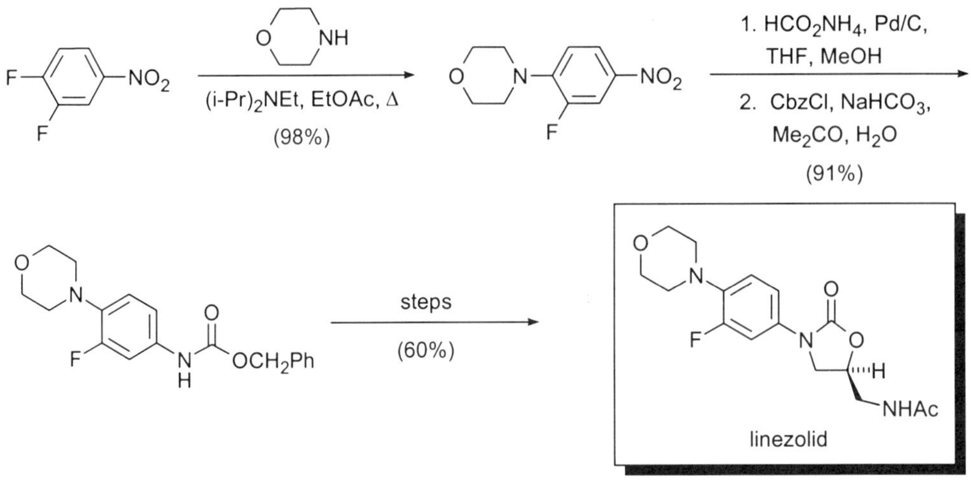

Scheme 3

al., 1996). In a departure from vancomycin, linezolid also displays modest activity against the fastidious gram-negative organisms *Haemophilus influenzae* and *Moraxella catarrhalis*, and has good activity versus anaerobic bacteria such as *Bacteroides fragilis*. Interestingly, linezolid is also quite active against *M. tuberculosis*, including isolates resistant to standard antitubercular agents.

The *in vitro* activity data for linezolid has correlated well with *in vivo* efficacy results (see Table 5) in experimental mouse models of bacteremia and skin and soft tissue infections (Ford et al., 1996). Orally (po) or subcutaneously (sq) administered linezolid demonstrated efficacy against staphylococcal infections comparable to that of vancomycin (sq). Good activity against vancomycin-resistant *E. faecium* (UC 15090) and penicillin- and cephalosporin-resistant *S. pneumoniae* (UC 15087) was also observed.

In phase I human clinical trials, orally or intravenously administered linezolid has been found to be well tolerated in single and multiple dose regimens (Pawsey, Daley-Yates, Wajszczuk and Stalker, 1996). No clinically significant adverse findings were observed at

Table 4. *In vitro* activity of linezolid

Organism	No. strains	MIC$_{90}$ (μg/mL)[1]	
		PNU-100766	Vancomycin
S. aureus, meth^S	12	4	1
S. aureus, meth^R	41	4	2
E. faecalis, Van^S	14	4	2
E. faecalis, VanB	10	4	>16
S. pneumoniae, Pen^R	10	1	≤0.25
H. influenzae	9	11.8[2]	>16
M. catarrhalis	10	4	>16
B. fragilis	10	4	>16
M. tuberculosis	10	0.5[3]	NT[4]

[1]Concentration of drug that inhibits 90% of the isolates
[2]weighted average
[3]MIC$_{80}$
[4]NT = not tested

Table 5. *In vivo* activity of linezolid

Organism	ED_{50} (mg/kg)	
	PNU-100766[1]	Vancomycin[2]
S. aureus UC9271[3]	2.9	13.2
S. aureus UC9213[4]	5.6	3.9
	2.0[2]	3.9
S. aureus UC6685[5]	3.8	2.6
E. faecium UC15090[6]	24.0	>100
S. pneumoniae UC15087[7]	3.8	>20[8]

[1]PO administration
[2]SC administration
[3]methicillin-susceptible
[4]MRSA
[5]multi-drug resistant MRSA
[6]vancomycin-resistant, immunocompromised mice
[7]penicillin- and cephalosporin-resistant
[8]penicillin G and cefaclor controls

oral doses of 400 mg/kg given three times per day (TID) for ten days (Pawsey, Daley-Yates, Wajszczuk and Stalker, 1996) or 625 mg dosed twice daily (BID) for 14.5 days (Stalker, Wajszczuk and Batts, 1997). Oral administration of 375 mg, 500 mg, or 625 mg of linezolid twice daily all afforded trough serum concentration levels above the MIC_{90} value of 4 µg/mL for *S. aureus* and steady-state concentrations remained above the MIC_{90} for 10 to 16 hours. Linezolid has recently entered phase III clinical trials.

Oxazolidinone Mechanism of Action

In early work at DuPont, the oxazolidinones were reported to be bacterial protein synthesis inhibitors, with inhibition uniquely occurring at the initiation phase of translation (Eustice, Feldman and Slee, 1988; Eustice, Feldman, Zajac and Slee, 1988). That is, the oxazolidinones do not block the elongation or termination steps of prokaryotic translation. However, the DuPont studies provided no experimental evidence of a direct interaction of an oxazolidinone with any component of the protein translation machinery. In ongoing mechanistic studies with eperezolid and linezolid at Pharmacia & Upjohn, workers have shown that the oxazolidinones inhibit protein synthesis by selectively binding to the 50S ribosomal subunit, thereby preventing formation of a functional initiation complex (Figure 4) (Lin, Murray, Vidmar and Marotti, 1997; Shinabarger, Marotti et al., 1997). The eperezolid/linezolid binding site is distinct from those of chloramphenicol and lincomycin, antibiotics that also have demonstrated evidence of binding to the 50S subunit.

Genesis of 1-Azetidinyl-, 1-Pyrrolidinyl-, and 1-Piperidinylphenyloxazolidinones

In contemplating potential bioisosteric replacements of the morpholinyl moiety of linezolid and piperazinyl subunit of eperezolid, we speculated that suitably functionalized

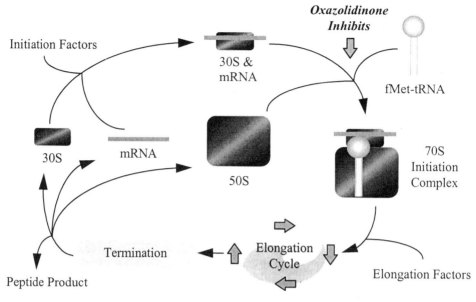

Figure 4. The ribosome cycle.

1-azetidinyl, 1-pyrrolidinyl, and 1-piperidinyl ring systems might have utility. Conceptually, we targeted compounds of generic structure **4** (Figure 5).

RESULTS AND DISCUSSION

Chemistry

The synthesis of the targeted oxazolidinones of generic structure **4** closely parallels that described for eperezolid and linezolid. A representative synthetic sequence leading to some 1-azetidinylphenyloxazolidinones is shown in Scheme 4. The starting azetidines **5** (Frigola et al., 1993) are deprotected and the resultant free azetidines condensed with 3,4-difluoronitrobenzene to furnish the adducts **6**. Reduction of the nitro group and conversion to the requisite benzyl carbamates **7** proceeded uneventfully. In the cases where R^2 = H, a *tert*-butyldimethylsilyl protecting group was installed via standard methodology. In what can be considered the key step in the reaction sequence, the carbamates **7** are deprotonated

R_1, R_2 = H, CH_3, CO_2R, OR, SR, NHR, =O, =NR   **Figure 5.** 1-Azetidinyl-, 1-pyrrolidinyl- and 1-pipe-
n, m = 1, 2   ridinylphenyloxazolidinones.

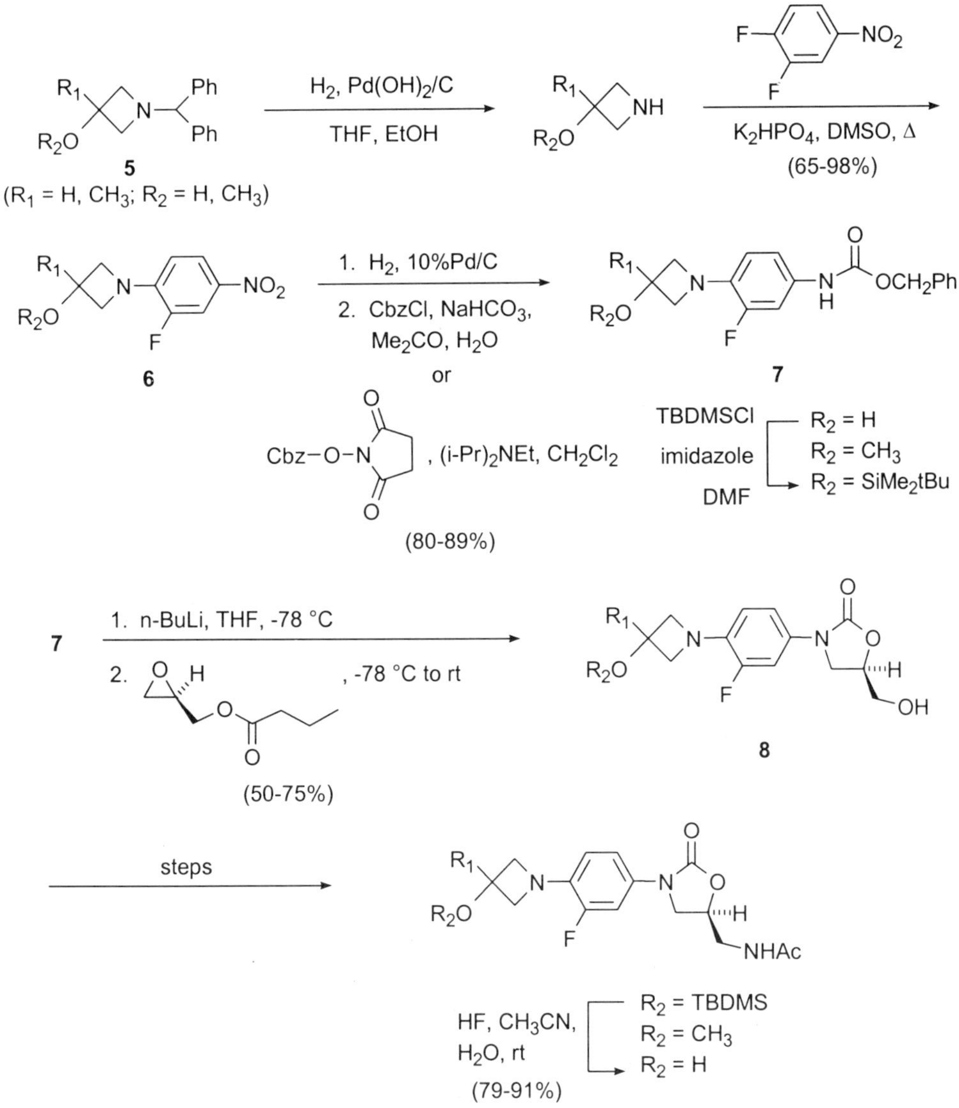

Scheme 4

with lithium base, typically *n*-butyllithium, and then reacted with commercially available
(*R*)-glycidyl butyrate to generate the important 5-(hydroxymethyl)oxazolidinones **8**
(Brickner, Manninen et al., 1993). The remaining synthetic steps directed at introduction
of the acetamido moiety of the C-5 sidechain closely parallels the chemistry described
previously (*vide supra*).

A number a pyrrolidinylphenyloxazolidinones have also been prepared. To illustrate
some variations on the usual synthetic theme, chemistry directed toward some
methylthiopyrrolidine derivatives is depicted in Scheme 5. The pyrrolidinol **9** was converted via a three-step sequence involving Mitsunobu dispacement, saponification, and
methylation to give the thioether **10**. Carbamate **10** was then subjected to the pivotal oxa-

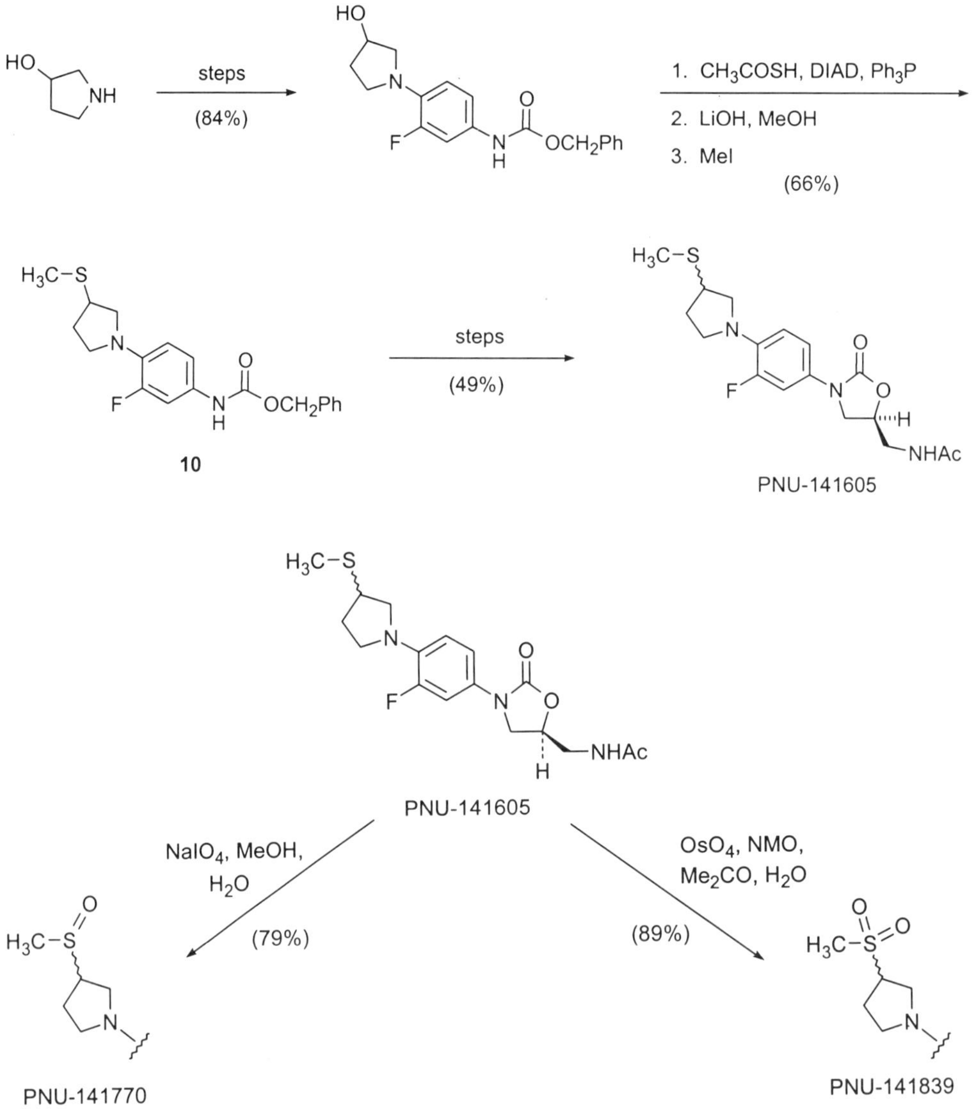

Scheme 5

zolidinone-forming reaction and subsequent sidechain functionalization to generate the targeted sufide PNU-141605. Thioether linkages are amenable to further elaboration. We were especially interested in oxidizing the sulfide to the corresponding sulfoxide or sulfone to probe the effect of such a modification on antibacterial activity. Oxidation of PNU-141605 to the sulfoxide PNU-141770 was smoothly accomplished through the action of sodium metaperiodate (Leonard and Johnson, 1962). The more highly oxygenated sulfone analog, PNU-141839, was prepared by the procedure described by Kaldor (1991).

A variety of piperidine starting materials are amenable to the general oxazolidinone synthetic protocol described previously. As shown in Scheme 6, the piperidine-substituted

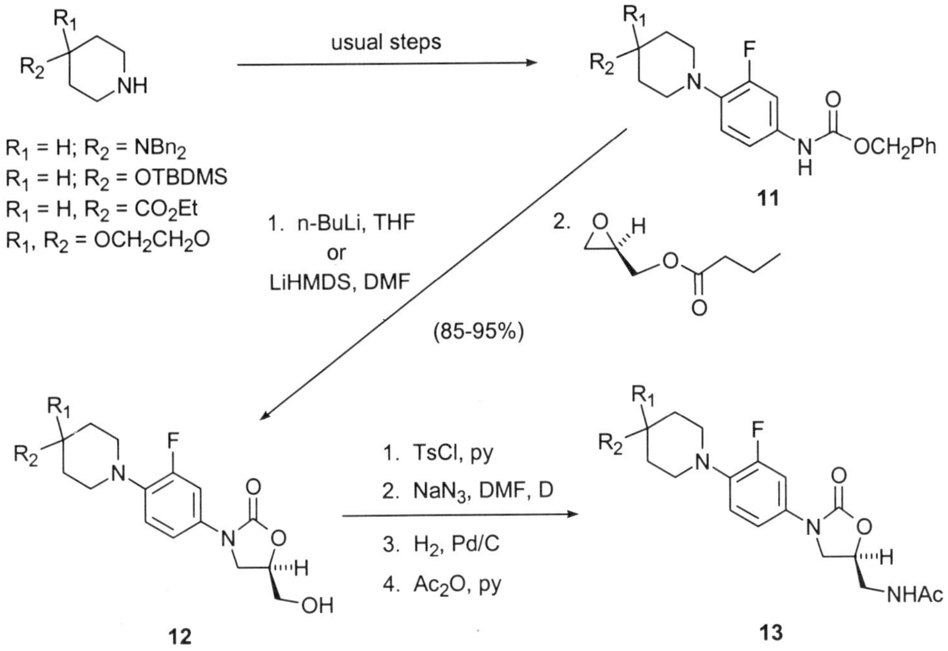

R$_1$ = H; R$_2$ = NBn$_2$
R$_1$ = H; R$_2$ = OTBDMS
R$_1$ = H, R$_2$ = CO$_2$Et
R$_1$, R$_2$ = OCH$_2$CH$_2$O

1. n-BuLi, THF
   or
   LiHMDS, DMF

(85-95%)

11

12

1. TsCl, py
2. NaN$_3$, DMF, D
3. H$_2$, Pd/C
4. Ac$_2$O, py

13

Scheme 6

carbamates **11** can be deprotonated with a suitable lithium base and then reacted with (R)-glycidyl butyrate to give the desired 5-(hydroxymethyl)oxazolidinones **12**. Further transformation of **12** then provides the targeted oxazolidinones **13**.

The product oxazolidinones, with their appended azetidine, pyrrolidine, or piperidine ring systems, are themselves amenable to additional synthetic modifications. For example, keto derivatives (see Scheme 7) can be prepared from the corresponding alcohols

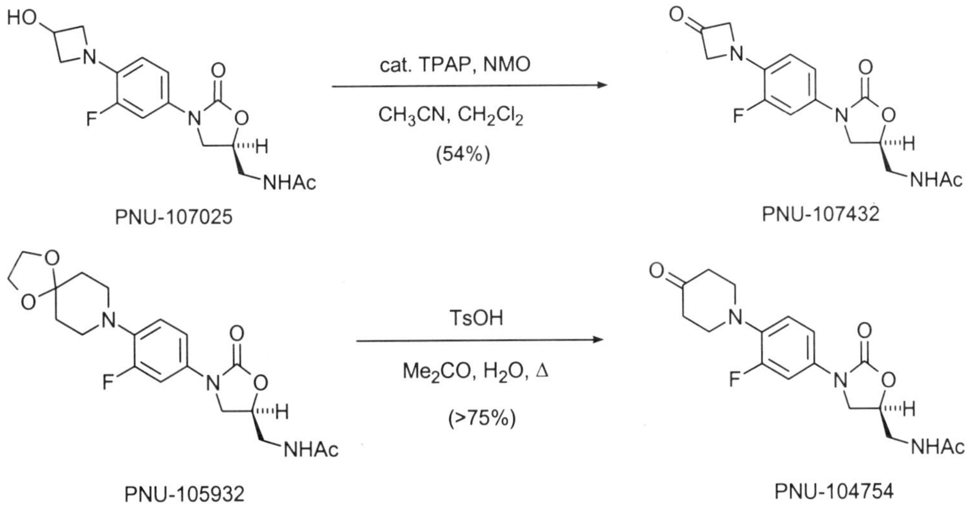

cat. TPAP, NMO

CH$_3$CN, CH$_2$Cl$_2$

(54%)

PNU-107025

PNU-107432

TsOH

Me$_2$CO, H$_2$O, Δ

(>75%)

PNU-105932

PNU-104754

Scheme 7

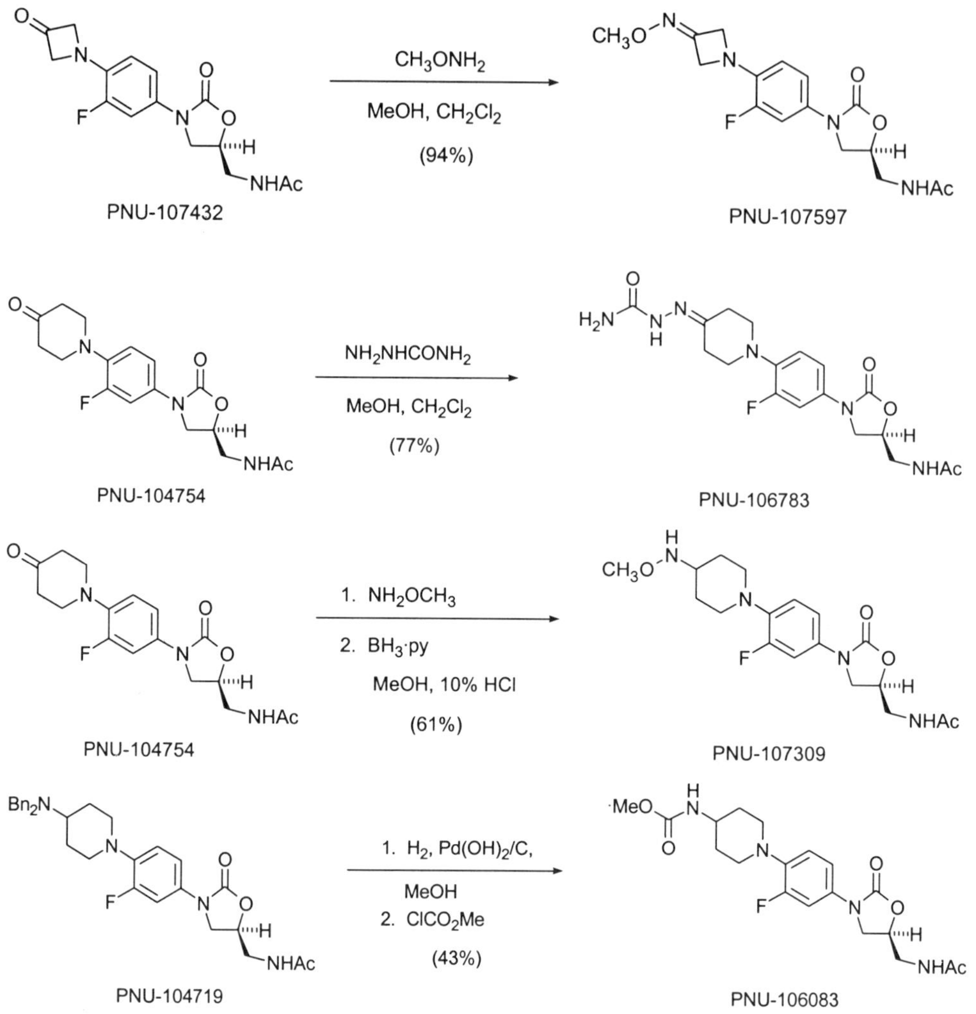

Scheme 8

through an appropriate oxidation process. For example, azetidinol PNU-107025 was sub-jected to a TPAP oxidation (Griffith and Ley, 1990) to furnish the azetidinone PNU-107432. In another approach, ketal derivatives such as PNU-105932 can be hydrolyzed with aqueous acid to generate the corresponding ketones, for example PNU-104754, in good yield.

The aforementioned ketone analogs are amenable to further synthetic manipulation (Scheme 8). For example, *O*-methylhydroxylamine was reacted with the azetidinone PNU-107432 to give the oxime PNU-107597 in excellent yield. In related chemistry, the piperidinone PNU-104754 was converted to the semicarbazone derivative PNU-106783. Reductive aminations are also viable synthetic options. In this way, the aminopiperidine congener PNU-107309 was prepared from PNU-104754. Such aminopiperidine deriva-tives are themselves suitable substrates for additional modification. For example, PNU-104719 was deprotected by hydrogenolysis and converted to the corresponding

Table 6. Effect of ring size on antibacterial activity

| | | | MIC (μg/mL)[1] | | | ED_{50} |
| | | | | | | (mg/kg)[5] |
PNU-no.	n	m	SA[2]	EF[3]	SP[4]	
107432	1	1	1	1	0.5	12.3 (1.3)[6]
105649	1	2	4	4	2	4.5 (2.8)[6]
104754	2	2	2	1	1	8.1 (2.8)[6]
141515	1	1	4	4	1	20.0 (1.4)[7]
141605	1	2	2	2	1	3.1 (2.9)[7]
140661	2	2	4	4	1	5.7 (1.3)[6]
linezolid			2	2	0.5	5.6 (3.9)[6]

[1]MIC = minimum inhibitory concentration
[2]SA = *Staphylococcus aureus* UC9213
[3]EF = *Enterococcus faecalis* UC9217
[4]SP = *Streptococcus pneumoniae* UC9912
[5]ED_{50} = effective dose$_{50}$ - dose that protects 50% of the animals - *S. aureus* UC9213; oxazolidinones administered orally
[6]subcutaneously administered vancomycin ED_{50} in parentheses
[7]eperezolid (PNU-100592) ED_{50} in parentheses

carbamate derivative PNU-106083. All of the synthetic chemistry described above should be considered merely representative.

Biological Activity: Structure-Activity Relationships

The effect of ring size on antibacterial activity was examined. As shown in Table 6, a comparison of 3-azetidinone (PNU-107432), 3-pyrrolidinone (PNU-105649), and 4-piperidinone (PNU-104754) derivatives reveals that the 4-membered ring system confers advantageous *in vitro* activity against representative gram-positive organisms, although the 5- and 6-membered congeners also demonstrate good activity levels. Interestingly, in the corresponding methylthio series (PNU-141515, PNU-141605, and PNU-140661), all three ring systems exhibit similar levels of *in vitro* activity against the test panel. In general, the observed *in vitro* activity levels are similar to those of linezolid. In a surprising but consistent finding, the 5-membered ring analogs usually display enhanced *in vivo* efficacy relative to their 4- and 6-membered ring counterparts. Employing a systemic mouse infection model, with *Staphylococcus aureus* as the infectious agent, the orally administered pyrrolidine analogs PNU-105649 and PNU-141605 were found to provide a protective effect comparable to those of the clinical comparators eperezolid, linezolid, and vancomycin. The reason for the consistently poor *in vivo* performance of the azetidine derivatives is unclear.

Table 7. Azetidine alkyl substitution and activity

PNU-no.	R_1	R2	MIC (μg/mL)[1]			ED_{50} (mg/kg)[5]
			SA[2]	EF[3]	SP[4]	
107025	H	H	4	8	2	>20.0
106798	H	Me	8	16	2	>20.0
105264	Me	H	4	8	2	13.8 (5.7)
106093	Me	Me	8	16	4	>20.0
linezolid			2	2	0.5	5.6 (3.9)

[1]MIC = minimum inhibitory concentration
[2]SA = *Staphylococcus aureus* UC9213
[3]EF = *Enterococcus faecalis* UC9217
[4]SP = *Streptococcus pneumoniae* UC9912
[5]ED_{50} = effective dose$_{50}$ - dose that protects 50% of the animals - *S. aureus* UC9213; oxazolidinones administered orally; subcutaneously administered vancomycin in parentheses

We also probed the effect of alkyl substitution on the activity of selected azetidinyl-phenyloxazolidinones (see Table 7). In general, the azetidinol analogs exhibited activity levels similar to those of the corresponding methyl ethers (PNU-107025 vis-à-vis PNU-105264). However, the addition of a methyl substituent at the C-3 position of the azetidine ring imparts reduced *in vitro* activity to the compounds (PNU-105264 vis-à-vis PNU-106093). The *in vivo* performance of these substituted azetidines was uniformly disappointing.

A number of azetidine, pyrrolidine, and piperidine analogs bearing methylthio appendages were prepared (*vide supra*). We examined the effect of sulfur oxidation state on the antibacterial activity of this series of oxazolidinones (see Table 8). In the piperidine subclass, the sulfone PNU-140847 was found to exhibit the most potent *in vitro* activity against *S. aureus*, followed by the sulfide PNU-140661, and then the sulfoxide PNU-140907. This relative ranking was mirrored in the *in vivo* efficacy test results. However, in the pyrrolidine series the sulfide PNU-141605 had the *in* vitro activity advantage over its more highly oxidized counterparts PNU-141770 and PNU-141839. Again, there was a good correlation between the *in vitro* activity and *in vivo* efficacy in this subset of analogs, with the sulfide congener giving superior results. On balance, and considering all of the comparative data, the sulfoxides emerge as the least interesting derivatives.

A wide range of substitution patterns are tolerated on the ring system distal to the oxazolidinone nucleus. An examination of a series of substituted piperidine derivatives effectively illustrates this point (see Table 9). Oxime, hydroxyl, semicarbazone, and various amino moieties confer interesting levels of *in vitro* antibacterial activity to the basic piperidin-1-ylphenyloxazolidinone template. The semicarbazone analog PNU-106783 most closely approximates the *in vitro* activity of linezolid. In terms of *in vivo* efficacy

Table 8. Effect of sulfur oxidation state on antibacterial activity

| PNU-no. | R | n | MIC (μg/mL)[1] | | | ED_{50} (mg/kg)[5] |
			SA[2]	EF[3]	SP[4]	
140661	A	0	4	4	1	5.7 (1.3)[6]
140907	A	1	8	4	1	17.3 (4.2)[7]
140847	A	2	2	2	<0.5	5.0 (1.3)[6]
141605	B	0	2	2	1	3.1 (2.9)[7]
141770	B	1	8	4	0.5	16.0 (5.2)[7]
141839	B	2	8	4	1	NT[8]
linezolid			2	2	0.5	5.6 (3.9)[6]

[1]MIC = minimum inhibitory concentration
[2]SA = *Staphylococcus aureus* UC9213
[3]EF = *Enterococcus faecalis* UC9217
[4]SP = *Streptococcus pneumoniae* UC9912
[5]ED_{50} = effective dose$_{50}$ - dose that protects 50% of the animals - *S. aureus* UC9213; oxazolidinones administered orally
[6]subcutaneously administered vancomycin ED_{50} in parentheses
[7]eperezolid (PNU-100592) ED_{50} in parentheses; [8]NT = not tested.

against *S. aureus*, the *O*-methyloxime derivative PNU-105955 exhibits the most gratifying activity, being directly comparable to the comparator vancomycin.

CONCLUSIONS

In summary, we have identified a number of bioisosteric replacements for the piperazine and morpholine subunits of the progenitor oxazolidinones eperezolid and line-zolid, respectively. Potent antibacterial activity was realized for phenyloxazolidinones with appended azetidine, pyrrolidine, and piperidine surrogates. However, on balance, the pyrrolidine and piperidine analogs exhibit more interesting and consistent activity levels than their azetidine congeners. Based on these and other results beyond the scope of this discussion, further work on these bioisosteric oxazolidinone analogs appears warranted.

ACKNOWLEDGMENTS

The authors are indebted to J. W. Allison, J. C. Hamel, J. K. Moerman, R. D. Schaadt, D. Stapert, D. M. Wilson and B. H. Yagi, all of Pharmacia Upjohn, for the *in vi-*

Table 9. Antibacterial activity of miscellaneous
piperidine derivatives

	MIC (μg/mL)[1]			ED$_{50}$
PNU-no.	SA[2]	EF3	SP[4]	(mg/kg)[5]
105955	4	4	1	5.0 (5.0)
104008	8	4	2	7.1 (3.4)
106083	4	4	1	9.2 (6.3)
107309	4	4	2	5.2 (1.5)
106783	2	2	1	10.0 (3.1)
linezolid	2	2	0.5	5.6 (3.9)

[1]MIC = minimum inhibitory concentration
[2]SA = *Staphylococcus aureus* UC9213
[3]EF = *Enterococcus faecalis* UC9217
[4]SP = *Streptococcus pneumoniae* UC9912
[5]ED$_{50}$ = effective dose$_{50}$ - dose that protects 50% of the animals; oxazolidinones administered orally; subcutaneously administered vancomycin in parentheses.

tro and *in vivo* test results. We also thank M. H. Cynamon and S. P. Klemens of the Veterans Affairs Medical center and SUNY Health Science Center, and S. E. Glickman and J. O. Kilburn of the Centers for Disease Control and Prevention, for the mycobacteria data.

REFERENCES

Ayliffe, G. A. J., 1997, The progressive intercontinental spread of methicillin-resistant *Staphylococcus aureus*, *Clin. Infect. Dis.* 24 (Suppl. 1): S74.

Barbachyn, M. R., Hutchinson, D. K., Brickner, S. J., Cleek, G. J., Garmon, S. A., Grega, K. C., Hendges, S. K., Lindberg, T. J., Manninen, P. R., Munesada, K., Reid, R. J., Thomas, R. C., Toops, D. S., and Ulanowicz, D. A., 1996, Synthesis and SAR of novel antibacterial oxazolidinones, *Abstracts of Papers*, 14th International Symposium on Medicinal Chemistry, Maastricht, The Netherlands, Abstract No. SL- 09.2.

Barbachyn, M. R., Hutchinson, D. K., Brickner, S. J., Cynamon, M. H., Kilburn, J. O., Klemens, S. P., Glickman, S. E., Grega, K. C., Hendges, S. K., Toops, D. S., Ford, C. W., and Zurenko, G. E., 1996, Identification of a novel oxazolidinone (U-100480) with potent antimycobacterial activity, *J. Med. Chem.* 39: 680.

Barbachyn, M. R., Toops, D. S., Grea, K. C., Hendges, S. K., Ford, C. W., Zurenko, G. E., Hamel, J. C., Schaadt, R. D., Stapert, D., Yagi, B. H., Buysse, J. M., Demyan, W. F., Kilburn, J. O., and Glickman, S. E., 1996, Synthesis and antibacterial activity of new tropone-substituted phenyloxazolidinone antibacterial agents. 2. Modification of the phenyl ring - the potentiating efect of fluorine substitution on *in vivo* activity., *Bioorg. Med. Chem. Lett.* 6: 1009.

Bloch, A. B., Simone, P. M., McCray, E., and Castro, K. G., 1996, Preventing multidrug-resistant tuberculosis, *JAMA* 275: 487.

Bloom, B. R., 1994, *Tuberculosis: Pathogenesis, Protection, and Control*, ASM Press: Washington, D.C.

Breiman, R. F., Butler, J. C., Tenover, F. C., Elliott, J. A., and Facklam, R. R., 1994, Emergence of drug- resistant pneumococcal infections in the United States, *JAMA* 271: 1831.

Brickner, S. J., 1996, Oxazolidinone antibacterial agents, *Cur. Pharm. Design* 2: 175.

Brickner, S. J., Hutchinson, D. K., Barbachyn, M. R., Manninen, P. R., Ulanowicz, D. A., Garmon, S. A., Grega, K. C., Hendges, S. K., Toops, D. S., Ford, C. W., and Zurenko, G. E., 1996, Synthesis and antibacterial activity of U-100592 and U-100766, two oxazolidinone antibacterial agents for the potential treatment of multidrug-resistant gram-positive bacterial infections, *J. Med. Chem.* 39: 673.

Brickner, S. J., Manninen, P. R., Ulanowicz, D. A., Lovasz, K. D., and Rohrer, D. C., 1993, Multicyclic fused-ring oxazolidinone antibacterial agents, *Abstracts of Papers*, 206th National Meeting of the American Chemical Society, Chicago, IL, American Chemical Society: Washington, D.C., ORGN 089.

Brumfitt, W. and Hamilton-Miller, J. M. T., 1992, Antibacterial oxazolidinones: in vitro activity of a new analogue, E3709, *Diagn. Microbiol. Infect. Dis.* 15: 621.

Carlson, R. K., Park, C.-H., and Gregory, W. A., 1990, Aminomethyloxooxazolidinyl arylbenzene derivatives useful as antibacterial agents, U.S. Patent 4,948,801.

Chopra, I., Hodgson, J., Metcalf, B., and Poste, G., 1996, New Approaches to the control of infections caused by antibiotic-resistant bacteria, *JAMA* 275: 401.

Chu, D. T. W. and Fernandes, P. B., 1989, Structure-activity relationships of the fluoroquinolones, *Antimicrob. Agents Chemother.* 33: 131.

Chu, D. T. W., Plattner, J. J., and Katz, L., 1996, New directions in antibacterial research, *J. Med. Chem.* 39: 3853.

Coque, T. M., Tomayko, J. F., Ricke, S. C., Okhyusen, P. C., and Murray, B. E., 1996, Vancomycin-resistant enterococci from nosocomial, community, and animal sources in the United States, *Antimicrob. Agents Chemother.* 40: 2605.

Eustice, D. C., Feldman, P. A., and Slee, A. M., 1988, The mechanism of action of DuP 721, a new antibacterial agent: effects on macromolecular synthesis, *Biochem. Biophys. Res. Commun.* 150: 965.

Eustice, D. C., Feldman, P. A., Zajac, I., and Slee, A. M., 1988, Mechanism of action of DuP 721: inhibition of an early event during initiation of protein synthesis, *Antimicrob. Agents Chemother.* 32: 1218.

Eustice, D. C.; Slee, A. M., 1987, *Abstracts of Papers*, 27th Interscience Conference on Antimicrobial Agents and Chemotherapy, New York, NY, ASM Press: Washington, D.C., Abstract No. 246.

Ford, C. W., Hamel, J. C., Wilson, D. M., Moerman, J. K., Stapert, D., Yancey, R. J., Jr., Hutchinson, D. K., Barbachyn, M. R., and Brickner, S. J., 1996, In vivo activities of U-100592 and U-100766, novel oxazolidinone antimicrobial agents, against experimental bacterial infections, *Antimicrob. Agents Chemother.* 40: 1508.

Frigola, J., Parés, J., Corbera, J., Vañó, M., Torrens, A., Más, J., and Valentí, E., 1993, 7- Azetidinylquinolones as antibacterial agents. Synthesis and structure-activity relationships., *J. Med. Chem.* 36: 801, and references cited therein.

Griffith, W. P. and Ley, S. V., 1990, TPAP: tetra-*n*-propylammonium perruthenate, a mild and convenient oxidant for alcohols, *Aldrichimica Acta* 23: 13.

Hiramatsu, K., Hanaki, H., Ino, T., Yabuta, K., Oguri, T., and Tenover, F. C., 1997, Methicillin-resistant *Staphylococcus aureus* clinical strain with reduced vancomycin susceptibility, *J. Antimicrob. Chemother.* 40: 135.

Kaldor, S. W. and Hammond, M., 1991, A mild, osmium tetraoxide-catalyzed method for the oxidation of sulfides to sulfones, *Tetrahedron Lett.* 32: 5043.

Klemens, S. P., Sharpe, C. A., and Cynamon, M. H., 1995, Activities of two novel oxazolidinones against *M. tuberculosis* (MTB) in a murine model, *Abstracts of Papers*, 35th Interscience Conference on Antimicrobial Agents and Chemotherapy, San Francisco, CA, ASM Press: Washington, D.C., Abstract No. F228.

Leonard, N. J. and Johnson, C. R., 1962, Periodate oxidation of sulfides to sulfoxides. Scope of the reaction., *J. Org. Chem.* 27: 282.

Leclercq, R., 1997, Enterococci acquire new kinds of resistance, *Clin. Infect. Dis.* 24 (Suppl. 1): S80.

Leclercq, R. and Courvalin, P., 1997, Resistance to glycopeptides in enterococci, *Clin. Infect. Dis.* 24: 545.

Lin, A. H., Murray, R. W., Vidmar, T. J., and Marotti, K. R., 1997, The oxazolidinone eperezolid binds to the 50S ribosomal subunit and competes with binding of chloramphenicol and lincomycin, *Antimicrob. Agents Chemother.* 41: 2127.

Martin, R., Wilcox, K. R., Campbell, C., and Ellis, H., 1997, Update: *Staphylococcus aureus* with reduced susceptibility to vancomycin - United States, 1997, *Morbidity and Mortality Weekly Report* 46: 813.

McCracken, G. H., 1996, Recent perspectives on drug-resistant *Streptococcus pneumoniae*, *Pediatr. Infect. Dis. J.*
15: 930.

McDonald, L. C., Kuehnert, M. J., Tenover, F. C., and Jarvis, W. R., 1997, Vancomycin-resistant enterococci outside the health-care setting: prevalence, sources, and public health implications, *Emerging Infectious Diseases* 3: 311.

Moreno, F., Crisp, C., Jorgensen, J. H., and Patterson, J. E., 1995, Methicillin-resistant *Staphylococcus aureus* as a
community organism, *Clin. Infect. Dis.* 21: 1308.

Nix, D. E. and Schentag, J. J., 1988, The quinolones: an overview and comparative appraisal of their pharmacokinetics and pharmacodynamics, *J. Clin. Pharmacol.* 28: 169.

Noble, W. C., Virani, Z., and Cree, R. G. A., 1992, Co-transfer of vancomycin and other resistance genes from *Enterococcus faecalis* NCTC 12201 to *Staphylococcus aureus*, *FEMS Microbiol. Lett.* 93: 195.

Park, C.-H., Brittelli, D. R., Wang, C. L.-J., Marsh, F. D., Gregory, W. A., Wuonola, M. A., McRipley, R. J.,
Eberly, V. S., Slee, A. M., and Forbes, M., 1992, Antibacterials. Synthesis and structure-activity studies of
3-aryl-2-oxazolidinones. 4. Multiply-substituted aryl derivatives., *J. Med. Chem.* 35: 1156, and references
cited therein.

Reuman, M., Daum, S. J., Singh, B., Coughlin, S. A., Sedlock, D. M., Rake, J. B., and Lesher, G. Y., 1989, Synthesis and antibacterial activity of some novel 1-substituted-7-pyridinyl-1,4-dihydro-4-oxoquinoline- 3-car-
boxylic acids, *Abstracts of Papers*, 29th Interscience Conference on Antimicrobial Agents and
Chemotherapy, Houston, TX, ASM Press: Washington, D.C., Abstract No. 1193.

Pawsey, S. D.; Daley-Yates, P. T.; Wajszczuk, C. P.; Stalker, D. J., 1996, *Abstracts of Papers*, First European Congress of Chemotherapy, Glasgow, Scotland, Abstract No. F151.

Pharmaprojects, April 12, 1995; PJB Publications, Ltd.: Richmond, Surrey, UK.

Pharmcast-International **1995**, February, 7-1-484, 487.

Piper, R. C., Platte, T. F., and Palmer, J. R., unpublished results, Pharmacia & Upjohn.

DuPont's new oxazolidinones, 1987, *Scrip*, 1250: 25.

Shinabarger, D. L., Marotti, K. R., Murray, R. W., Lin, A. H., Melchior, E. P., Swaney, S. M., Dunyak, D. S., Demyan, W. F., and Buysse, J. M., 1997, Mechanism of action of oxazolidinones: effects of linezolid and
eperezolid on translation reactions, *Antimicrob. Agents Chemother.* 41: 2132.

Silver, L. L. and Bostian, K. A., 1993, Discovery and development of new antibiotics: the problem of antibiotic resistance, *Antimicrob. Agents Chemother.* 37: 377.

Slee, A. M., Wuonola, M. A., McRipley, R. J., Zajac, I., Zawada, M. J., Bartholomew, P. T., Gregory, W. A., and
Forbes, M., 1987, *Abstracts of Papers*, 27th Interscience Conference on Antimicrobial Agents and Chemotherapy, New York, NY, ASM Press: Washington, D.C., Abstract No. 244.

Spangler, S. K., Jacobs, M. R., and Appelbaum, P. C., 1996, Activities of RPR 106972 (a new oral streptogramin),
ceditoren (a new oral cephalosporin), two new oxazolidinones (U-100592 and U- 100766), and other oral
and parenteral agents against 203 penicillin-susceptible and -resistant pneumococci, *Antimicrob. Agents
Chemother.* 40: 481.

Stalker, D. J., Wajszczuk, C. P., and Batts, D. H., 1997, Linezolid safety, tolerance, and pharmacokinetics following oral dosing twice daily for 14.5 days *Abstracts of Papers* 37th Interscience Conference on Antimicrobial Agents and Chemotherapy, Toronto, Ontario, Canada, ASM Press: Washington, D.C., Abstract No.
A115.

Stalker, D. J., Wajszczuk, C. P., and Batts, D. H., 1997, Linezolid safety, tolerance, and pharmacokinetics after in-
travenous dosing twice daily for 7.5 days *Abstracts of Papers*, 37th Interscience Conference on Antimicrobial Agents and Chemotherapy, Toronto, Ontario, Canada, ASM Press: Washington, D.C., Abstract A116.

Tomasz, A., 1997, Antibiotic resistance in *Streptococcus pneumoniae*, *Clin. Infect. Dis.* 24 (Suppl. 1): S85.

Tomasz, A., 1994, Multiple-antibiotic-resistant pathogenic bacteria, *N. Engl. J. Med.* 330: 1247.

Voss, A., Milatovic, D., Wallrauch-Schwarz, C., Rosdahl, V. T., and Braveny, I., 1994, Methicillin-resistant
Staphylococcus aureus in Europe, *Eur. J. Clin. Microbiol. Infect. Dis.* 13: 50.

Zamkoff, J. P., Cline, K., Klemens, S. P., and Cynamon, M. H., 1995, Activity of U-100480, an oxazolidinone,
against *M. avium* complex (MAC) infection in beige mice. *Abstracts of Papers*, 35th Interscience Conference on Antimicrobial Agents and Chemotherapy, San Francisco, CA, ASM Press: Washington, D.C., Abstract No. F229.

Zurenko, G. E., Yagi, B. H., Schaadt, R. D., Allison, J. W., Kilburn, J. O., Glickman, S. E., Hutchinson, D. K.,
Barbachyn, M. R., and Brickner, S. J., 1996, In vitro activities of U-100592 and U-100766, novel oxazolidinone antibacterial agents, *Antimicrob. Agents Chemother.* 40: 839.

CONCEPT, DESIGN, AND PRECLINICAL EVALUATION OF QUINOLONYL LACTAM ANTIBACTERIALS

Paul M. Hershberger and Thomas P. Demuth, Jr

Procter & Gamble Pharmaceuticals
Health Care Research Center
Mason, Ohio 45040

INTRODUCTION

The issue of bacterial resistance to current classes of antibiotics is now well known and widely published (Levy, 1998; Chin and Marx, 1994). Indeed, untreatable contagious infectious diseases have already generated significant medical crises in localized environments. Such crises may become more widespread, perhaps in the not too distant future. Laboratories worldwide have responded with highly creative research programs, many of which are reviewed in this book. Nonetheless, the successful discovery, development, and commercialization of new therapies that address bacterial resistance have proved challenging.

Approaches to overcoming resistance were summarized by Silver and Bostian (1993). Many research programs may be considered molecular biology based approaches that are focused on the discovery and exploitation of new targets. It is widely believed that resistant organisms will be susceptible to new classes of drugs that attack new targets. The multifunctional antibacterial approach, on the other hand, is more typically a chemistry based initiative that combines multiple existing mechanisms of action in a single unique drug. The successful design of a multifunctional antibacterial results in a compound with potency against resistant organisms. Furthermore, some of these compounds may experience a slower rate of resistance development than molecules acting via a single mechanism. This chapter reviews the conceptualization, design, and preclinical evaluation of quinolonyl lactam multifunctional antibacterials.

THE MULTIFUNCTIONAL ANTIBIOTIC CONCEPT

Previous reviews of Roche's work on quinolonyl lactams (Albrecht et al., 1990, Albrecht and Christenson, 1992; Dax, 1992; Keith et al., 1993) provide a description of the

Resolving the Antibiotic Paradox, edited by Rosen and Mobashery.
Kluwer Academic / Plenum Publishers, New York, 1998.

239

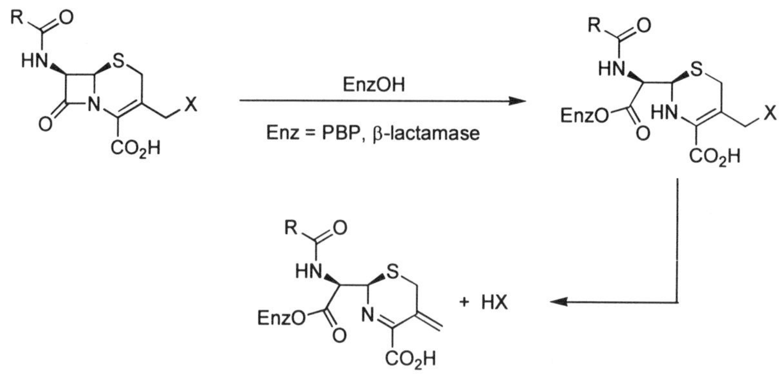

Figure 1. Dual action concept.

"dual action" concept. A brief summary is shown in Figure 1. Bacterial enzymes react with β-lactams via a ring opening nucleophilic attack. Resistant organisms produce β-lactamase enzymes that cleave the pharmacophore in an essentially irreversible fashion. It is documented (Hamilton-Miller et al., 1970; Hamilton-Miller et al., 1970; Boyd et al., 1975; Boyd and Lunn, 1979; Page and Proctor, 1984; Page, 1984; Faraci and Pratt, 1984) that suitably functionalized β-lactams may eliminate a leaving group "X" via enzymatic processes, such as those mediated by penicillin-binding proteins (PBPs) and β-lactamases. Accordingly, multifunctional β-lactams were envisioned whereby "X" is actually a second antibacterial. Importantly, "X" is potentially delivered at the site of the infection, perhaps as a direct consequence of the organism's resistance mechanism. It was therefore hypothesized that multifunctional β-lactams would be useful against both sensitive and resistant organisms. Moreover, it was noted that an organism would have to undergo two distinct mutations to resist such a compound, and that this attribute may actually slow the rate of new resistance development.

Implementation of the Multifunctional β-Lactam Concept

Attempts to exploit this concept have been active in various laboratories for more than 25 years. Typically, antimicrobial agents have been attached to the C-3' (C-10) position of cephalosporins. Examples are noted in Figure 2. Russell and Fountain (1971) described cephalosporin 7/30, which supported the release mechanism shown in Figure 1 by exhibiting the properties of dimethyldithiocarbamate. O'Callaghan et al. (1976) reported MCO, which exhibited the combined properties of both pharmacophores and even maintained activity against certain β-lactamase producing bacteria. The cephalosporin dipeptides **1** and **2** (Mobashery et al., 1986; Mobashery and Johnston, 1986; Mobashery and Johnston, 1987) reinforced the notion that suitably functionalized lactams could inhibit the growth of β-lactamase producing organisms. More recently, Perrone et al. (1992) reported a series of penems linked to nitrofuranyl, quinolinyl, and cycloserinyl substituents that further supported the dual-action concept. The following year, Kim et al. (1993) disclosed a series of cephalosporins linked to thiones derived from quinolonyl intermediates. These compounds exhibited broad spectrum antibacterial properties. Additionally, Hwu et al. (1997) described a set of cephalosporin 3'-phloroglucide esters, and reported activity profiles superior to the independent parts.

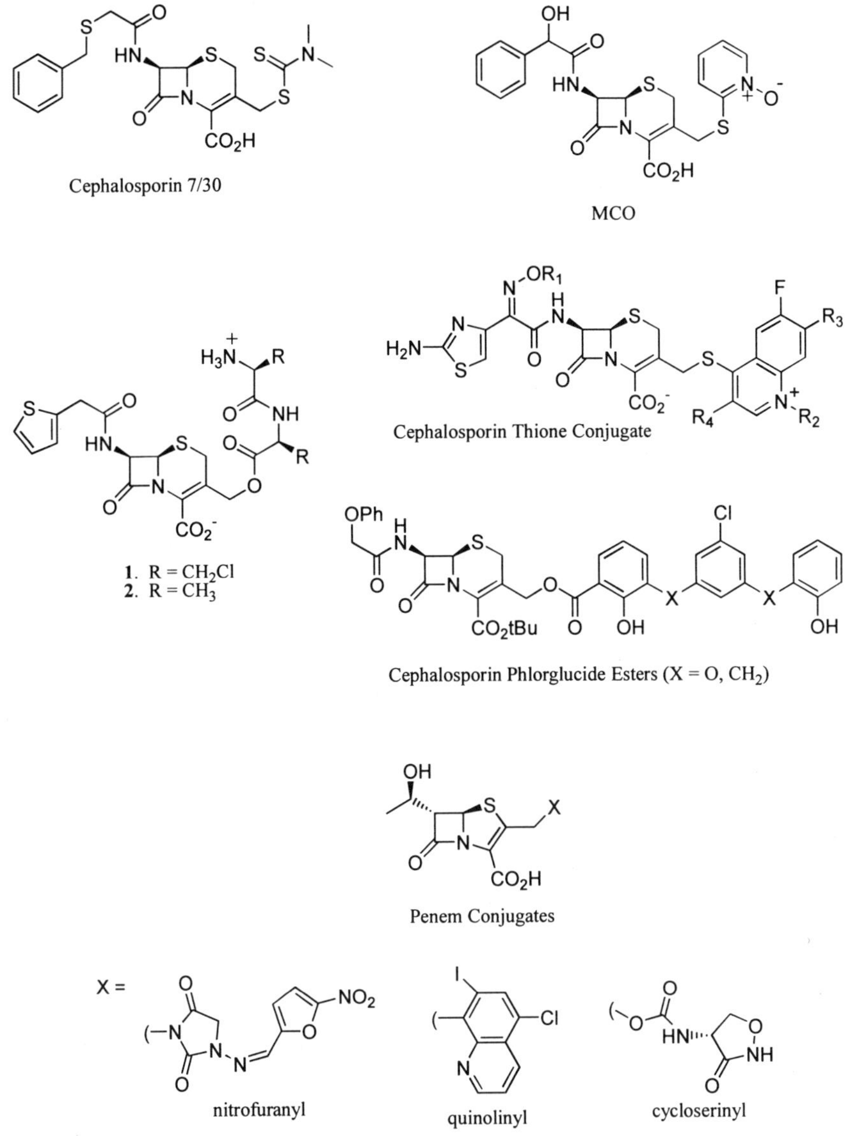

Figure 2. Examples of antimicrobial multifunctional β-lactams.

Research in this field extends to the anticancer and elastase inhibitor fields. In the anticancer area, cephalosporin prodrugs have been reported that target tumors via catalytic interaction with monoclonal antibody β-lactamases. Alexander et al. (1991) and Svensson et al. (1992) described cephalosporins linked to nitrogen mustards. At about the same time, Meyer et al. (1992) published on a cephalosporin prodrug linked to desacetylvinblastine-3-carboxylic acid. This prodrug was less cyctotoxic than the parent compound. The following year, Hanessian and Wang (1993) described a cephalosporin-carboplatinum prodrug activatable by β-lactamase. More recently, Alexander et al. (1996) reported on a N-nitrososchloroethyl-cephalosporin prodrug. Last year, Veinberg et al. (1997) extended the multifunctional concept into the elastase inhibitor field. These workers prepared cephalosporin 1,1-dioxides linked to aspirin or diclofenac, and reported that the new compounds were potent elastase inhibitors and stimulators of NO biosynthesis in macrophages.

THE QUINOLONYL LACTAM CONCEPT

Quinolonyl-lactams are the class of multifunctional β-lactams where the group "X" (Figure 1) is a quinolonyl antibacterial compound. In the 1980s at Procter & Gamble, quinolones were chosen as "X" for some of the same reasons summarized in the aforementioned Roche reviews. Generally, P&G's basis for interest in quinolonyl lactams included the following points:

1. β-lactams and quinolones of the 1980s possessed somewhat complementary potency profiles.
2. The mechanisms of action (inhibition of penicillin-binding proteins for β-lactams, inhibition of DNA-gyrase for quinolones) are distinct and were not expected to interfere with one another. Two distinct mutations may therefore be required to confer drug resistance.
3. The solubility of the conjugated molecule was expected to exceed that of the quinolone.
4. Quinolone related toxicity might be attenuated in the conjugated molecule.
5. The release mechanism might impart overall potency and resistance development properties superior to a physical mixture ("cocktail") of the individual drugs.
6. Both pharmacophores could potentially be operative in the intact molecule.

In addition to the programs at P&G and Roche, scientists at Farmitalia (Perrone et al., 1992; Jabes et al., 1993) initiated a quinolonyl lactam program during the 1980s. More recently, scientists at Bayer have disclosed results from a quinolonyl lactam program (Mielke et al., 1996; Petersen et al., 1994; Petersen et al., 1994). Academic laboratories have also published results in this field. These include very recent work at the Univerisity of Notre Dame, as reported by Stocksdale et al. (1998), and earlier work reported (La et al., 1993; La et al., 1993) from Chungham National University.

DESIGN OF QUINOLONYL LACTAMS

The design of quinolonyl lactams focused on the three key structural variables; namely, the *lactam*, the *quinolone*, and the *link* between them. Lactams have included various cephalosporins, penems, carbapenems, and recently carbacephems. A wide assortment of quinolones and related naphthyridines have been utilized. Links have included various types of carbamates, amines, esters, and ethers. Roche has also reported thioester (Dax, 1992; Keith et al., 1993), quaternary ammonium(Albrecht et al., 1991), and tetrazole links (Dax et al., 1993). The remainder of this chapter reviews the impact of these three key structural variables on potency, the synthetic routes used to prepare most quinolonyl lactams, and the key properties of some lead quinolonyl lactams.

The Lactam Variable

Carbamate-Linked Quinolonyl Lactams Derived from Ciprofloxacin. Figure 3 shows a list of quinolonyl lactams that were all derived from ciprofloxacin (**3**) and a carbamate link. Only the lactam variable is different among this set. Comparison of these compounds

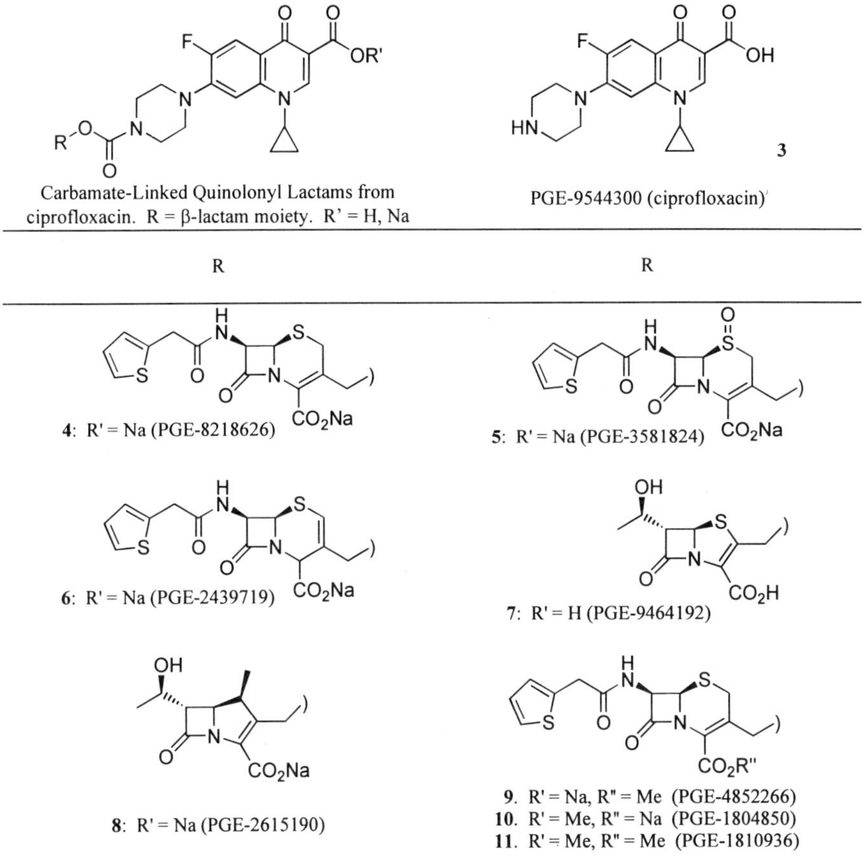

Carbamate-Linked Quinolonyl Lactams from ciprofloxacin. R = β-lactam moiety. R' = H, Na

PGE-9544300 (ciprofloxacin)

4: R' = Na (PGE-8218626)

5: R' = Na (PGE-3581824)

6: R' = Na (PGE-2439719)

7: R' = H (PGE-9464192)

8: R' = Na (PGE-2615190)

9. R' = Na, R'' = Me (PGE-4852266)
10. R' = Me, R'' = Na (PGE-1804850)
11. R' = Me, R'' = Me (PGE-1810936)

Figure 3. Carbamate quinolonyl lactams derived from ciprofloxacin.

allows the role of the lactam to be addressed. This set includes a cephalosporin, a cephalosporin sulfoxide, a Δ2 cephalosporin, a penem, a carbapenem, and three cephalosporin controls with either the lactam, the quinolonyl moiety, or both groups protected as the ester.

These quinolonyl lactams were typically prepared from the corresponding hydroxymethyl lactam, ciprofloxacin, and a phosgene-equivalent reagent. The schemes below are representative of the methods for preparing the molecules shown in Figure 3. A preparation of the carbapenem **8** has been reported by Corraz et al. (1992).

Figure 4 shows the preparation of **4**, as reported by Demuth et al. (1990). This synthesis began with the controlled hydrolysis of commercial 7-amino cephalosporanic acid **12**. Acylation with thienylacetyl chloride followed by treatment with diphenyldiazomethane provided **13**. In this case, tetrachloroethyl chloroformate proved to be an effective phosgene equivalent primarily because the carbonate intermediate **14** could be reacted directly with the quinolone ciprofloxacin under basic aqueous conditions. This minimized the need for protecting groups in the synthesis. This particular carbonate (**14**) was sufficiently stable to be chromatographed and stored. Removal of the DPM ester with TFA afforded **4**.

Figure 5 shows the synthesis of the corresponding penem carbamate **7**, as reported by Rourke et al. (1992). The 2-hydroxymethyl penem starting material **15** was previously

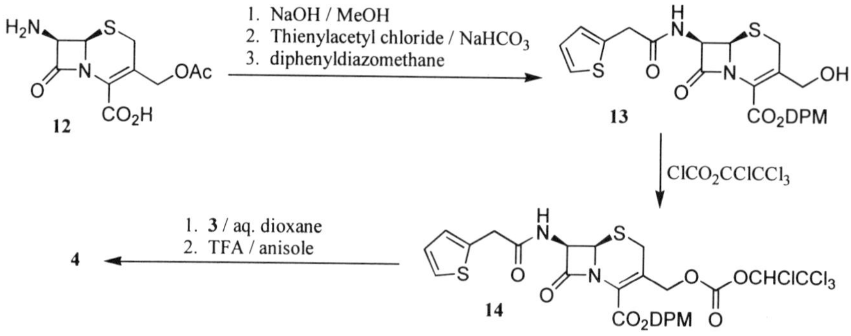

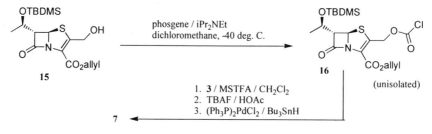

Figure 4.   Preparation of **4**.

reported by Alpegiani et al. (1985). This molecule did not react efficiently with the tetrachloroethyl chloroformate reagent system shown in Figure 4. Instead, **15** was treated with phosgene to obtain the expected chloroformate intermediate **16** *in situ*. This was successfully reacted by direct treatment with ciprofloxacin pretreated with N-methyl-N-(trimethylsilyl)trifluoroacetamide) (MSTFA). This reagent silylated the unprotected quinolone, thereby solubilizing it in dichloromethane. Removal of the protecting groups furnished **7**.

Secondary Amine-Linked Quinolonyl Lactams Derived from 17. Figure 6 shows another list of quinolonyl lactams derived from **17**, the 6,8-difluoroquinolone described by Sanchez et al. (1988). These compounds also have the link variable held constant, in this case as a 2° amine. Each member of this set has a variation of a cephem as the lactam. These compounds provide additional insight on the lactam variable. Albrecht et al. (1994) reported a similar set of 3° amine-linked quinolonyl cephems derived from ciprofloxacin.

Gray et al. (1995) described the procedures for making these compounds. The cephalosporin starting materials used to make **18** (R = thienylacetyl) and **19** (R = aminothiazolyl(methoximo)acetyl) were obtained commercially. The other three N-acyl cephem starting materials (for making **20**: phenoxyacetyl, for making **21**: phenylacetyl, and for making **22**: hydroxyphenylacetyl) were prepared according to literature procedures (Cocker et al., 1965; Nishimura et al., 1991). As indicated in Figure 7, the 10-acetoxy group for all five cases was converted to an iodo intermediate **23** using the procedure described by Bonjouklian and Phillips (1981). The quinolone **17** was prepared according to the procedure published by Sanchez et al. (1988). Coupling of **17** to the various io-

Figure 5.   Preparation of **7**.

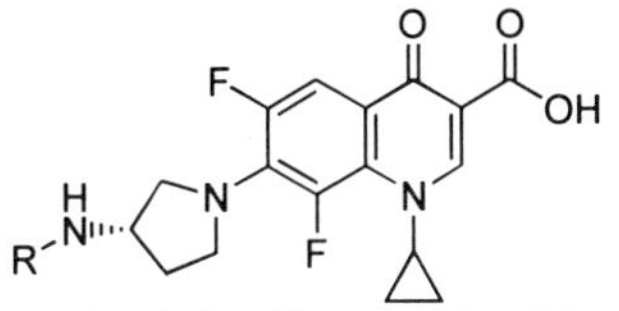

2° Amine-Linked Quinolonyl Lactams: R = β-lactam moiety.

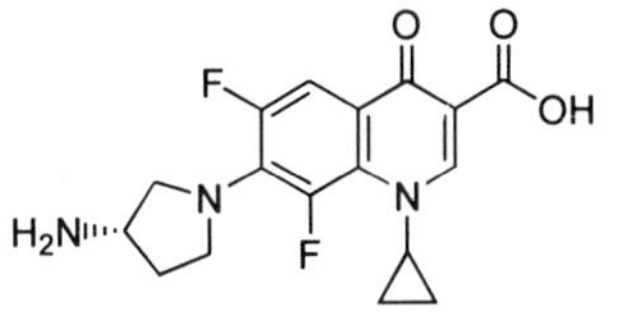

17: PGE-1842612 (quinolone control)

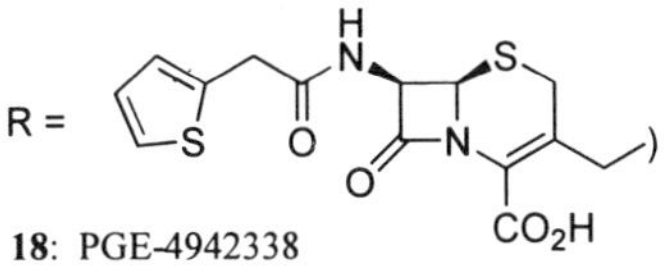

18: PGE-4942338

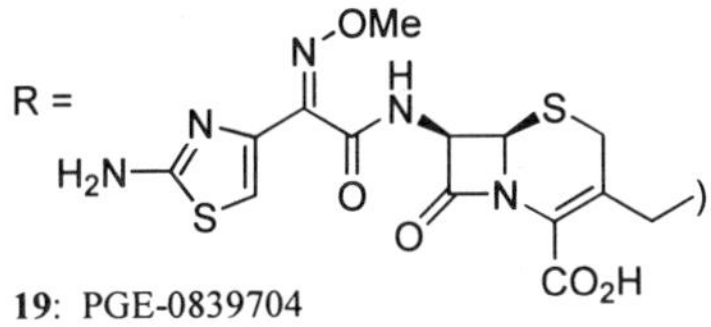

19: PGE-0839704

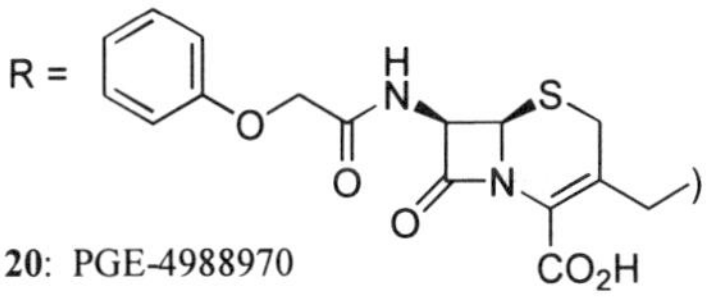

20: PGE-4988970

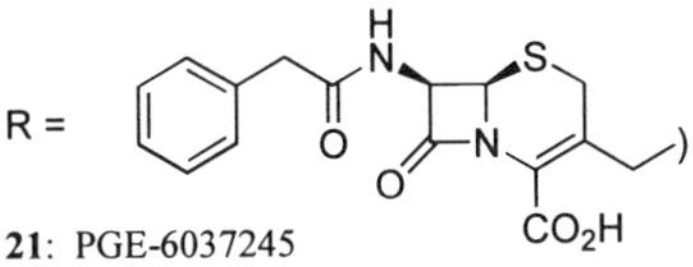

21: PGE-6037245

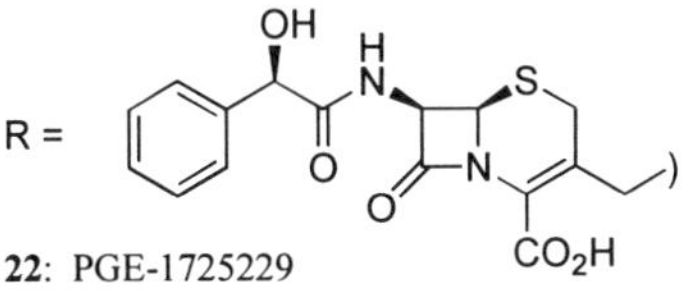

22: PGE-1725229

Figure 6. Secondary amine-linked quinolonyl lactams derived from 17.

domethyl cephems followed by removal of protecting groups gave the quinolonyl lactams shown in Figure 6.

Impact of the Lactam on Potency and Enzyme Inhibition. Table 1 summarizes the growth inhibition studies for the set of compounds shown in Figure 3. The importance of the β-lactam is most easily observed against the MI345 strain of *S. aureus*, which is resistant to ciprofloxacin but sensitive to methicillin. In this case, inhibition of this organism specifically requires an active lactam pharmacophore. The cephalosporin 4, the penem 7 and the carbapenem 8 all inhibited MI345 with good potency. The potencies of these three compounds against the four strain array of *S. aureus* (ATCC 29213, MI300, MI345, and MI339) indicate that the quinolonyl lactam exhibits the combined properties of both pharmacophores, giving it a better spectrum of activity than either the lactam or the quinolone. Specifically, these compounds were active against the wild type *S. aureus*, the MSCR

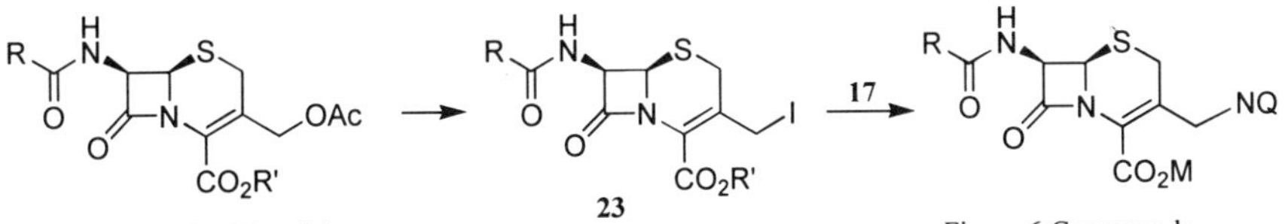

Cephem Starting Material

23

Figure 6 Compounds

Figure 7. Synthesis of 2° amine-linked quinolonyl cephems derived from quinolone 17.

Table 1. Minimum inhibitory concentration data (μg/mL) for carbamate-linked quinolonyl lactams

Organism	Strain	3	24	4	5	6	7	8	9	10	11
Gram positive											
Staphylococcus aureus MSCS	ATCC 29213	0.25	≤0.12	0.25	2	4	0.06	0.12	0.5	0.12	>128
Staphylococcus aureus MRCS	MI300	0.25	4	1	1	0.5	0.25	0.5	1	32	>128
Staphylococcus aureus MSCR	MI345	16	0.25	0.25	32	16	0.25	0.12	4	0.5	>128
Staphylococcus aureus MRCR	MI339	32	>64	32	>64	>128	32	16	>128	>128	>128
Staphylococcus saprophyticus	MI276	0.25	0.5	1	NT	16	0.5	0.5	2	1	>128
Enterococcus faecalis	ATCC 29212	0.25	32	8	NT	16	4	1	4	16	>128
Streptococcus pyogenes	STA2	0.5	≤0.12	≤0.016	NT	2	0.02	<0.06	≤0.12	≤0.12	>128
Streptococcus pneumoniae	STP1	0.5	0.5	0.06	NT	8	0.03	<0.06	2	0.06	>128
viridans streptococcus	STV1	2	0.25	NT	NT	NT	0.06	<0.06	0.25	0.06	>128
Gram Negative											
Escherichia coli	ATCC 25922	≤0.016	16	0.06	NT	0.12	0.12	<0.06	≤0.12	64	>128
Pseudomonas aeruginosa CS	ATCC 27853	0.25	>64	1	NT	8	2	1	4	>128	>128
Pseudomonas aeruginosa CR	PS314	32	>64	NT	NT	NT	>128	>64	>128	>128	>128
Proteus mirabilis	PR91	≤0.016	32	1	NT	2	0.5	0.25	1	128	>128
Klebsiella pneumoniae CS	KL21	≤0.016	>64	0.25	NT	0.06	0.03	NT	2	64	>128
Klebsiella pneumoniae CR	KL328	2	>64	NT	NT	NT	64	16	>128	>128	>128
Enterobacter cloacae	AE63	≤0.016	>64	≤0.016	NT	0.5	0.06	<0.06	1	4	>128

Data reported by Demuth et al. (1990) and Rourke et al. (1992). MS: methicillin sensitive. CS: ciprofloxacin sensitive. MR: methicillin resistant. CS: ciprofloxacin resistant NT: not tested. Compound **24**: deasacetyl-cephalothin control. Compound **3**: quinolone control (ciprofloxacin).

Table 2. Minimum inhibitory concentration data (μg/mL) for 2° amine-linked quinolonyl lactams

Organism	Strain	17	18	19	20	21	22
Gram positive							
Staphylococcus aureus MSCS	ATCC 29213	0.008	0.25	1	0.12	0.12	0.12
Staphylococcus aureus MRCS	MI300	0.016	≤0.06	0.25	0.12	≤0.016	≤0.06
Staphylococcus aureus MSCR	MI345	0.5	2	16	1	1	2
Staphylococcus aureus MRCR	MI339	0.5	16	32	4	4	4
Staphylococcus saprophyticus	MI276	0.03	1	4	0.25	0.12	0.5
Enterococcus faecalis	ATCC 29212	0.03	8	2	2	2	1
Streptococcus pyogenes	STA2	0.03	≤0.06	≤0.06	0.12	≤0.016	≤0.06
Streptococcus pneumoniae	STP1	0.06	0.25	0.25	0.5	0.25	0.5
viridans streptococcus	STV1	0.03	0.12	0.25	0.25	0.03	≤0.06
Gram negative							
Escherichia coli	ATCC 25922	≤0.002	0.5	0.25	0.12	0.12	0.12
Pseudomonas aeruginosa CS	ATCC 27853	0.03	4	4	4	2	1
Pseudomonas aeruginosa CR	PS314	2	>64	>64	>64	>16	32
Proteus mirabilis	PR91	0.016	2	2	4	0.5	0.5
Klebsiella pneumoniae CS	KL21	≤0.002	≤0.06	≤0.06	≤0.06	0.03	0.12
Klebsiella pneumoniae CR	KL328	0.5	32	>64	32	16	8
Enterobacter cloacae	AE63	≤0.002	≤0.06	0.12	≤0.06	≤0.016	≤0.06

Data reported by Gray et al. (1995). Compound 17: Quinolone control. MS: methicillin sensitive. CS: ciprofloxacin sensitive. MR: methicillin resistant. CR: ciprofloxacin resistant

strain, and the MRCS strain. They only failed against the MRCR strain, although the carbapenem retained some activity (16 μg/mL). When the activity of the lactam pharmacophore was compromised, either as the sulfoxide **5**, the Δ2 isomer **6**, or as the ester **9**, a significant loss in potency was observed against the MSCR *S. aureus*. Clearly, activity against this organism depended on the β-lactam pharmacophore. Similarly, when the quinolonyl part was esterified **10**, the potency was lost against the MRCS *S. aureus*, but retained against the MSCR strain. Predictably, the diester control compound **11** was inactive. Overall, the penem and carbapenem were somewhat more potent than the cephalosporin in this set. The carbapenem also stood out as the preferred compound against the CR strain of *K. pneumoniae*. Additionally, it was noted that the cephalosporin, the penem, and the carbapenem were similarly potent against organisms sensitive to ciprofloxacin but resistant to desacetyl-cephalothin (**24**), such as *S. aureus* MI300 and the gram negatives. This suggested that the contribution of the quinolonyl pharmacophore was not highly affected by the nature of the lactam.

The secondary amine-linked quinolonyl cephalosporins shown in Figure 6 had similar potency profiles (Table 2). The cefotaxime related compound **19** was somewhat less potent than the others against gram positive bacteria, most notably the MSCR *S. aureus*. Against gram negatives, the phenyl-acetyl **21** and the hydroxyphenyl-acetyl **22** compounds were better overall than the others. The quinolone **17** was active against the cipro-resistant *S. aureus*, and this activity was partially retained in the quinolonyl lactam molecules, particularly the phenoxy-, the phenyl-, and the hydroxyphenyl-acetyl compounds. This effect was retained to a lesser extent against the CR gram negative *K. pneumoniae*.

Several of the quinolonyl lactams from Figures 3 and 6 inhibited both PBPs and DNA-gyrase, as shown in Table 3. The compounds inhibited PBPs efficiently, with IC_{50} values typically close to the MICs and comparable to the cephalothin and cefotaxime controls. Compounds with the compromised lactam pharmacophore still inhibited PBPs, but

Table 3. Inhibition of PBPs and DNA-gyrase (IC$_{50}$, μg/mL)

Compound	PBP-1	PBP-2	PBP-3	MIC (μg/mL)	DNA-gyrase
β-lactams					
Cephalothin	0.1	0.1	0.1	0.25	NT
Cefotaxime	0.3	0.1	2	1	NT
Quinolonyl lactams					
4	0.26	0.33	0.13	0.33	22
5	2	2	2	2	NT
6	3	5	2	4	NT
7	<0.31	<0.31	<0.31	0.12	15
9	1	1	0.7	0.5	NT
19	0.2	0.4	5	1	5
Quinolones					
3	NT	NT	NT	NT	1.4
17	NT	NT	NT	NT	0.2

Data reported by Demuth et al., (1993), Gray et al., (1995), Koenigs et al., (1997). NT: not tested.
PBPs: from *S. aureus* ATCC29213. DNA-gyrase: from *E. coli*.

with less efficiency. Inhibition of DNA-gyrase was less efficient for quinolonyl lactams than for the parent quinolones. For the quinolonyl lactams, the gyrase inhibition was better for the amine **19** than for the two carbamates (**4** and **7**). The carbamates decrease the basicity of the the R7 quinolonyl substituent, whereas the amine link preserves it. The DNA-gyrase inhibition data exhibited by the quinolonyl lactams were consistent with quinolone SAR, which prefers basicity in this group.

Summary Discussion of the Lactam Variable. Overall, both Tables 1 and 2 support the supposition that the β-lactam makes an important contribution to the quinolonyl lactams' spectrum of activity, and that modification of the lactam attenuates the potency against key organisms. In the carbamate set, the penem and the carbapenem gave somewhat better potency than the cephalosporin. In the secondary amine set, some differences in activity were observed for the various cephalosporin side chains. Overall, the phenylacetyl and the hydroxyphenyl-acetyl side chains exhibited advantages relative to the others. The function of the lactam variable was confirmed by the PBP enzyme inhibition studies (Table 3). Optimization of the lactam to maximize the PBP binding affinity therefore became a high priority in the design of broad spectrum quinolonyl lactams. The quinolonyl pharmacophore was also active in these compounds, as evidenced by their potencies against methicillin resistant strains and gram negatives, as well as by the inhibition of bacterial DNA-gyrase. The apparent quinolonyl contribution was not highly dependent on the nature of the lactam variable.

The Quinolone Variable

Carbamate-Linked Quinolonyl Penems. Figure 8 illustrates a set of carbamate-linked quinolonyl penems derived from 10 different quinolones. A comparison of this set puts in perspective the relevance of the quinolone variable.

Carbamate-Linked Quinolonyl Penems

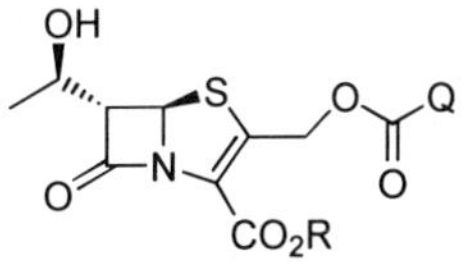

7, 25, 27, 29, 30, 32, 34, 36, 38, 40
Q = quinolonyl moiety. R = H or Na

Quinolones

Q-H

3, 17, 26, 28, 31, 33, 35, 37, 39, 41

Q	Q

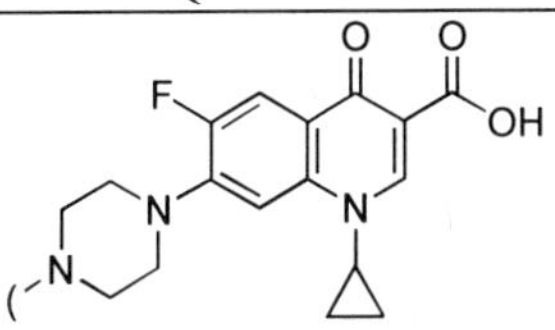

7: R = H (PGE-9464192)
3: ciprofloxacin (PGE-9544300)

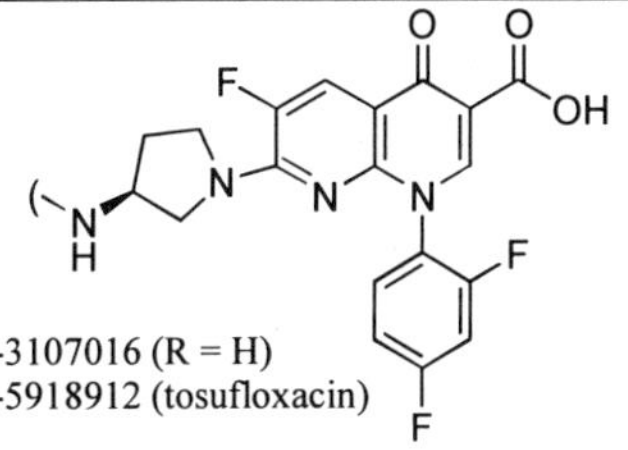

25: PGE-3107016 (R = H)
26: PGE-5918912 (tosufloxacin)

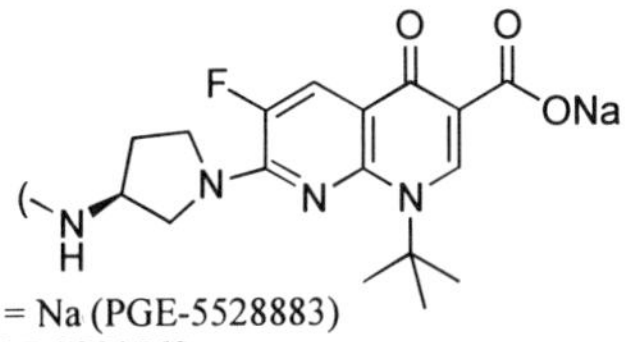

27: R = Na (PGE-5528883)
28: PGE-2291563

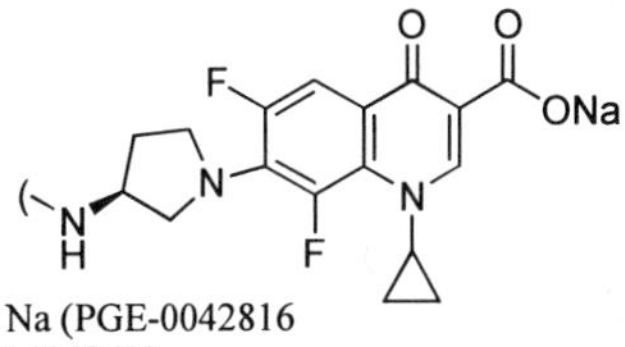

29: R = Na (PGE-0042816
17: PGE-1842612

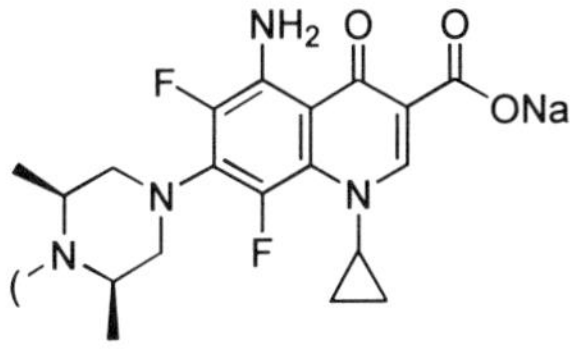

30: R = Na (PGE-9218983)
31: sparfloxacin (PGE-5762076)

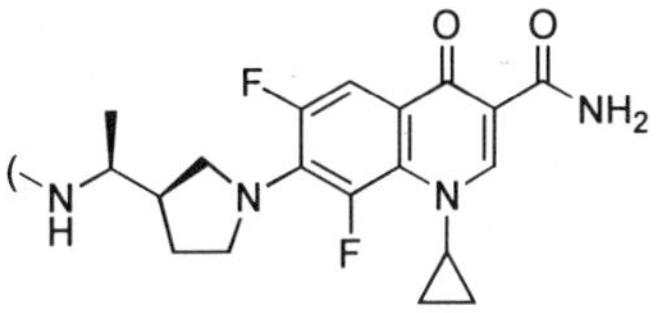

32: R = H (PGE-5261691
33: PGE-9914565

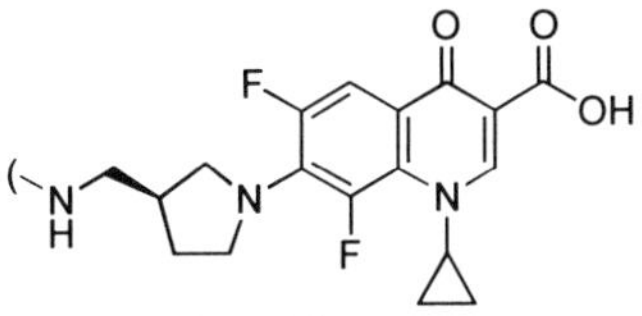

34: R = H (PGE-1821706)
35: PGE-3941527

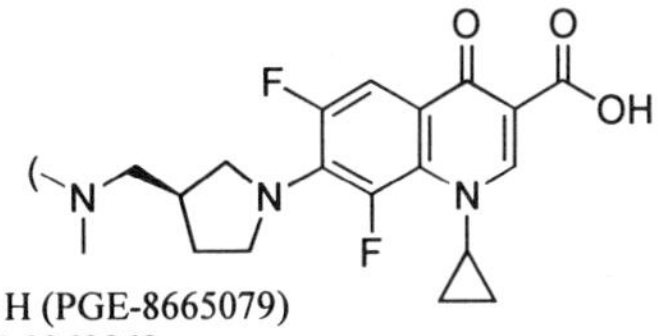

36: R = H (PGE-8665079)
37: PGE-0269868

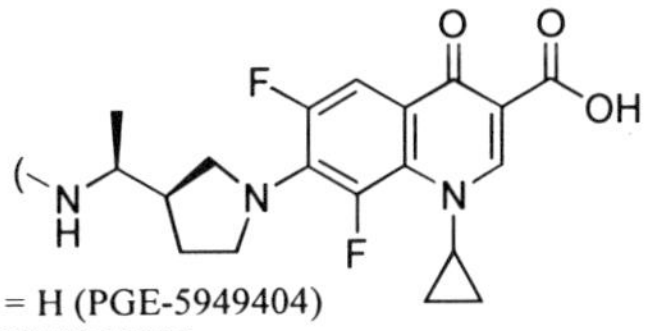

38: R = H (PGE-5949404)
39: PGE-9215875

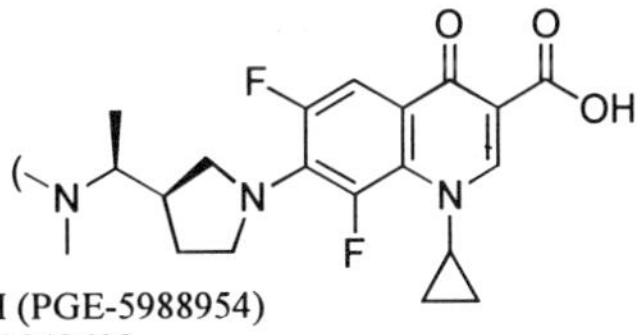

40: R = H (PGE-5988954)
41: PGE-3842608

Figure 8. Carbamate-linked quinolonyl penems and quinolone controls.

The synthesis of **7** was described in Figure 5. The other carbamate-linked quinolonyl penems in Figure 8 were prepared from the hydroxymethyl intermediate **15** using essentially the same coupling conditions. The quinolones used to prepare this set of molecules are also illustrated in Figure 8. Compound **25** was prepared from the naphthyridine tosufloxacin (**26**), which was reported by Rosen et al. (1988). Compound **27** was prepared from the 1-t-butyl-naphthyridine (**28**) described by Bouzard et al. (1990). Compound **29** was prepared from the 6,8-difluoroquinolone reported by Sanchez et al. (1988) **17**. Compound **30** was prepared from sparfloxacin (**31**), a quinolone reported by Miyamoto et al. (1990). Domagala et al. (1993) reported on the four quinolones (**35, 37, 39,** and **41**) used to prepare **34, 36, 38,** and **40**. The quinolone carboxamide **33** used to prepare **32** was prepared by amidation of the corresponding BOC-protected quinolone.

Impact of the Quinolone on Potency and Enzyme Inhibition. Table 4 shows the MIC results for the 10 carbamate-linked quinolonyl penems, and Table 5 shows the MICs for the quinolone controls. The columns are synchronized in these tables so that each quinolonyl penem can be compared with its quinolone control. These data confirmed that the ciprofloxacin resistant bacteria can be inhibited by newer more potent quinolones (Table 5). Importantly, carbamate-linked quinolonyl penems derived from such quinolones also gained potency against these bacteria. Thus, the compounds in Table 4 achieved an outstanding spectrum of activity; however, with somewhat less potency than the corresponding quinolones, especially against gram negative organisms and the MRCR *S. aureus*. In these cases, the conjugated molecules were typically about 8 fold less active than the quinolone, itself. Overall, the best potency was achieved by quinolonyl penems derived from the three 8-methoxy quinolones. A related series of amine-linked quinolonyl penems described by Ma et al. (1996) produced a similar activity trend. Because of the very high potency associated with the quinolonyl pharmacophore in many of these examples, the contribution of the β-lactam was difficult to observe via the MIC against MSCR *S. aureus*. Nonetheless, the carbamate-linked quinolonyl penems generally inhibited PBPs as efficiently as the 2-hydroxymethyl penem control (Table 6), which suggested that the compounds were capable of utilizing this mechanism as a key weapon against the bacteria. These compounds also inhibited bacterial DNA-gyrase, although somewhat less efficiently than typical quinolones.

Summary Discussion of the Quinolone Variable. The potency of quinolones increased dramatically since the initiation of quinolonyl lactam programs in the 1980s. Incorporation of the newer quinolonyl moieties into quinolonyl lactams resulted in a corresponding increase in the potency and spectrum of activity for the conjugated molecules. In fact, the overall potency of the quinolonyl lactams was related to the potency of the quinolonyl moiety. The quinolone variable was recognized as crucial for the incorporation of broad spectrum potency, especially against ciprofloxacin resistant and gram negative bacteria.

The Link Variable

Quinolonyl Lactams Derived from Cephalothin and Ciprofloxacin. Figure 9 shows a set of four compounds that focus on the link between the β-lactam and the quinolone. For these compounds, the lactam was cephalothin and the quinolone was ciprofloxacin. The links were carbamate, ester, tertiary amine, and dithiocarbamate.

The synthesis of carbamate **4** was discussed in Figure 4. Demuth et al. (1990) published the preparation of the ester **43**. Iodomethyl cephalosporin **16** was treated with the

Table 4. Minimum inhibitory concentration data (µg/mL) for carbamate-linked quinolonyl penems

Organism	Strain	7	25	27	29	30	32	34	36	38	40
Gram Positive											
Staphylococcus aureus MSCS	ATCC 29213	0.06	0.06	0.06	≤0.06	0.06	0.06	≤0.06	0.06	0.03	0.12
Staphylococcus aureus MRCS	MI300	0.25	0.06	0.12	≤0.06	0.12	0.25	≤0.06	≤0.03	0.016	≤0.06
Staphylococcus aureus MSCR	MI345	0.25	0.06	NT	0.25	NT	0.06	0.12	0.25	0.12	1
Staphylococcus aureus MRCR	MI339	32	8	NT	4	NT	16	0.25	2	0.5	1
Staphylococcus saprophyticus	MI276	0.5	0.5	0.5	0.25	0.25	0.25	≤0.06	0.25	0.03	0.12
Enterococcus faecalis	ATCC 29212	4	0.5	1	0.5	1	1	≤0.06	0.25	0.12	0.5
Streptococcus pyogenes	STA2	0.02	0.03	0.03	≤0.06	0.002	≤0.03	≤0.06	0.12	0.016	≤0.06
Streptococcus pneumoniae	STP1	0.03	0.06	0.25	0.12	0.06	≤0.03	≤0.06	0.06	0.016	≤0.06
viridans streptococcus	STV1	0.06	0.06	0.06	≤0.06	0.03	≤0.03	≤0.06	0.06	0.016	0.12
Gram Negative											
Escherichia coli	ATCC 25922	0.12	0.02	0.016	≤0.06	0.016	16	0.12	0.25	0.25	1
Pseudomonas aeruginosa CS	ATCC 27853	2	1	1	1	4	>32	2	8	>1	16
Pseudomonas aeruginosa CR	PS314	>128	NT	NT	64	NT	>32	>64	>32	>1	>64
Proteus mirabilis	PR91	0.5	0.5	1	0.25	2	>32	1	4	>1	8
Klebsiella pneumoniae CS	KL21	0.03	0.004	NT	≤0.06	NT	2	≤0.06	≤0.03	0.016	≤0.06
Klebsiella pneumoniae CR	KL328	64	8	16	>16	32	>32	>64	32	>1	>64
Enterobacter cloacae	AE63	0.06	0.02	0.03	≤0.06	0.06	16	≤0.06	0.06	≤0.12	0.5

Data assembled from the reports of Hu et al. (1996), Demuth et al. (1993), Rourke et al. (1993) MS: methicillin sensitive. CS: ciprofloxacin sensitive. MR: methicillin resistant. CS: ciprofloxacin resistant.
NT: not tested

Table 5. Minimum inhibitory concentration data (μg/mL) for quinolone controls

Organism	Strain	3	26	28	17	31	33	35	37	39	41
Gram Positive											
Staphylococcus aureus MSCS	ATCC 29213	0.25	0.06	0.008	0.008	0.03	0.12	≤0.008	≤0.03	≤0.008	≤0.008
Staphylococcus aureus MRCS	MI300	0.25	0.02	0.004	0.016	0.03	0.12	≤0.008	≤0.03	≤0.008	≤0.008
Staphylococcus aureus MSCR	MI345	16	NT	NT	0.5	NT	1	0.06	0.5	0.016	0.03
Staphylococcus aureus MRCR	MI339	32	NT	NT	0.5	NT	2	0.06	0.25	0.06	0.03
Staphylococcus saprophyticus	MI276	0.25	0.06	0.03	0.03	0.5	2	≤0.008	≤0.03	≤0.008	≤0.008
Enterococcus faecalis	ATCC 29212	0.25	0.06	0.06	0.03	0.25	0.12	≤0.008	≤0.03	≤0.008	≤0.008
Streptococcus pyogenes	STA2	0.5	0.06	0.03	0.03	0.5	0.016	≤0.008	≤0.03	≤0.008	≤0.008
Streptococcus pneumoniae	STP1	0.5	0.06	0.03	0.06	0.25	0.03	≤0.008	≤0.03	≤0.008	≤0.008
viridans streptococcus	STV1	2	0.12	0.06	0.03	0.25	0.03	≤0.008	≤0.03	≤0.008	≤0.008
Gram Negative											
Escherichia coli	ATCC 25922	≤0.016	0.06	0.0005	≤0.002	0.008	4	≤0.008	≤0.03	≤0.008	≤0.008
Pseudomonas aeruginosa CS	ATCC 27853	0.25	0.25	0.12	0.03	0.5	>4	0.25	1	0.25	1
Pseudomonas aeruginosa CR	PS314	32	NT	NT	2	NT	>4	8	16	8	>8
Proteus mirabilis	PR91	≤0.016	0.12	0.12	0.016	0.5	>4	0.06	0.12	0.06	0.06
Klebsiella pneumoniae CS	KL21	≤0.016	0.06	NT	≤0.002	NT	0.12	≤0.008	≤0.03	0.008	≤0.008
Klebsiella pneumoniae CR	KL328	2	NT	NT	0.5	NT	>4	4	4	1	4
Enterobacter cloacae	AE63	≤0.016	0.03	0.0005	≤0.002	0.016	>4	≤0.008	≤0.03	0.008	≤0.008

Data assembled from the reports of Hu et al., (1996), Demuth et al., (1993), Rourke et al., (1993) MS: methicillin sensitive. CS: ciprofloxacin sensitive. MR: methicillin resistant. CS: ciprofloxacin resistant. NT: not tested.

Table 6. Enzyme inhibition (IC_{50}, µg/mL) for
carbamate-linked quinolonyl penems

Enzyme	7	29	32	36	38	42
PBP-1	0.6	0.2	1	0.04	0.5	0.1
PBP-2	0.4	0.1	0.3	≤0.04	≤0.06	0.05
PBP-3	0.4	0.1	0.2	≤0.04	≤0.1	0.1
DNA-Gyrase	15	4	25.6	NT	8	NT

Data reported by Hu et al., (1996), Demuth et al., (1993), Koenigs et al., (1997)
PBPs from *S. aureus* ATCC29213. **42**: 2-hydroxymethyl penem control. NT: not
tested

allyl ester of ciprofloxacin in the key coupling step. The solvent system was 50% DMF in dioxane. The use of a less polar co-solvent to prevent double bond isomerization in the cephem was published by Mobashery and Johnston (1986). Compound **44** was prepared as described by Ma et al. (1994), as summarized in Figure 10. The cephalosporin starting material **46** was prepared according to the procedure of Yamanaka et al. (1985). The key coupling step was achieved by pretreating **3** with MSTFA to promote dissolution, thereby making additional protecting group chemistry unnecessary. The preparation of the dithio-carbamate **45**, reported by Demuth et al. (1992), is outlined in Figure 11. Unlike most other quinolonyl lactams, this compound was prepared without any protecting group chemistry via intermediate **47**.

Impact of the Link Variable on Potency. The antimicrobial potencies of the four compounds shown in Figure 9 are summarized in Table 7. Once again, these quinolonyl

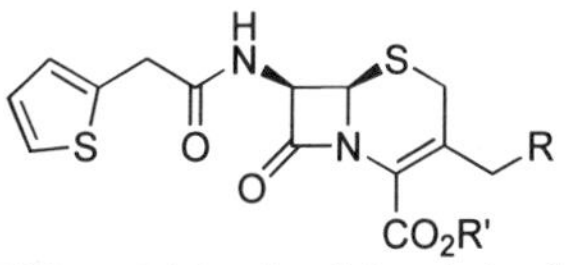

Quinolonyl Lactams With Different Links: R = link and ciprofloxacinmoiety. R' = H, Na

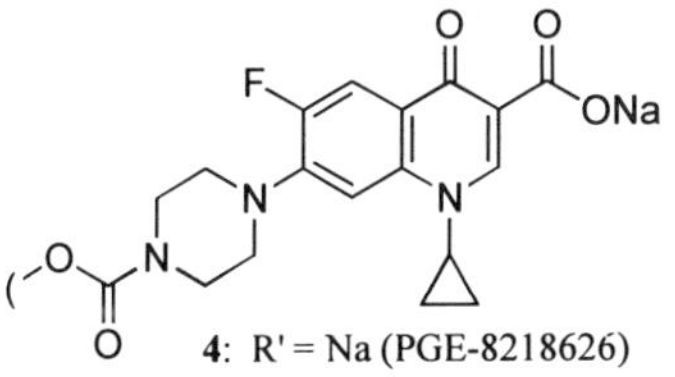

4: R' = Na (PGE-8218626)

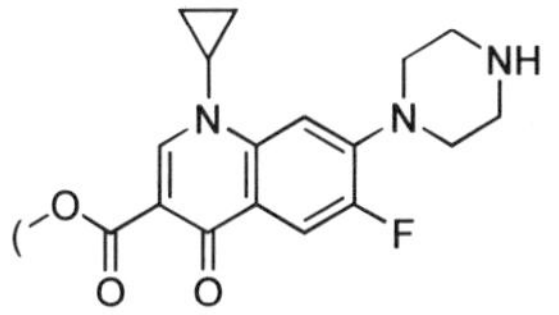

43: R' = H (PGE-0923160)

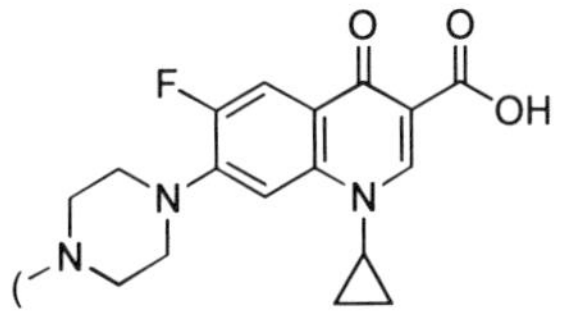

44: R' = H (PGE-8039005)

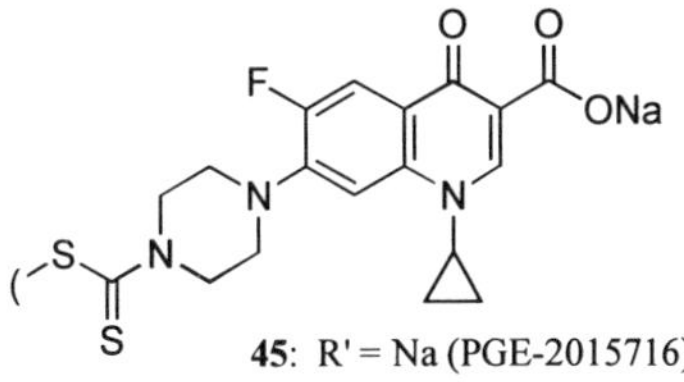

45: R' = Na (PGE-2015716)

Figure 9. Quinolonyl lactams derived from cephalothin and ciprofloxacin.

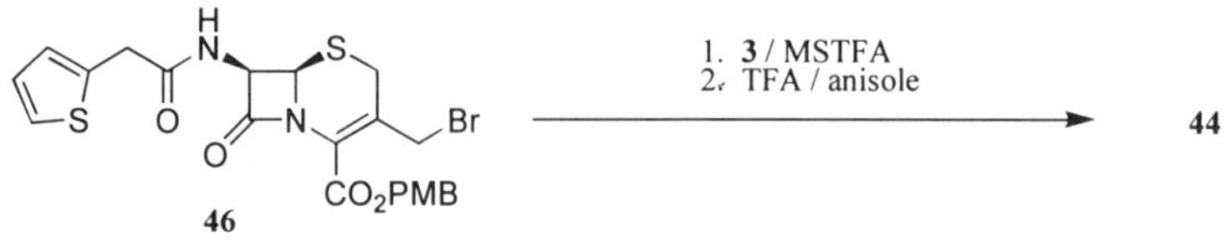

Figure 10. Preparation of **44**.

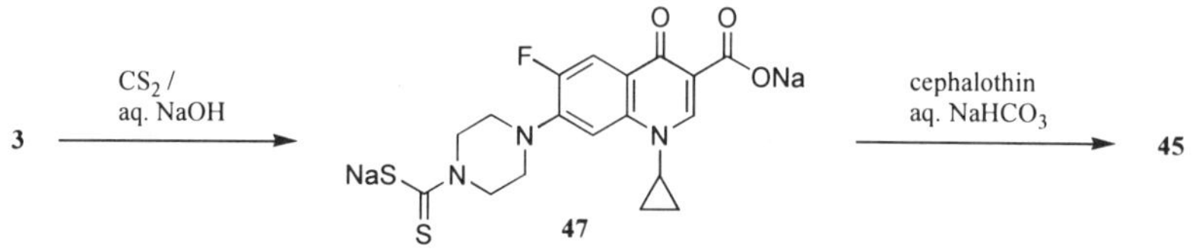

Figure 11. Preparation of **45**.

lactams exhibited a spectrum of activity better than the independent cephem and quinolone. The conjugated molecules also displayed advantages relative to an equimolar mixture of ciprofloxacin and desacetyl-cephalothin against gram positive organisms,
especially the streptococci. This fascinating result is discussed in more detail later in this
chapter. With respect to potency, these four links gave similar results overall.

Thioether-Linked Quinolonyl Carbapenems. The two carbapenems **48** and **49** shown
in Figure 12 provided further insight on the link variable. These compounds were specifically designed to maximize the stability of the link between the two pharmacophores.
Since it was believed that such a link might have a deleterious effect on potency, the β-

Table 7. Minimum inhibitory concentration data (μg/mL) for quinolonyl lactams with different links

Organism	Strain	24	3	Cocktail	4	43	44	45
Gram positive								
Staphylococcus aureus MSCS	ATCC 29213	≤0.12	0.25	0.25	0.25	0.5	1	1
Staphylococcus aureus MRCS	MI300	4	0.25	1	1	4	1	2
Staphylococcus aureus MSCR	MI345	0.25	16	NT	0.25	NT	2	0.25
Staphylococcus aureus MRCR	MI339	>64	32	NT	32	NT	>64	32
Staphylococcus saprophyticus	MI276	0.5	0.25	2	1	1	1	8
Enterococcus faecalis	ATCC 29212	32	0.25	1	8	8	16	8
Streptococcus pyogenes	STA2	≤0.12	0.5	0.25	≤0.016	≤0.01	0.03	0.01
Streptococcus pneumoniae	STP1	0.5	0.5	2	0.06	0.06	0.25	0.01
viridans streptococcus	STV1	0.25	2	2	NT	0.06	NT	0.01
Gram negative								
Escherichia coli	ATCC 25922	16	≤0.016	≤0.02	0.06	0.25	0.25	0.25
Pseudomonas aeruginosa CS	ATCC 27853	>64	0.25	0.5	1	2	16	16
Pseudomonas aeruginosa CR	PS314	>64	32	NT	NT	NT	NT	NT
Proteus mirabilis	PR91	32	≤0.016	0.12	1	1	2	1
Klebsiella pneumoniae CS	KL21	>64	≤0.016	0.02	0.25	0.06	0.03	0.06
Klebsiella pneumoniae CR	KL328	>64	2	NT	NT	NT	NT	NT
Enterobacter cloacae	AE63	>64	≤0.016	0.03	≤0.016	0.03	0.03	0.12

Data reported by Demuth et al., (1993).MS: methicillin sensitive. CS: ciprofloxacin sensitive. MR: methicillin resistant. CS:
ciprofloxacin resistant. NT: not tested. The cocktail was a 1:1 molar ratio of ciprofloxacin and desacetyl-cephalothin. Compound
24: desacetyl-cephalothin control. Compound **3**: quinolone control (ciprofloxacin).

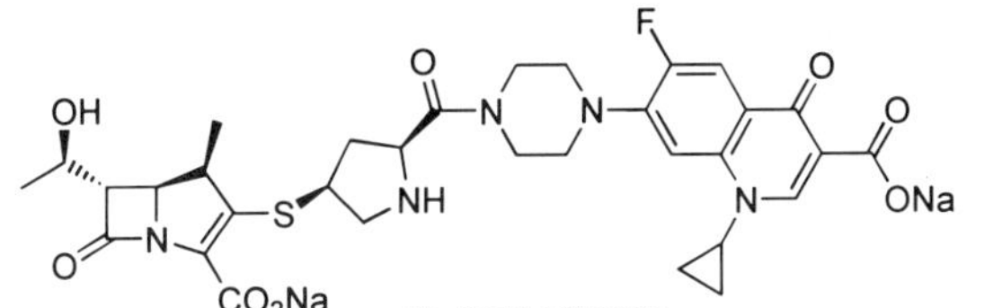

48: PGE-5428060

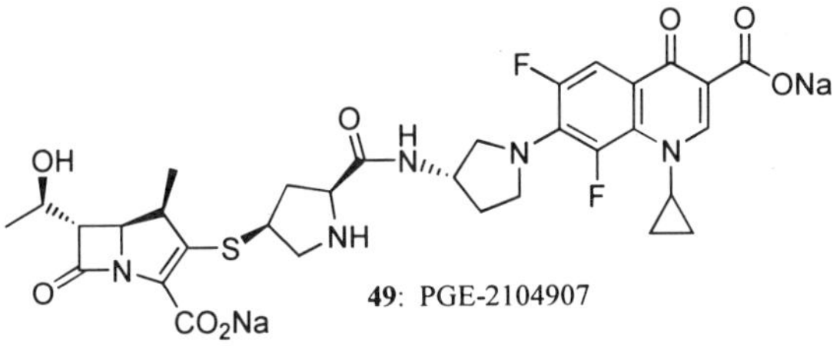

49: PGE-2104907

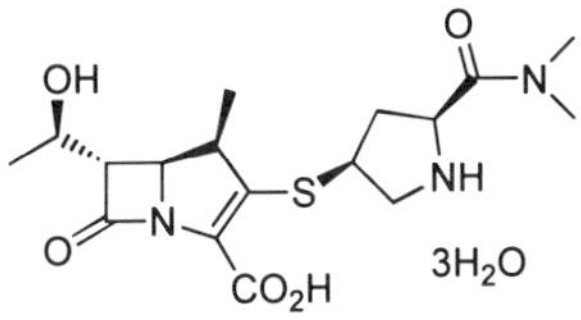

50: Meropenem Trihydrate

Figure 12. Thioether-linked quinolonyl carbapenems, and meropenem.

lactam moiety was designed to resemble the potent antibacterial meropenem (Figure 12, **50**), described by Sunagawa et al. (1990), to maximize the probability of achieving an acceptable spectrum of activity. These compounds were synthesized according the route reported by Hershberger et al. (1996), which is summarized in Figure 13. The acid **51** is an intermediate in the meropenem procedure published by Sunagawa et al. (1990). This compound was coupled to the p-nitrobenzyl ester of a quinolone to give **52**. Conversion of the thioacetate to the corresponding thiol was achieved with pyrrolidine. No disulfide oxidation was observed. Coupling of the thiol with the carbapenem **53**, a compound reported by Shih et al. (1984), followed by simultaneous removal of all three protecting groups gave the desired thioether linked quinolonyl carbapenems. Table 8 shows the potencies of these compounds. Although they exhibited broad spectrum potency, the impact of the quinolone

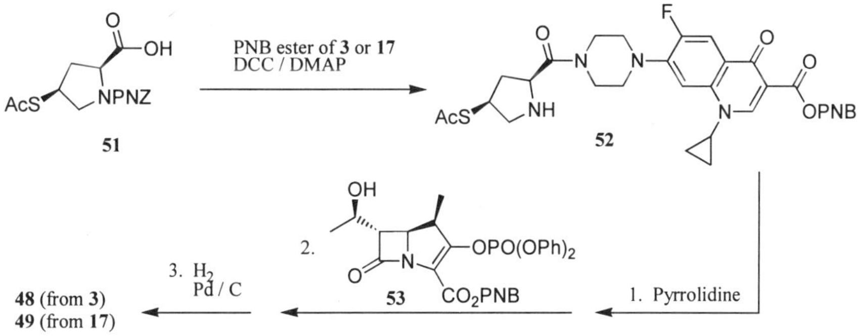

Figure 13. Synthesis of thioether linked quinolonyl carbapenems.

Table 8. Minimum inhibitory concentration data (μg/mL) for thioether-linked quinolonyl carbapenems

Organism	Strain	3	17	48	49	50
Gram positive						
Staphylococcus aureus MSCS	ATCC 29213	0.25	0.008	0.25	0.5	≤0.06
Staphylococcus aureus MRCS	MI300	0.25	0.016	2	8	1
Staphylococcus aureus MSCR	MI345	16	0.5	0.25	1	≤0.06
Staphylococcus aureus MRCR	MI339	32	0.5	64	>64	32
Staphylococcus saprophyticus	MI276	0.25	0.03	1	4	0.25
Enterococcus faecalis	ATCC 29212	0.25	0.03	8	8	4
Streptococcus pyogenes	STA2	0.5	0.03	≤0.06	≤0.06	≤0.06
Streptococcus pneumoniae	STP1	0.5	0.06	≤0.06	0.25	≤0.06
viridans streptococcus	STV1	2	0.03	≤0.06	≤0.06	≤0.06
Gram negative						
Escherichia coli	ATCC 25922	≤0.016	≤0.002	8	8	≤0.06
Pseudomonas aeruginosa CS	ATCC 27853	0.25	0.03	>64	>64	0.25
Pseudomonas aeruginosa CR	PS314	32	2	>64	>64	2
Proteus mirabilis	PR91	≤0.016	0.016	64	64	≤0.06
Klebsiella pneumoniae CS	KL21	≤0.016	≤0.002	0.5	4	≤0.06
Klebsiella pneumoniae CR	KL328	2	0.5	64	64	≤0.06
Enterobacter cloacae	AE63	≤0.016	≤0.002	8	8	≤0.06

Data reported by Hershberger et al. (1996). MS: methicillin sensitive. CS: ciprofloxacin sensitive. MR: methicillin resistant. CS: ciprofloxacin resistant. Compounds 3 and 17: Quinolone controls. Compound 50: meropenem control, supplied by Zeneca Pharmaceuticals

was significantly less than in other quinolonyl lactams. Generally, quinolonyl lactams derived from **17** were more potent than those derived from **3**; however, in this case, the more potent quinolonyl moiety offered no advantage in the in vitro growth inhibition assay. Both thioether-linked compounds were less potent than either the corresponding quinolone or meropenem. Compound **48** was an efficient inhibitor of PBPs ($IC_{50} = 0.2$ μg/mL) and a poor inhibitor (>100 μg/mL) of bacterial DNA-gyrase.

Comparison of Quinolonyl Lactams with Quinolone / Lactam Cocktails. Quinolonyl lactams clearly reinforced the multifunctional hypothesis by displaying the positive attributes of both pharmacophores. Their spectrum of activity is consistent with what is typically envisioned for future antibiotics, especially with respect to resistant organisms. Nonetheless, the fundamental value of the covalently linked molecule vs. a physical mixture of the two components remained an outstanding question. This section reviews in vitro results showing that the conjugated molecules have unique properties that are superior to either the independent lactam or quinolone, or even the *sum* of those parts.

Table 9 summarizes the potency benefit of ciprofloxacin-derived quinolonyl cephalosporins relative to an equimolar cocktail of the two substructures. Remarkably, all four compounds were better than the cocktail against the gram positive organisms, especially the streptococci. The cocktail remained better against the gram negatives due to the relatively high potency of the quinolone.

Serial passage resistance experiments were run to evaluate the potential rate of resistance development for several quinolonyl lactams. Figure 14 illustrates the results of these studies where **7** (the carbamate-linked penem molecule derived from ciprofloxacin) was compared with the corresponding 2-hydroxymethylpenem (**42**), quinolone (**3**), and the

Table 9. Potency comparison of quinolonyl
cephalosporins vs. a cocktail

Bacteria set	4	43	44	45	Cocktail
7 Gram pos.	0.27	0.33	0.61	0.25	0.91
3 Streptococci	0.04	0.03	0.12	0.01	1
5 Gram neg.	0.20	0.25	0.43	0.5	0.05

Values are the geometric mean MICs (µg/mL). Cocktail: 1:1 molar mixture of desacetyl-cephalothin and ciprofloxacin. The quinolonyl moiety
was derived from ciprofloxacin.

cocktail of both parts. The comparisons were made against three strains of *S. aureus* having different types of resistance, and against *P. aeruginsosa*. The experiment using the sensitive *S. aureus* is shown in the upper left quadrant of Figure 14. This organism developed
resistance to the ciprofloxacin after only three to four passages. Sensitivity to the penem
42 was lost after about 7 passages. As expected, the cocktail tended to track the more effective of the two parts, in this case the penem. However, the conjugated molecule **7** retained potency throughout the experiment and did not begin to experience significant
resistance until the ninth passage. Similar observations were made against resistant *S.
aureus*, with the conjugated molecule typically remaining more potent for more passages
than the cocktail. This effect was also observed against the gram negative *P. aeruginosa*
organism. Overall, these data suggest that quinolonyl lactams might succumb to resistance
mechanisms more slowly than independent β-lactams and quinolones, or cocktails.

Summary Discussion of the Link Variable. The link variable did not have a large
overall impact on potency, except for the case of the thioethers which rendered the quinolonyl moiety a poor leaving group. Most importantly, a suitable link offered advantages
relative to a cocktail, with potential implications on both potency and resistance development. The potency benefit of the conjugates relative to the individual parts was most easily observed for compounds derived from quinolones that are not significantly more potent
than the β-lactam. Nonetheless, even in cases where the quinolonyl pharmocophore may
be the dominant force with respect to potency, the possibility of a slower rate of new resistance development for the conjugated molecule remains a powerful incentive for the continued development of quinolonyl lactam antibacterials. Pace et al. (1991) at Roche also
reported data suggesting that a quinolonyl lactam was effective in cases where its components were not, such as in certain *E. coli* strains. This group has further reported (Georgopapadakou et al., 1989) mechanism of action studies relating to this effect, in addition
to results indicating that carbamate- and amine-linked compounds may exhibit activity
from both the lactam and the quinolonyl moiety in the intact molecule (Georgopapadakou
and Bertasso, 1993). The impact of the link on quinolonyl penems has been further investigated at Creighton University, as reported by by Ehrhardt and Saunders (1997). The general collection of positive attributes associated with linked compounds strongly suggested
the potential therapeutic utility of the quinolonyl lactam concept. The link also had a big
impact on the stability of the compounds. For example, White et al. (1993) reported that
the aqueous stabilities ($t_{1/2}$) of **4** (carbamate) and **44** (amine) were 12 hours and >100
hours, respectively. Likewise, Albrecht and Christenson (1992) of Roche reported $t_{1/2}$ values of 3 hours and 12.5 hours for two related ester-linked compounds, and 48–72 hours for
a quaternary ammonium-linked compound. For the purpose of compound design, the link

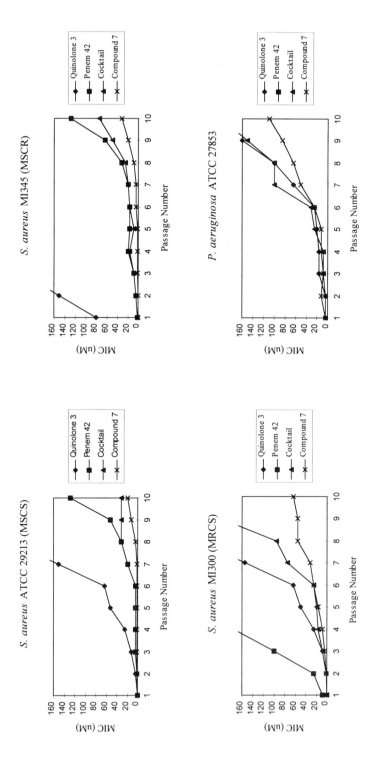

Figure 14. Serial passage resistance development of a quinolonyl penem.

MS: methicillin sensitive. CS: ciprofloxacin sensitive. MR: methicillin resistant. CR: ciprofloxacin sensitive.
Quinolone **3**: ciprofloxacin. Penem **42**: 2-hydroxymethylpenem. Cocktail: equimolar mixture of **3** and **42**.

variable was therefore recognized as a means for developing attributes superior to a cock-tail, and for attenuating the hydrolytic stability in quinolonyl lactams.

QUINOLONYL LACTAM LEADS

As the impact of various structural features became clear, quinolonyl lactam pro-grams moved quickly on the preclinical development of increasingly promising com-pounds. Generally, lactam selection was based primarily on potency and PBP binding affinity, the quinolonyl moieties were selected based primarily on potency and toxicity profiles, and the links were selected with improved stability as a key goal. This resulted in many compounds with desirable properties. The groups at Procter & Gamble and Roche have published most extensively in the field.

Examples of Leads

Figure 15 shows a representative set of lead molecules. Compounds **7** and **29** are penem carbamates with different quinolones. Compounds **54** and **55** are cephalosporin-derived compounds with variations of the amine-link. The quinolonyl moiety in these two compounds was derived from the 8-methoxy series published in the Domagala (1993) manuscript. The Roche compound Ro 23-9424 (**56**), derived from cefotaxime and fleroxacin, was widely investigated (Keith et al., 1993) and was well tolerated in Phase I clinical trials, as related by Squires and Christenson (1991). Albrecht et al. (1991) also reported on Ro24-4383 (**57**), a carbamate-linked compound derived from cefotaxime and ciprofloxacin.

Table 10 summarizes the key preclinical data reported for the quinolonyl lactams shown in Figure 15. The quinolonyl lactams derived from ciprofloxacin (**7** and **57**) and the compound derived from fleroxacin (**56**) gave disappointing results against resistant *S. aureus*. Better results against this organism were achieved by modifying the quinolonyl moiety, as in **29**, **54**, and **55**. The latter two compounds were also effective against van-comycin resistant *Enterococcus faecium* (VRE). Generally, good potency was observed against the streptococci, including strains resistant to penicillin, and against *E. coli*. Com-pound **29** was the most effective member of the group against *P. aeruginosa*; however, this compound exhibited photoxicity similar to the quinolonyl moiety. In vivo efficacy studies confirmed the quinolonyl lactams' broad spectrum of utility.

Aqueous stability remained a central issue. For example, the ester-linked compound **56**, exhibited a relatively short half life in aqueous solution. The carbamates **57**, **7**, and **29** showed a significant improvement in aqueous stability, as did the amine-lnked compound **54**. The propenyl 2° amine-linked compound **55** was considerably better than any of the others. It exhibited a half life of more than 8 days in pH 7.4 aqueous buffer.

Half life was also evaluated in vivo. In the rat model, the ester **56** and the car-bamates (**7** and **29**) all had half lives of 20 minutes or less. In the dog model, these car-bamates were signficantly better than the ester. The 2° amine **54** was better than either the ester or the carbamates in both the rat and the dog models. The propenyl 2° amine-linked compound **55** was even better than the 2° amine, based on comparison in the rat and the primate models.

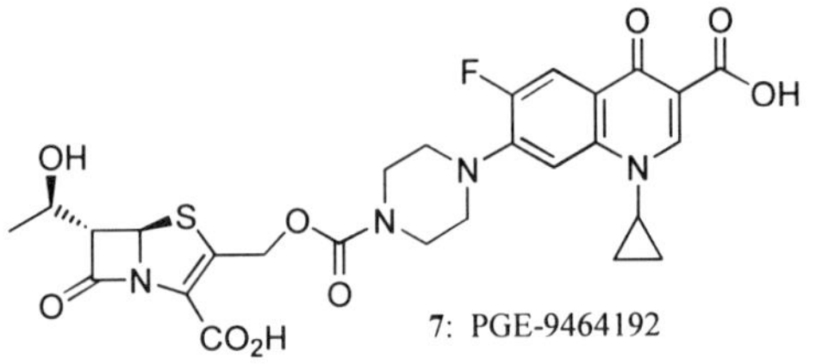

7: PGE-9464192

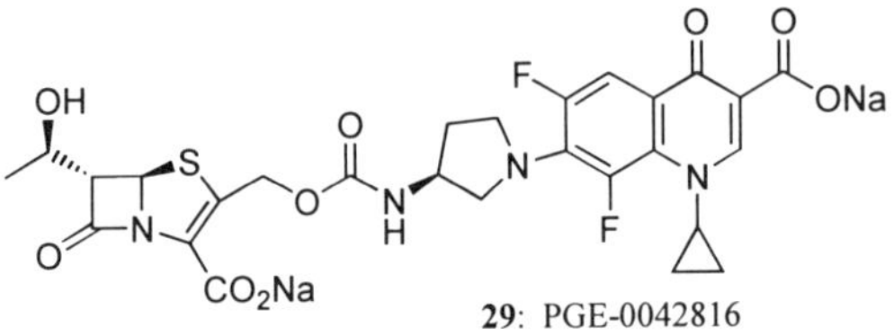

29: PGE-0042816

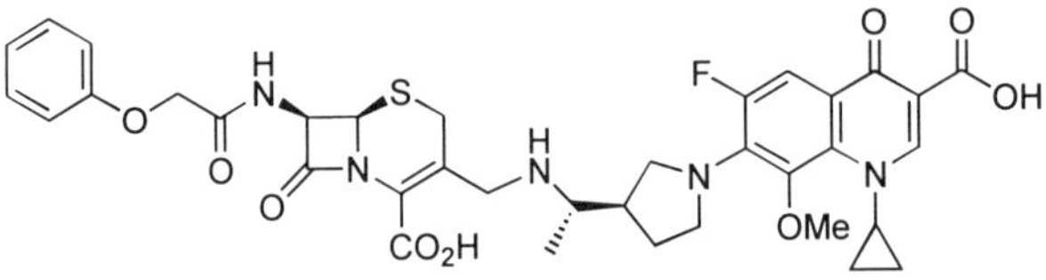

54: PGE-7594630

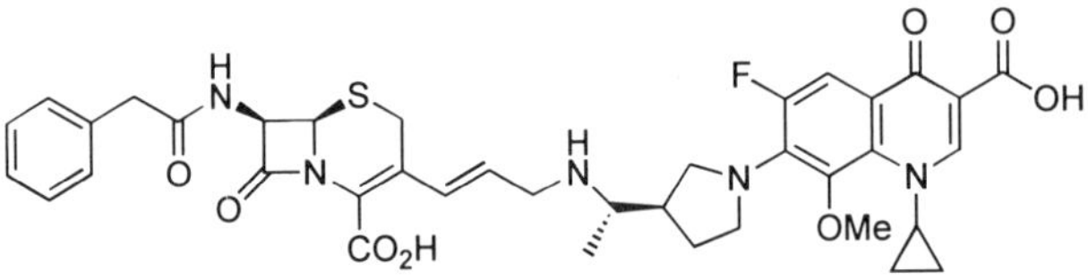

55: PGE-9576326

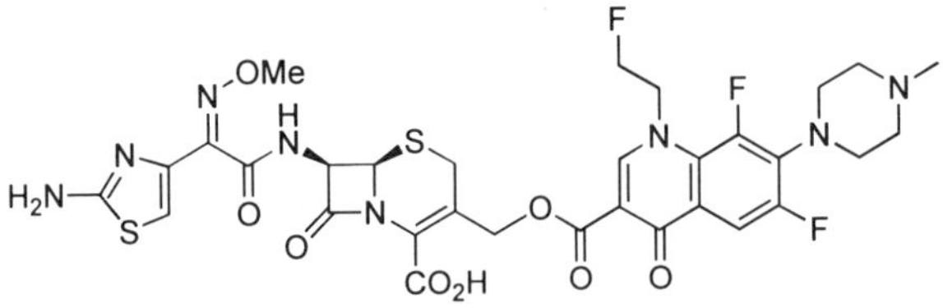

56: Ro 23-9424

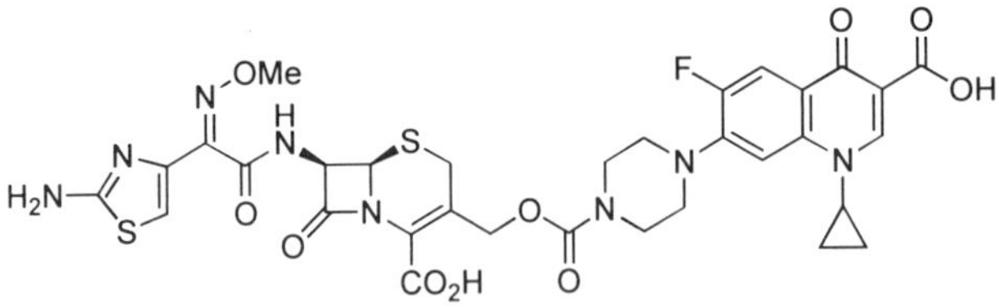

57: Ro 24-4383

Figure 15. Initial quinolonyl lactam leads.

Table 10. Summary of reported biological results for initial quinolonyl lactam leads

Assay	7	29	54	55	56	57
MIC90 (µg/mL)						
Staphylococcus aureus resistant	>64	4	2	2	16	8
Streptococcus pneumoniae	0.06	0.016	NT	NT	0.25	NR
Streptococcus pneumoniae PR	NT	0.016	0.03	0.12	0.25	NR
Enterococcus faecium	NT	NT	4 (VR)	1 (VR)	>16	8
Enterococcus faecalis	8	1	1	1	16	8
Escherichia coli	0.125	0.5	>2	2	0.5	0.063
Pseudomonus aeruginosa	4	2	16	32	8	4
Bacteroides fragilis	16	4	4	8	32	NR
PD50 (mg/kg)						
Streptococcus pneumoniae	23	9.0	2.5	1.5	<1	10
Staphylococcus aureus	9.2	0.88	1.5	2.8	5.6	12
Staphylococcus aureus MRSA	12	0.87	29	96	11	28
Escherichia coli	0.4	0.36	5.6	16	1.8	1.4
Aqueous Stability (hr)						
$(t_{1/2})$, pH 7.4 buffer	70.3	59.7	54.8	>200	2.7	10.5
In Vivo Serum Half-Life (hr)						
$(t_{1/2})$, Rat	0.28	0.16	2.07	6.34	0.30	0.58
$(t_{1/2})$, Dog	2.47	3.44	11.04	NT	0.60	NR
$(t_{1/2})$, Primate	NT	NT	1.75	5.60	1.25	NR

Data assembled from the reports of Mallalieu et al. (1997), Bierman et al. (1997), Mallalieu et al. (1997), Kraft et al. (1997), Gu and Neu (1990), Beskid et al. (1991), Beskid et al. (1990), Jones et al. (1989), Christenson et al. (1990), Christenson et al. (1990), and Rolston et al., (1992). Perrone et al. (1992) of Farmitalia also reported PD50 data on **29**. MR: methicillin resistant. CR: ciprofloxacin resistant. PR: penicillin resistant. OR: oxacillin resistant. VR: vancomycin resistant. NT: not tested. NR: not reported. Resistant *S. aureus* used for MIC 90s was MRCR for **7, 29, 54**, and **55**, MR for **56**, and OR for **57**. MIC 90 data for Ro 23-4383 against the enterococci reflected a combination of *E. faecalis* and *E. faecium*. MRSA in the PD50 assay was sensitive to ciprofloxacin for **7** and **29**. MRSA used for **56** and **57** in the PD50 assay was OR.

Quinolonyl Carbacephems

While the compounds shown in Figure 15 exhibited very good overall properties, more robust preclinical leads remain under investigation. White et al. (1997) of Procter & Gamble recently reported on the synthesis and biological properties of new quinolonyl carbacephems that represent a significant improvement over the first generation of leads. The compounds **58** and **59** shown in Figure 16 are representative of this new series.

The preparation of the quinolonyl carbacephems is illustrated in Figure 17. The quinolone **60** was reported in the Domagala (1993) paper. The carbacephems **61** and **62**, reported in the Cook et al. (1989) manuscript, were employed as starting materials. The 3-vinyl compound **61** was ozonized to the corresponding formyl compound, which was then reduced to the alcohol and captured *in situ* as the carbonate **63**. Reaction with **60** in the presence of pyridine, followed by deprotection and conversion to the disodium salt, gave the carbamate-linked quinolonyl carbacephem **58**. The triflate **62** was coupled with the appropriate organostannane alcohol (Jung and Light, 1982) to give a propenyl hydroxy intermediate which was oxidized to the aldehyde **64**. Reductive amination with **60**, and deprotection followed by salt formation provided the propenyl 2° amine-linked quinolonyl carbacephem **59**.

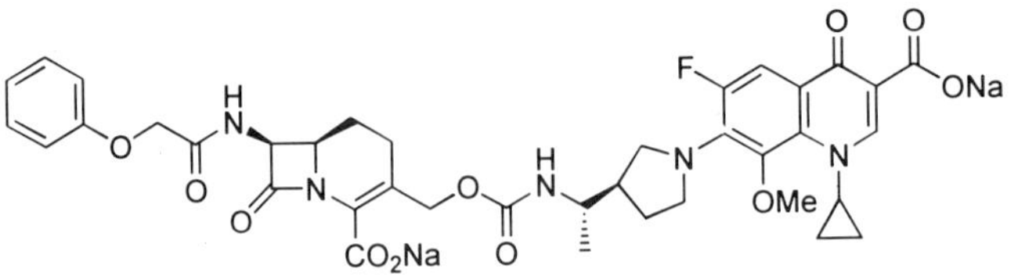

58: PGE-1818689

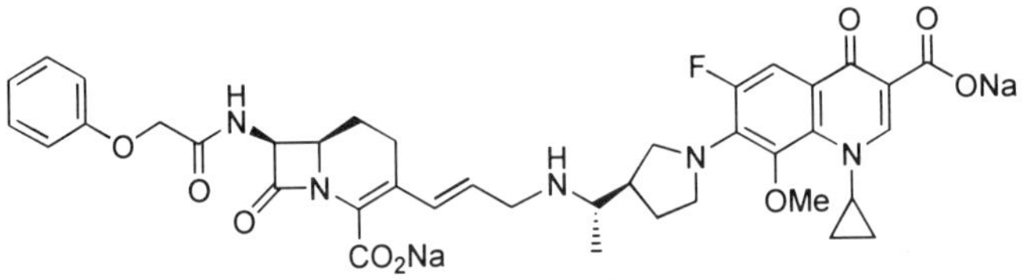

59: PGE-7119699

Figure 16. Quinolonyl carbacephem leads.

Preclinical data for the quinolonyl carbacephems are summarized in Table 11. These compounds exhibited very good broad spectrum potency in vitro. Perhaps the most unique attributes reported for this class were observed in stability studies. The carbamate-linked compound **58** had half lives of 9.5 hours in aqueous buffer and, more impressively, 2 and 3 days in rat and dog plasma, respectively. However, the corresponding 2° amine-linked molecule **59** gave even better results. This compound exhibited a remarkable half life of

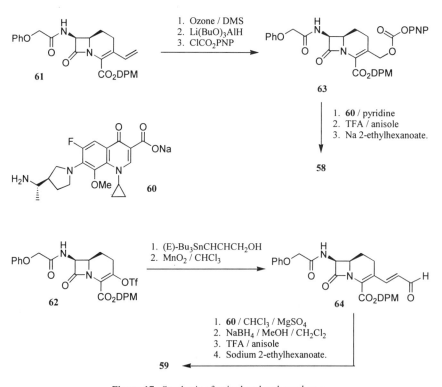

Figure 17. Synthesis of quinolonyl carbacephems.

Table 11. Biological results for quinolonyl carbacephems

Assay	58	59
MIC 90 (μg/mL)		
Staphylococcus aureus MSCS (32)	≤0.004	0.06
Staphylococcus aureus MRCR (32)	0.5	4
Streptococcus pneumoniae (16)	0.008	0.06
Escherichia coli (23)	0.12	2
Klebsiella pneumoniae (24)	0.5	4
Pseudomonus aeruginosa (23)	4	>64
Aqueous Stability (hr)		
($t_{1/2}$), pH 7.4 buffer	9.5	403
Plasma Stability (hr)		
($t_{1/2}$), Rat	47.8	129
($t_{1/2}$), Dog	72.3	169

Data published by White et al. (1997).

nearly 17 days in aqueous solution. The values measured in rat and dog plasma were 5 and 7 days.

CLOSING REMARKS

Quinolonyl lactam programs have greatly broadened the multifunctional antibiotic concept. The current generation of leads indeed have impressive and unique properties. These include:

1. High potency and broad spectrum of antibacterial activity against a range of clinically significant bacterial pathogens.
2. Activity against newly emerging strains of quinolone and β-lactam resistant bacteria, e.g., methicillin resistant ciprofloxacin resistant (MRCR) *Staphylococcus aureus*, penicillin resistant *Streptococcus pneumoniae*, and vancomycin resistant *Enterococcus faecium*
3. Pharmacokinetic properties which include high serum levels that were sustained over a long period of time
4. Good aqueous solution stability at physiological pH, with half-life at 37°C greater than 60 hours

These properties support the continued evaluation of quinolonyl lactams as clinical progression candidates.

ACKNOWLEDGMENTS

The authors acknowledge their many colleagues at Procter & Gamble who have participated in the quinolonyl lactam program, as well as the scientists working at other organizations who have conducted and published results in this field.

REFERENCES

Albrecht, H.A., Beskid, G., Chan, K., Christenson, J.G., Cleeland, R., Deitcher, K.H., Georgopapadakou, N.H., Keith, D.D., Pruess, D.L., Sepinwall, J., Specian, Jr., A.C., Then, R.L., Weigele, M., West, K.F., Yang, R., 1990, Cephalosporin 3'-quinolone esters with a dual mode of action, *J. Med. Chem.*, 33:77–86.

Albrecht, H.A., Beskid, G., Christenson, J.G., Deitcher, K.H., Georgopapadakou, N.H., Keith, D.D., Konzelmann, F.M., Pruess, D.L., and Wei, C.C., 1994, Dual-action cephalosporins incorporating a 3'-tertiary-amine-linked quinolone, *J. Med. Chem.*, 37:400–7.

Albrecht, H.A., Beskid, G., Christenson, J.G., Durkin, J.W., Fallat, V., Georgopapadakou, N.H., Keith, D.D., Konzelmann, F., Lipschutz, E.R., McGarry, D.H., Siebelist, J.A., Wei, C.-C., Weigele, M., and Yang, R., 1991, Dual-action cephalosporins:cephalosporin 3'-quaternary ammonium quinolones, *J. Med. Chem.*, 34:669–75.

Albrecht, H.A., Beskid, G., Christenson, J.G., Georgopapadakou, N.H., Keith, D.D., Konzelmann, F.M., Pruess, D.L., Rossman, P.L., and Wei, C.-C., 1991, Dual-action cephalosporin 3'-quinolone carbamates, *J. Med. Chem.*, 34:2857–64.

Albrecht, H.A., and Christenson, J.G., 1992, Mechanism-based dual-action cephalosporins, *Adv. Med. Chem.*, 1:207–34.

Alexander, R.P., Bates, R.W., Pratt, A.J., and (in part) Kraunsoe, J.A.E., 1996, A N-nitrosochloroethyl-cephalosporin carbamate prodrug for antibody-directed enzyme prodrug therapy (ADEPT), *Tetrahedron*, 52(16):5983–8.

Alexander, R.P., Beeley, N.R.A., O'Driscoll, M., O'Neill, F.P., Millican, T.A., Pratt, A.J., and Willenbrock, F.W., 1991, Cephalosporin nitrogen mustard carbamate prodrugs for ADEPT, *Tetrahedron Lett.*, 32(27):3269–72.

Alpegiani, M., Bedeschi, A., Perrone, E., Zarini, F., and Franceschi, G., 1985, 2-(Heteroatom-substituted)methyl penems. I. Sulphur derivatives, *Heterocycles*, 23:2255–70.

Beskid, G., Albrecht, H.A., Fallat, V., Keith, D.D., Lipschutz, E.R., McGarry, S.M., McGarry, D.H., Rossman, P., and Siebelist, J.A., 1991, In vitro and in vivo activity of carbamate-linked dual-action antibacterial Ro 24–4383, *J. Chemother.*, 37:310–7.

Beskid, G., Siebelist, J.A., McGarry, C.M., Cleeland, R., Chan, K., and Keith, D.D., 1990, In vivo evaluation of a dual-action antibacterial, Ro 23–9424, compared to cefotaxime and fleroxacin, *Chemother.*, 36:109–16.

Bierman, J.C., Mallalieu, N.L., Walling, M.A., Kuzmak, B.R., Emig, J.E., Dirr, M.K., Tirey, D.A., Zoutendam, P.H., White, R.E., Gray, J.L., Matson, P.A., Ma, X., Kraft, W.G., Demuth, Jr., T.P., and Leunk, R.D., 1997, In vivo efficacy and pharmacodynamics of four quinolonyl-lactam antibacterial agents in mice, *37th Interscience Conf. Antimicrobial Agents Chemother.*, Abstr. No. F197, Toronto, Canada.

Bonjouklian, R., and Phillips, M.L., 1981, Reactions of TMSI with cephalosporin esters, *Tetrahedron Lett.*, 22:3915–8.

Bouzard, D., Cesare, P.D., Essiz, M., Jacquet, J.P., Kiechel, J.R., Remuzon, P., Weber, A., Oki, T., Masuyoshi, M., Kessler, R.E., Fung-Tomc, J., and Desiderio, J., 1990, Fluoronaphthyridines and quinolones as antibacterial agents. 2. Synthesis and structure-activity relationships of new 1-*tert*-butyl 7-substituted derivatives, *J. Med. Chem.*, 33:1344–52.

Boyd, D.B., Hermann, R.B., Presti, D.E., and Marsh, M.M., 1975, Electronic structures of cephalosporins and penicillins. 4. Modeling acylation by the β-lactam ring, *J. Med. Chem.*, 18(4):40617.

Boyd, D.B., and Lunn, W.H.W., 1979, Electronic structures of cephalosporins and penicillins. 9. Departure of a leaving group in cephalosporins, *J. Med. Chem.*, 22(7):778–84.

Chin, G.J., and Marx, J., 1994, Resistance to antibiotics, *Science*, 264:359.

Christenson, J.G., Beskid, G., Cleeland, R., Farrish, Jr., H.H., Holzknecht, B.D., Keith, D.D., Pruess, D.L., and Talbot, M.K., 1990, Pharmacokinetic and mechanistic differences between ester- and carbamate-linked dual-action cephalosporins, *30th Interscience Conf. Antimicrob. Agents Chemother.*, Abstr. No. 405, Atlanta, GA.

Christenson, J.G., Chan, K.K., Cleeland, R., Dix-Holzknecht, B., Farrish, Jr., H.H., Patel, I.H., and Specian, A., 1990, Pharmacokinetics of Ro 23–9424, a dual-action cephalosporin, in animals, *Antimicrob. Agents Chemother.*, 34(10):1895–1900.

Cocker, J.D., Cowley, B.R., Cox, J.S.G., Eardley, S., Gregory, G.I., Lazenby, J.K., Long, A.G., Sly, J.C.P., and Somerfield, G.A., 1965, Cephalosporin acids. Part II. Displacement of the acetoxy group by nucleophiles, *J. Chem. Soc.*, 5015–31.

Cook, G.K., Hornback, W.J., Jordan, C.L., McDonald III, J.H., and Munroe, J.E., 1989, Palladium-catalyzed chemistry of β-lactam vinyl triflates: coupling with organostannanes and alkoxycarbonylation, *J. Org. Chem.*, 54:5828–30.

Corraz, A.J., Dax, S.L., Dunlap, N.K., Georgopapadakou, N.H., Keith, D.D., Pruess, D.L., Rossman, P.L., Then, R., Unowsky, J., and Wei, C.-C., 1992, Dual-action penems and carbapenems, *J. Med. Chem.*, 35:1828–39.

Dax, S.L., 1992, Dual-action β-lactam antibacterials, *Current Opinion in Therapeutic Patents, Antimicrobials*, September:1375–84.

Dax, S.L., Pruess, D.L., Rossman, P.L., and Wei, C.-C., 1993, Synthesis and mechanistic studies of a 'tetrazole-tethered' cephalosporin-quinolone hybrid, *Bioorg. Med. Chem. Lett.*, 3(2):209–14.

Demuth, Jr., T.P., Berk, J.D., Davis, B.W., Koenigs, P.M., Kraft, W.G., McOsker, C.C., Rourke, F.J., Shinabarger, D.L., Tietjen, R.A., and White, R.E., 1993, Preclinical evaluation of quinolonyl-lactam antibacterials: compounds designed to combat drug-resistance in bacteria, *Eastern Pennsylvania Branch of American Society of Microbiology Symposium*, Nov. 11–12, Philadelphia, PA.

Demuth, Jr., T.P, White, R.E., Tietjen, R.A., Ebetino, F.H., Kraft, W.G., Andersen, J.A., McOsker, C.C., Walling, M.A., Davis, B.W., and Rourke, F.J., 1990, C-10 Quinolonyl-cephem carbamates: synthesis, and evaluation of a new class of antibacterial agents, *200th ACS Meeting*, Abstr. No. MEDI-154.

Demuth, Jr., T.P., White, R.E., Tietjen, R.A., Pollack, J.R., Kraft, W.G., Davis, B.W., and Rourke, F.J., 1992, Preparation and antimicrobial activity of novel C-10 quinolonyl-cephem dithiocarbamates, *32nd Interscience Conf. Antimicrob. Agents Chemother.*, Abstr. No. 773, Anaheim, CA.

Demuth, Jr., T.P., White, R.E., Tietjen, R.A., Storrin, R.J., Skuster, J.R., Andersen, J.A., McOsker, C.C., Freedman, R., and Rourke, F.J., 1991, Synthesis and antibacterial activity of new C-10 quinolonyl-cephem esters, *J. Antibiotics*, 44:200–9.

Domagala, J.M., Hagen, S.E., Joannides, T., Kiely, J.S., Laborde, E., Schroeder, M.C., Sesnie, J.A., Shapiro, M.A., Suto, M.J., and Vanderroest, S., 1993, Quinolone antibacterial containing the new 7-[3-(1-aminoethyl)-1-pyrrolidinyl] side chain: the effects of the 1-aminoethyl moiety and its stereochemical configurations on potency and in vivo efficacy, *J. Med. Chem.*, 36:871–82.

Ehrhardt, A.F., and Saunders, C., 1997, Structure-activity studies of quinolone-penems in genetically defined strains of *Escherichia coli*, *Antimicrob. Agents Chemother.*, 41(11):2570–2.

Faraci, W.S., and Pratt, R.F., 1984, Elimination of a good leaving group from the 3'-position of a cephalosporin need not be concerted with β-lactam ring opening: TEM-2 β-lactamase-catalyzed hydrolysis of pyridine-2-azo-4'-(N',N'-dimethylaniline) cephalosporin (PADAC) and of cephaloridine, *J. Am. Chem. Soc.*, 106:1489–90.

Perrone, E., Jabes, D., Alpegiani, M., Andreini, B.P., Bruna, C.D., Nero, S.D., Rossi, R., Visentin, G., Zarini, F.,and Franceschi, G., 1992, Dual-action penems, *J. Antibiotics*, 45(4):589–94.

Georgopapadakou, N.H., and Bertasso, A., 1993, Mechanisms of action of cephalosporin 3'-quinolone esters, carbamates, and tertiary amines in *Escherichia coli*, *Antimicrob. Agents Chemother.*, 37(3):559–65.

Georgopapadakou, N.H., Bertasso, A., Chan, K.K., Chapman, J.S., Cleeland, R., Cummings, L.M., Dix, B.D., and Keith, D.D. 1989, Mode of action of the dual-action cephalosporin Ro 23–9424, *Antimicrob. Agents Chemother.*, 33(7):1067–71.

Gray, J.L., Shrum, G.P., Gasparski, C.M., Wang, A.M., Ramberger, N.R., Davis, B.W., McKeever, H.D., Koenigs, P.M., Paule, S.M., Twinem, T.L., Kraft, W.G., Rourke, F.J., and Demuth, Jr., T.P., 1995, Antibacterial activity of multifunctional quinolonyl-cephem 2°-amines, *35th Interscience Conf. Antimicrob. Agents Chemother.*, San Francisco, CA.

Gu, J.-W., and Neu, H.C., 1990, In vitro activity of Ro 23–9424, a dual-action cephalosporin, compared with activities of other antibiotics, *Antimicrob. Agents Chemother.*, 34(2):189–95.

Hamilton-Miller, J.M.T., Newton, G.G.F., and Abraham, E.P., 1970, Products of aminolysis and enzymic hydrolysis of the cephalosporins, *Biochem. J.*, 116:371–84.

Hamilton-Miller, J.M.T., Richards, E., and Abraham, E.P., 1970, Changes in proton-magnetic-resonance spectra during aminolysis and enzymic hydrolysis of cephalosporins, *Biochem J.*, 116:385–95.

Hanessian, S., and Wang, J., 1993, Design and synthesis of a cephalosporin-carboplatinum prodrug activatable by a β-lactamase, *Can. J. Chem.*, 71:896–906.

Hershberger, P.M., Switzer, A.G., Yelm, K.E., Coleman, M.C., DeVries, C.A., Rourke, F.J., Davis, B.W., Kraft, W.G., Twinem, T.L., Koenigs, P.M., Paule, S.M., Siehnel, R.J., Zoutendam, P.H., Imbus, R., and Demuth, Jr., T.P., 1996, Synthesis and biological evaluation of 2-thioether-linked quinolonyl carbapenems, *36th Interscience Conf. Antimicrob. Agents Chemother.*, Abstr. No. F170, New Orleans, LA.

Hu, X.E., Morgan, J.D., Hershberger, P.M., White, R.E., Gasparski, C.A., Kim, N., Shrum, G.P., Ramberger, N.R., Ma, X., O'Hara, T.L., Prohotsky, D.L., Anthony, D.R., Matson, P.A., Davis, B.W., DeVries, C.A., Koenigs, P.M., Paule, S.M., Twinem, T.L., Zoutendam, P.H., Imbus, R., Leunk, R.D., and Demuth, Jr., T.P., 1996, Multifunctional quinolonyl-penem carbamates and their antibacterial activities, *36th Interscience Conf. Antimicrob. Agents Chemother.*, Abstr. No. F168, New Orleans.

Hwu, J.R., Moshfegh, A.A., Tsay, S.-C., Lin, C.C., Tseng, W.N., Azaripour, A., Mottaghian, H., and Hakimelahi, G.H., 1997, Cephalosporin 3'-phloroglucide esters and 7-(phloroglucamido)cephalosporins as novel antibacterial agents, *J. Med. Chem.*, 40:3434–41.

Jabes, D., Rossi, R., Bruna, C.D., Perrone, E., Alpegiani, M., Andreini, B.P., Visentin, G., Zarini, F., and Franceschi, G., 1993, Activity of new penems against defined MRSA strains, *Bioorg. Med. Chem. Lett.*, 3(11):2165–70.

Jones, R.N., Barry, A.L., and Thornsberry, C., 1989, Antimicrobial activity of Ro 23–9424, a novel ester-linked co-drug of fleroxacin and desacetylcefotaxime, *Antimicrob. Agents Chemother.*, 33(6):944–50.

Jung, M.E., and Light, L.A., 1982, Preparation of iodoallylic alcohols via hydrostannylation: spectroscopic proof of structures, *Tetrahedron Lett.*, 23(38):3851–4.

Keith, D.D., Albrecht, H.A., Beskid, G., Chan, K.K., Christenson, J.G., Cleeland, R., Deitcher, K., Delaney, M., Georgopapadakou, N.H., Konzelmann, F., Okabe, M., Pruess, D., Rossman, P., Specian, A., Then, R., Wei, C.-C., and Weigele, M., 1993, Mechanism-based dual-action cephalosporins, *Spec. Publ. - R. Soc. Chem.*, 119 (Recent Advances in the Chemistry of Anti-Infective Agents):79–92.

Kim, K.W., Kang, J.H., and Park, C.-H., 1993, Novel cephalosporin compounds, WO 9315084.

Koenigs, P., Paule, S., Shah, S., DeVries, C., Davis, B., Hu, X.E., White, R.E., Ma, X., Shrum, G.P., Stanton, K., Demuth, Jr., T.P., and Kraft, W.G., 1993, Structure-activity relationships for quinolonyl-lactam antibacterial binding to *Staphylococcus aureus* penicillin-binding proteins, *37th Interscience Conf. Antimicrob. Agents Chemother.*, Abstr. No. F194, Toronto, Canada.

Kraft, W.G., Leunk, R.D., McKeever, H.D., DeVries, C.A., Gray, J.L., Gasparski, C.M., Ma, X., Matson, P.A., Shrum, G.P., and Demuth, Jr., T.P., 1997, In vitro activity of quinolonyl-cephem amines, *37th Interscience Conf. Antimicrob. Agents Chemother.*, Abstr. No. F195, Toronto, Canada.

La, S., Jung, M., Kim, W., and Jee, U., 1993, Synthesis and antibacterial activity of cephalosporin 3'-quinolone dithiocarbamate, *Yakhak Hoechi*, 37(2):136–42.

La, S., Kong, J., Kim, W., and Jee, U., 1993, Physicochemical properties, stabilities, and pharmacokinetics of cephalosporin 3'-quinolone dithiocarbamate, *Yakhak Hoechi*, 37(6):638–46.

Levy, S.B., 1998, The challenge of antibiotic resistance, *Scientific American*, March:46–53.

Ma, X., Davis, B.W., O'Hara, T.L., Anthony, D.R., Billings, D.M., Matson, P.A., White, R.E., Krauss, H.J., Berk, J.D., Wood, N.A., Loenigs, P.M., Shah, S.K., Shinabarger, D.L., Twinem, T.L., McOsker, C.C., Kraft, W.G., Rourke, F.J., and Demuth, Jr., T.P., 1994, Synthesis and multifunctional antibacterial activity of new quinolonyl-cephem 3°-amines, *34th Interscience Conf. Antimicrob. Agents Chemother.*, Orlando, FL.

Ma, X., White, R.E., Matson, P.A., DeVries, C.A., Switzer, A.G., Hu, X.E., Hershberger, P.M., Prohotsky, D.L., Anthony, D.R., O'Hara, T.L., Koenigs, P.M., Davis, B.W., Twinem, T.L., Kraft, W.G., Leunk, R.D., and Demuth, Jr., T.P., 1996, Synthesis and multifunctional antibacterial activity of amine-linked quinolonyl penems, *36th Interscience Conf. Antimicrob. Agents Chemother.*, Abstr. No. F167, New Orleans, LA.

Mallalieu, N.L., Bierman, J.C., Emig, J.E., Dirr, M.K., Baker, T.R., Tirey, D.A., Zoutendam, P.H., Demuth, Jr., T.P., Hu, X.E., Gray, J.L., Shrum, G.P., Matson, P.A., Ma, X., White, R.E., and Leunk, R.D., 1997, Prediction of the pharmacokinetics and dosing schedule of quinolonyl-lactam (QL) antibacterials in humans from data obtained in animals, *37th Interscience Conf. Antimicrob. Agents Chemother.*, Abstr. No. F196, Toronto, Canada.

Mallalieu, N.L., Dorsey, J.S., Emig, J.E., Bierman, J.C., Dirr, M.K., Tirey, D.A., Zoutendam, P.H., Demuth, Jr., T.P., and Leunk, R.D., 1997, Comparison of the pharmacokinetics of penem versus cephem quinolonyl-lactam (QL) antibacterials in three mammalian species, *Pharmaceutical Research*, 14(11):S-363, Abstr. No. 2453.

Meyer, D.L., Jungheim, L.N., Mikolajczyk, S.D., Shephard, T.A., Starling, J.J., and Ahlem, C.N., 1992, Preparation and characterization of a β-lactamase-Fab' conjugate for the site-specific activation of oncolytic agents, *Bioconjugate Chem.*, 3:42–8.

Mielke, B., Philipps, T., Bremm, K., and Endermann, R., 1996, Beta-lactam derivatives of quinolonecarboxylic acids as bactericides, DE 4435478.

Miyamoto, T., Matsumoto, J., Chiba, K., Egawa, H., Shibamori, K., Minamida, A., Nishimura, Y., Okada, H., Kataoka, M., Fujita, M., Hirose, T., and Nakano, J., 1990, Synthesis and structure-activity relationships of 5-substituted 6,8-difluoroquinolones, including sparfloxacin, a new quinolone antibacterial agent with improved potency, *J. Med. Chem.*, 33:1645–56.

Mobashery, S., and Johnston, M., 1987, Inactivation of alanine racemase by β-chloro-L-alanine released enzymatically from amino acid and peptide C_{10}-esters of desacetylcephalothin, *Biochemistry*, 26:5878–84.

Mobashery, S., and Johnston, M., 1986, Reactions of *Escherichia coli* TEM β-lactamase with cephalothin and with C_{10}-dipeptidyl cephalosporin esters, *J. Biol. Chem.*, 261:7879–87.

Mobashery, S., and Johnston, M., 1986, Preparation of ceph-3-em esters unaccompanied by $\Delta^2 \rightarrow \Delta^3$ isomerization of the cephalosporin, *J. Org. Chem.*, 51:4723.

Mobashery, S., Lerner, S.A., and Johnston, M., 1986, Conscripting β-lactamase for use in drug delivery. Synthesis and biological activity of a cephalosporin C_{10}-ester of an antibiotic dipeptide, *J. Am. Chem. Soc.*, 108:1685–86.

Nishimura, T., Yoshimura, Y., Yamaoka, M., Kawai, T., and Miyake, A., 1991, Studies on condensed-heterocyclic azolium cephalosporins, *J. Antibiotics*, 44:1371–93.

O'Callaghan, C.H., Sykes, R.B., and Staniforth, S.E., 1976, A new cephalosporin with a dual mode of action, *Antimicrob. Agents Chemother.*, 10:245–8.

Pace, J., Bertasso, A., and Georgopapadakou, N.H., 1991, *Escherichia coli* resistant to cephalosporins and quinolones is still susceptible to the cephalosporin-quinolone ester Ro 23–9424, *Antimicrob. Agents Chemother.*, 35(5):910–15.

Page, M.I., 1984, The mechanisms of reactions of β-lactam antibiotics, *Acc. Chem. Res.*, 17:144–51.

Page, M.I., and Proctor, P., 1984, Mechanism of β-lactam ring opening in cephalosporins, *J. Am. Chem. Soc.*, 106:3820–25.

Petersen, U., Schrock, W., Haebich, D., Krebs, A., Schenke, T., Philipps, T., Grohe, K., Endermann, R., Bremm, K., and Metzger, K.G., 1994, Quinolonecarboxylic acid beta-lactam antibiotics, EP 591808.

Petersen, U., Schrock, W., Haebich, D., Krebs, A., Schenke, T., Philipps, T., Grohe, K., Endermann, R., Bremm, K., and Metzger, K.G., 1994, Preparation of penemylmethyl and cephalosporinylmethyl 7-(diazabicyclonono)quinolonecarboxylates as bactericides, DE 4234330.

Rolston, K.V.I., Nguyen, H.T., Ho, D.H., LeBlanc, B., and Bodey, G., 1992, In vitro activity of Ro 23–9424, a dual action antibacterial agent, against bacterial isolates from cancer patients compared with those of other agents, *Antimicrob. Agents Chemother.*, 36(4):879–82.

Rosen, T., Chu, D.T.W., Lico, I.M., Fernandes, P.B., Shen, L., Borodkin, S., and Pernet, A.G., 1988, Asymmetric synthesis and properties of the enantiomers of the antibacterial agent 7-(3-aminopyrrolidin-1-yl)-1-(2,4-difluorophenyl)-1,4-dihydro-6-fluoro-4-oxo-1,8-naphthyridine-3-carboxylic acid hydrochloride, *J. Med. Chem.*, 31:1586–90.

Rourke, F.J., Davis, B.W., Kraft, W.G., White, R.E., McOsker, C.C., O'Hara, T.L., and Demuth, Jr., T.P., 1993, In vitro activity of two new quinolonyl-penem carbamates, *33rd Interscience Conf. Antimicrob. Agents Chemother.*, Abstr. No. 1489, New Orleans.

Rourke, F.J., Davis, B.W., Kraft, W.G., White, R.E., McOsker, C.C., Walling, M.A., Andersen, J.A., Salvagno, A.M., Fitzpatrick, P.M., Jamieson, L.A., and Demuth, Jr., T.P., 1992, Evaluation of new quinolonyl penem carbamates, *32nd Interscience Conf. on Antimicrob. Agents Chemother.*, Abstr. No. 772, Anaheim, CA.

Russell, A.D., and Fountain, R.H, 1971, Aspects of the mechanism of action of some cephalosporins, *J. Bacteriol.*, 106:65–69.

Sanchez, J.P., Domagala, J.M., Hagen, S.E., Heifetz, C.L., Hutt, M.P., Nichols, J.B., and Trehan, A.K., 1988, Quinolone antibacterial agents. Synthesis and structure-activity relationships of 8-substituted quinoline-3-carboxylic acids and 1,8-naphthyridine-3-carboxylic acids, *J. Med. Chem.*, 31:983–91.

Shih, D.H., Baker, F., Cama L., and Christensen, B.G., 1984, Synthetic carbapenem antibiotics I. 1-β-methylcarbapenem, *Heterocycles*, 21(1):29–40.

Silver, L.L, and Bostian, K.A., 1993, Discovery and Development of new antibiotics: the problem of antibiotic resistance, *Antimicrob. Agents Chemother.*, 37(3):377–83.

Squires, E., and Christenson, J.G., 1991, Ro 23–9424, *Drugs of the Future*, 16:620–3.

Stocksdale, M.G., Ramurthy S., and Miller, M.J., 1998, Asymmetric total synthesis of an important 3-(hydroxymethyl)carbacephalosporin, *J. Org. Chem.*, 63:1221–25.

Sunagawa, M., Matsumura, H., Inoue, T., Fukasawa M., and Kato, M., 1990, A novel carbapenem antibiotic, SM-7338 structure-activity relationships, *J. Antibiotics*, 43(5):519–32.

Svensson, H.P., Kadow, J.F., Vrudhula, V.M., Wallace, P.M., and Senter, P.D., 1992, Monoclonal antibody-β-lactamase conjugates for the activation of a cephalosporin mustard prodrug, *Bioconjugate Chem.*, 3:176–81.

Veinberg, G., Shestakova, I., Petrulanis, L., Grigan, N., Musel, D., Zeile, D., Kanepe, I., Domrachova, I., Kalvinsh, I., Strakovs, A., and Lukevics, E., 1997, Synthesis and evaluation of dual action cephalosporins as elastase inhibitors, *Bioorg. Med. Chem. Lett.*, 7(7):843–6.

White, R.E., Demuth, Jr., T.P., Berk, J.D., Tietjen, R.A., Jamieson, L.A., Kraft, W.G., McOsker, C.C., Davis, B.W., Rourke, F.J., Koenigs, P., Shah, S., Shinabarger, D.L., Shrum, G.P., Walling, M.A., and White, A.H., 1993, Preparation and comparative antibacterial activity of quinolonyl-cephem amines and carbamates, *33rd Interscience Conf. Antimicrob. Agents Chemother.*, Abstr. No. 1491, New Orleans, LA.

White, R.E., Gasparski, C.M., Kim, N., Hu, X.E., Shrum, G.P., Lockhart, N.R., Switzer, A.G., Hershberger, P.M., Koenigs, P.M., Paule, S.M., Twinem, T.L., DeVries, C.A., Zoutendam, P.H., Imbus, R., Kraft, W.G., Leunk, R.D., and Demuth, Jr., T.P., 1997, Synthesis and biological evaluation of quinolonyl-carbacephalosporin antibacterials, *37th Interscience Conf. Antimicrob. Agents Chemother.*, Abstr. No. F193, Toronto, Canada.

Yamanaka, H., Chiba, T., Kawabata, K., Takasugi, H., Masugi, T., and Takaya, T., 1985, Studies on β-lactam antibiotics, *J. Antibiotics.*, 38(12):1738–51.

14

BACTERIAL TWO-COMPONENT SIGNALLING AS A THERAPEUTIC TARGET IN DRUG DESIGN

Inhibition of NRII by the Diphenolic Methanes (Bisphenols)

John M. Domagala,[1*] Diane Alessi,[2] Maxwell Cummings,[4]
Stephen Gracheck,[3] Liren Huang,[4] Michael Huband,[3] Gregg Johnson,[3]
Eric Olson,[2] Martin Shapiro,[2] Rajeshwar Singh,[4] Yuntao Song,[1]
Ruth Van Bogelen,[2] Dean Vo,[4] and Sara Wold[3]

[1]Chemistry Department
[2]Molecular Biology Department
[3]Infectious Disease Department
Parke-Davis Pharmaceutical Research
2800 Plymouth Road
Ann Arbor, Michigan 48105
[4]SynPhar Laboratories, Inc.
Edmonton Alberta
Canada T6E 5U2

INTRODUCTION

The Problem of Bacterial Resistance

Bacterial resistance to the currently available antibiotics is a worldwide problem with catastrophic potential (Kunin, 1993; Berkowitz, 1995; Domagala and Sanchez, 1997). In the US, overall mortality from infectious diseases has increased 58% with deaths from respiratory infections and septicemia up 20 and 83% respectively (Pinner et al., 1996). Increased resistance has been documented for every major group of pathogens with methicillin resistant *Staphyloccus aureus* (MRSA), vancomycin resistant enterococci (VRE) and β-lactam resistant streptococci causing the greatest alarm (Cormican and Jones, 1996; Howe et al., 1996). In fact, VRE has been described as the most feared nosocomial pathogen today (Hagman and Strausbaugh, 1996). The fear of vancomycin resis-

---

[*] Author to whom all correspondence should be addressed.

Resolving the Antibiotic Paradox, edited by Rosen and Mobashery.
Kluwer Academic / Plenum Publishers, New York, 1998.

tant MRSA has sparked calls for stringent preemptive controls (Edmund et al., 1996). Equally alarming is the dramatic increase in resistance among the gram negative organisms (Jones, 1996). Nosocomial pneumonias (often with resistant organisms) occur in 0.5–5% of all hospitalized patients with a mortality of 20–70%, and an added annual cost of $2.5 billion for increased care and treatment (Gaynes and Lynch, 1991; Swartz, 1994). So great and urgent is the problem that the prestigious journal Science has devoted two issues to bacterial resistance (Travis, 1994; Koshland, 1992), and the American Society for Microbiology formed a Task Force to define the problem and make recommendations. Their insightful report, issued in 1995 (Report 1995), called for an increased effort in the discovery of new drugs and new drug targets in bacteria.

Response to the Problem of Resistance: New Drugs

In response to the bacterial resistance alarms, pharmaceutical companies and academic labs alike have refocussed their research efforts toward the discovery of new antibacterial agents (Stinson, 1996). Several approaches are being followed. The most obvious approach is to modify existing drugs for additional potency or to devise drugs to directly combat resistance development (Chu et al., 1996). A second approach is to target the resistance mechanisms themselves. This approach seeks to design new or modified drugs that attack an enzyme or protein that causes a particular resistance. Examples would include inhibitors of β-lactamases, aminoglycoside modifying enzymes, ribosomal modifying enzymes, the MecA or Fem proteins which confer methicillin resistance, or any of the proteins leading to high level vancomycin resistance (Setti et al., 1997; Chu, 1996). A third approach is to use modern screening technologies to identify novel inhibitors of well known processes such as DNA replication and cell wall synthesis, or not so well known processes such as envelope function, protein secretion, adherence, or two-component signalling (Desnottes, 1996).

We at Parke-Davis were particularly interested in bacterial two-component signalling. Herein we describe our selection of the target, the mass screening, and a detailed study of one class of inhibitors.

TWO-COMPONENT SIGNALLING AS A TARGET

Bacteria must constantly respond to an often hostile and precarious environment, and accordingly, they have evolved an elaborate network of environmental sensors and adaptive output devices. The most common of these are the two-component signalling pathways, which include the sensor (first component) and a response regulator (second component). The process is depicted in Figure 1.

The sensor protein has an N-terminal domain that is usually associated with the membrane. This sensor domain receives the signal. The C-terminal portion of the sensor protein is a histidine kinase (HK), which autophosphorylates at a highly conserved histidine as the signal is received. The response regulator (RR) also contains two functional domains. The N-terminal response domain contains a highly conserved aspartate, which receives the phosphate from the kinase. The C-terminal region is the output domain. Generally a change in the conformation of the response domain, upon phosphorylation, triggers the output domain. The output domain usually contains a DNA or RNA binding motif, and acts at the transcriptional level to ultimately produce the proteins that will mediate the appropriate response to the signal. In one case which governs chemotaxis, the response regulator modulates bacterial swimming by a direct interaction with the flagella

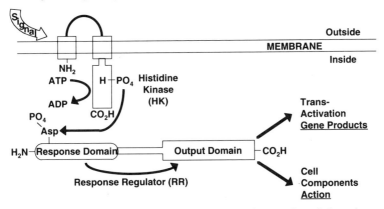

Figure 1. Diagram of a typical two-component regulatory pathway in bacteria.

apparatus. The sensor and output domains vary widely according to function, but the HK and RR are highly conserved in most HK/RR pairs. Some HKs are not associated with membranes and receive their signals from within the cytoplasm.

There are over 80 characterized two-component systems which govern such diverse processes as nutrient uptake, motility, virulence, and resistance. Table 1 lists several

HK/RR pairs and the functions they regulate. A single *Escherichia coli* (E. coli) is estimated to contain at least 50 HK/RR pairs (Haldiman et al., 1996). The highly feared vancomycin resistant enterococci utilize the two-component pathway (VanS/VanR) to sense the presence of vancomycin and to respond by producing all the Van proteins that confer resistance to the drug. The two-component signalling pathways have been the subject of several excellent reviews (Parkinson and Kofoid, 1992; Bourret et al., 1991; Stock et al., 1989; Swanson et al., 1994).

Clearly, the bacterial two-component signalling pathways would appear to be an ideal target for antibacterial development: the pathways are widely distributed among all bacteria; the pathways are thought to be specific to bacteria although sequence analysis suggests a presence in eukaryotes too (Koshland, 1993); there is high homology in the two phosphorylation sites; and the pathways govern numerous vital processes required for bacterial survival. Yet, in spite of this latter fact, most of the HK/RR pairs are not individually essential proteins. Their knock-out mutations are generally not lethal, but instead lead to

Table 1. A listing of several two-component systems and their histidine kinase/response regulator pairs

Process	Histidine kinase	Response regulator
Chemotaxis	CheA	CheY, CheB
Nitrogen regulation	NRII	NRI
Vanco resistance	VanS	VanR
Membrane porins	EnvZ	OmpR
Phosphate Assimilation	PhoR	PhoB
Virulence	VirA, BvgS	VirG, BvgA
Alginate (capsule)	AlgR2	AlgR1
Degradative enz.	DegS	DegU
Nitrogen fixation	FixL	FixJ
Dicarboxylate transport	DctB	DctD
Sporulation	KinA	SpoOF

organisms that are not as fit or versatile. Thus, a compound that inhibited one of the pathways might not be cidal. Alternatively, one might try to design an agent that would inhibit multiple HK/RR pairs.

Part of the reason that histidine kinases and their response regulators are not individually essential may lie in the redundant backup pathways that bacteria possess. Small molecule phosphates are able to phosphorylate certain response regulators in the absence of their HK partners (Lukat et al., 1992; McCleary and Stock, 1994). Cross talk may also play a role. Certain RRs may be phosphorylated by other histidine kinase partners as part of their general regulation (Wanner, 1992). Even if these alternate phosphorylation pathways could be overcome, as is possible, the level of experimental complexity might make it more difficult to define the precise actions of an inhibitor.

KNOWN HK/RR INHIBITORS

While two-component signalling has been suggested as a potential target for antibacterial drug design in multiple reviews, there have been few reports describing actual inhibitors of these pathways. Roychoudhury and colleagues (1993) employed a screening library to discover inhibitors of the alginate two-component pathway (AlgR2/AlgR1), which regulates the formation of the exopolysaccharide, alginate, in *Pseudomonas aeruginosa*. This exopolysaccharide encapsulates the bacteria and likely plays a significant role in its pathogenicity. These workers screened at the transcriptional level using a reporter gene inserted into the promoter gene AlgD. Active compounds were those that inhibited the production of the reporter protein (spectrophotometric monitoring). This assay would identify inhibitors of the histidine kinase or the response regulator or any other protein that governed transcription. From 25,000 compounds, two classes were discovered represented by the isothiazalone **1** and the quaternary imidazole **2**. Both compounds were inhibitory in the primary screen at 0.2–0.4 μg/ml. Compound **1** was shown to inhibit the autophosphorylation of the histidine kinase AlgR2, while compound **2** inhibited transcription by interfering with the binding of AlgR1 to its DNA promoter site (gel shift assays). When tested against other soluble HKs such as CheA, NRII, and KinA, **1** was not inhibitory; however, **2** inhibited NRII very effectively. This report did not reveal if the inhibitors actually reduced capsule formation, and no antibacterial activity was given.

In a second report, cis-fatty acids were found to inhibit the autophosphorylation of purified KinA (sporulation) pathway (Strauch, 1992). Trans and branched acids were not active. The inhibitors were non-competitive with ATP, and no antibacterial activity was reported.

Several initial communications (meeting abstracts) regarding other inhibitors of KinA/SpoOF have just appeared from one research group. Two of the compounds revealed were the amidines **3a** and **3b** (Demers et al., 1997, Licata et al., 1997) and the salicylamide **4** (Macielag et al., 1997). All were low μM inhibitors at the KinA/SpoOF enzyme level and all displayed good gram positive antibacterial activity of 1–4 μg/ml. An analog of **4** was also active in inhibiting initiation of the VanS/VanR vancomycin resistance pathway in whole cell assays. The compounds reported did not exhibit animal efficacy.

3a   3b

4

IDENTIFICATION OF THE DIPHENOLIC METHANES AS INHIBITORS OF THE HISTIDINE KINASE NRII

The Assay

In our research, we chose to study the well characterized and soluble histidine kinase NRII, which regulates the nitrogen pool within *E. coli* (Atkinson and Ninfa, 1993). We specifically chose not to assay at the transcription level so as to avoid complications with DNA binders and intercalators.

Purified NRII (300 nM) was incubated with labelled ATP (50 μM total concentration) for five minutes in Tris buffer at pH 8 containing $MgCl_2$ and KCl at room temperature. The NRII was collected onto filters and was washed, dried, and counted. The level of reduced counts relative to control determined the % inhibition.

The Inhibitors

Over 150,000 compounds were screened and several novel classes were identified (Classes 1–5), which were highly potent inhibitors of NRII autophosphorylation at the 100 μM test concentration. It is notable that 4/5 of the classes are phenolic in nature. The close structural relationship between Classes 2 and 4 was also noted. The Class 5 compounds were reminiscent of the quaternary imidazoles that were identified, as cited earlier (Roychoudhary, 1993). Classes 2, 4 and 5 had the largest number of representative actives from the screening.

Class 1   **Class 2**

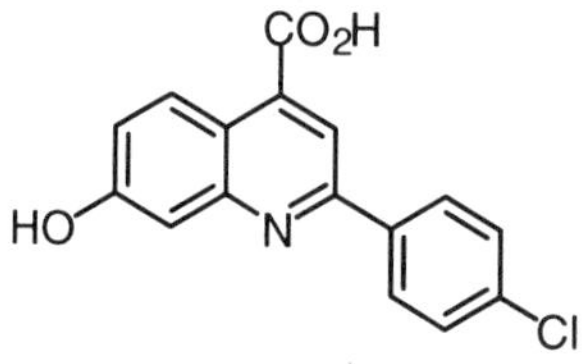

Class 3

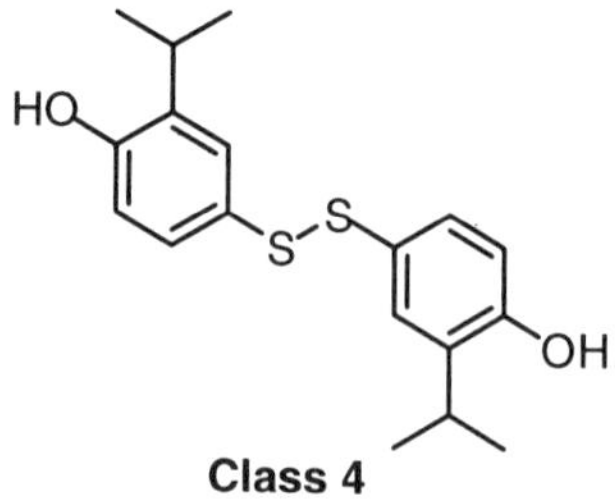

Class 4

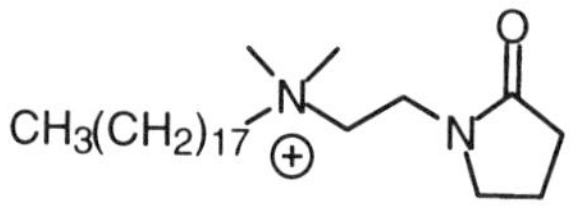

Class 5

The Diphenolic Methanes

We were attracted to the Class 2 diphenolic methanes (bisphenols) because there were many members of this class in our compound library and a full range of NRII inhibition was displayed (0–100%, inhibition at 100 μM) providing a good initial structure activity relationship (SAR). Moreover, the disulfides of Class 4 contained the same structural elements suggesting that the diphenolic groups constituted a particularly good pharmacophore. One member of the class, compound **5**, was selected and shown to be equally inhibitory vs the histidine kinases EnvZ and VanS while displaying no inhibition vs mammalian tyrosine kinases. Thus, the Class 2 compounds were broadly active and selective for the bacterial histidine kinases. Finally, the diphenolic methanes were relatively easy to prepare. All of these facts persuaded us to study the diphenolic methanes in depth.

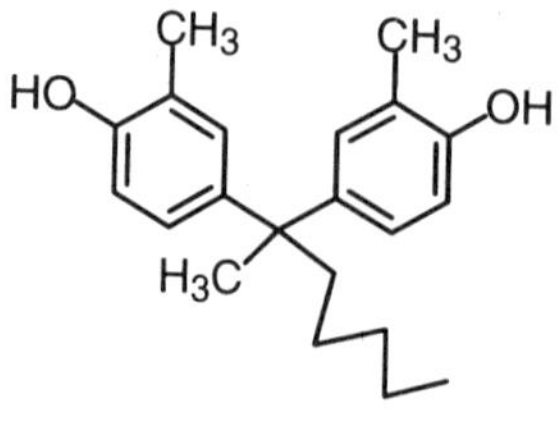

5 (PD009094)

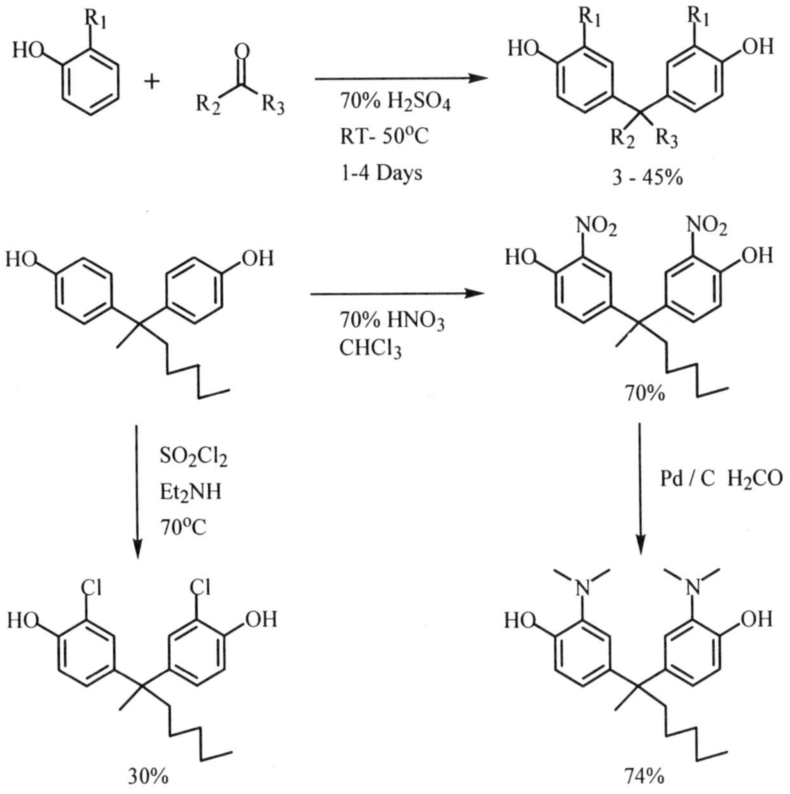

Scheme 1

Synthesis

The diphenolic methanes were readily prepared according to Scheme 1. The substituted phenols could be directly condensed with the appropriate ketone or aldehyde. Alternatively, the diphenolic methanes could be substituted by typical electrophilic chemistry to give the desired products.

Previous History of the Diphenolic Methanes

Certain diphenolic methanes have been previously described. Bisphenol A is a widely used monomer in the production of plastics and coatings (Spivack et al., 1989) and has been shown to possess mild antibacterial and antifungal properties (Subramaniam et al., 1989). The diisopropyl analog of bisphenol A (**7**) was reported as a cell wall synthesis inhibitor with moderate activity vs gram positive pathogens (Shimi et al., 1976). Finally, certain diphenolic cyclohexanes were reported to have mild antibacterial activity. The mini-SAR revealed the phenolic groups to be essential and the preferred R_1 substituent was H or CH_3 (Garchar et al., 1993). In our hands, bisphenol A and compound **8** (R_1=H or

CH$_3$) did not inhibit NRII and only compound **8** (R$_1$=CH$_3$) displayed any antibacterial activity (Minimum Inhibitory Concentrations, MICs, $\geq$ 8 μg/ml).

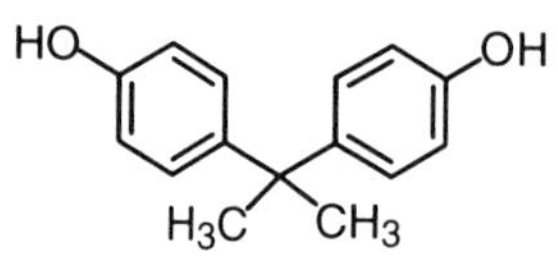

6

Bisphenol A   **7** 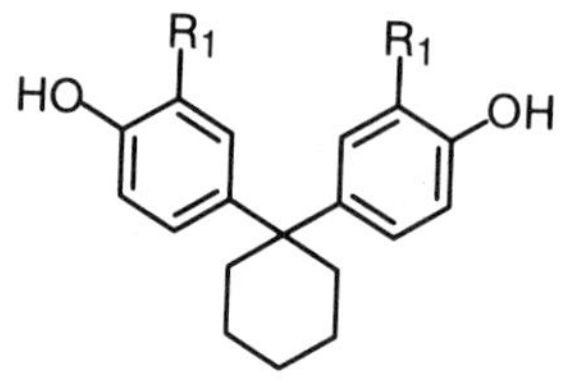   **8**

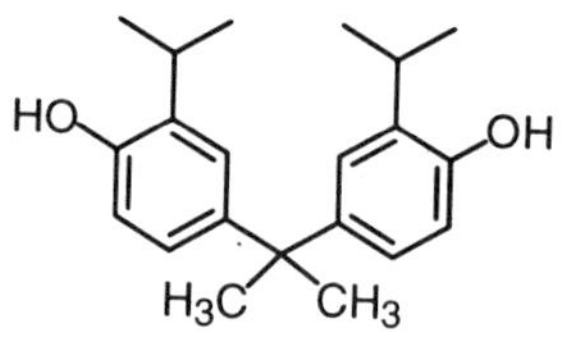

SAR OF THE DIPHENOLIC METHANES

Efforts to optimize the activity of the diphenolic methanes were performed at two levels. The first involved the identification of structural features that controlled the % inhibition vs the NRII kinase. Compounds were tested for % inhibition at 100 μM. Selected agents were also titrated and plotted to record the concentration of drug producing 50% inhibition of autophosphorylation (IC$_{50}$, μM). Secondly, we attempted to optimize antibacterial potency. Compounds were tested using standard microtitration techniques (Cohen et al., 1985) vs a panel of organisms, which included *E. coli, Bacillus subtilis, Staphylococcus aureus, Streptococcus pyogenes*, and a cell wall permeable (imp minus) *E. coli* (*E. coli* LKY). This strain permits the evaluation of the drugs in a gram negative organism without an intact permeability barrier.

The diphenolic methanes offered several possible sites for optimization as depicted in the generic structure **9**. In addition to the ortho and methylene substituents (R$_1$-R$_3$) we also sought to explore the importance of the phenols and their optimal relative positions in the rings. The results are shown in Tables 2–5.

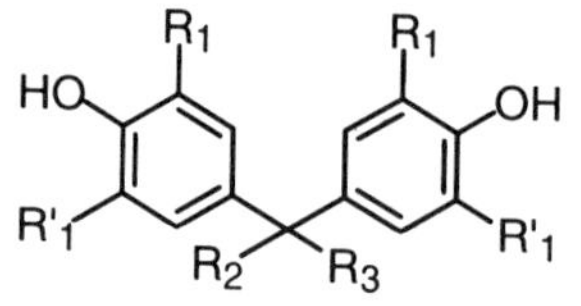

9

Variation of R$_2$, R$_3$

The % inhibition of NRII increases with chain length of R$_3$ (Table 2) with no inhibition where R$_3$ is propyl. The inhibition is 48% when R$_3$ is pentyl (PD009094) and is optimal when R$_2$ is ethyl and R$_3$ is pentyl (PD163892). The MICs show the same trend, except that some antibacterial activity is observed (8 μg/ml) even when the % inhibition of NRII is non-existent. This observation might imply alternate mechanisms of action or the inhibition of other histidine kinases other than NRII. The MICs peak when R$_2$ is ethyl and R$_3$ is pentyl as seen with the NRII inhibition.

Table 3 summarizes the results obtained when R$_2$ and R$_3$ form a ring. The trends parallel the observations in Table 2. The cyclooctyl and substituted cyclohexyl are the most

Table 2. Structure activity of the diphenolic methanes: Variation R_2 and R_3

Structure			Enzyme (μM or %) NRII IC$_{50}$ (% Inh)	Antibacterial data MICs (μg/mL)				
R_2	R_3			E. coli	E. coli LKY	B. subtilis	S. aureus	S. pyogenes
H	H		(0)	>64	>64	>64	>64	>64
CH$_3$	CH$_3$		(12)	>64	32	32	32	32
CH$_3$	Et		(0)	>64	32	16	16	8
CH$_3$	Pr		(0)	64	32	8	8	8
CH$_3$	Pent	PD009094	77 (48)	>64	4	2	2	2
CH3	Hept		(80)	>64	16	2	4	1
Et	Pent	PD163892	7(100)	>64	2	0.5	1	1
Pent	Pent		3 (94)	64	32	2	8	1

Table 3. Structure activity of the diphenolic methanes: Variation where R_2 and R_3 form a ring

Structure Cyclo Alkyl	Enzyme (μM or %)NRII IC$_{50}$ (%Inh)	Antibacterial data MICs (μg/mL)				
		E. coli	E. coli LKY	B. subtilis	S. aureus	S. pyogenes
	>200 (0)	>64	32	32	32	32
	200 (30)	>64	32	16	16	8
	(17)	>64	16	8	8	8
	20 (60)	>64	4	2	2	2
(PD 164592)	43 (97)	>64	2	1	0.5	0.5

Table 4. Structure activity of the diphenolic methanes: Variation at R_1

Structure		Enzyme (μM or %) NRII IC$_{50}$ (% Inh)	Antibacterial Data MICs (μg/mL)				
R_1	R_1		E. coli	E. coli LKY	B. subtilis	S. aureus	S. pyogenes
H	H	(39)	>64	8	4	8	4
CH$_3$	H	(48)	>64	4	2	2	2
E	H	(98)	>64	8	2	2	1
i Pr	H	9 (97)	64	8	2	4	2
t Bu	H	12 (78)	>64	32	4	64	2
Cl	H	<30 (98)	64	2	1	1	0.5
Cl	Cl	<30 (98)	>64	4	1	1	0.5
CH$_3$	Cl	20 (99)	>64	64	4	8	1
Br	H	-	>64	8	4	4	2
F	H	-	>64	4	4	4	4
OMe	H	200 (11)	>64	32	16	16	16
NMe$_2$	H	200 (0)	>64	32	32	32	32
NO$_2$	H	140 (50)	>64	64	64	64	16

Table 5. Structure activity of the dipenolic methanes: The essentialness of the phenolic groups

Structure	Enzyme (μM or %) NRII IC$_{50}$ (% Inh)	Antibacterial data MICs (μg/mL)				
		E. coli	E. coli LKY	B. subtilis	S. aureus	S. pyogenes
R=OH	(47)	>64	16	8	8	8
R=NH$_2$	>200 (25)	>256	>256	>256	>256	>256
RR'=OH	(48)	>64	4	2	2	2
RR'=OMe	>200	>64	>64	>64	>64	>64
RR'=OMe R'=OH	100	>64	64	4	8	2
RR'=H	>200	>256	>256	>256	>256	>256
	200 (0)	64	8	4	4	4

inhibitory of NRII and bacterial growth, while rings larger than 8 atoms began to diminish activity (data not shown). The effect of adding the *t*-butyl group to the unsubstituted cyclohexane is noteworthy.

Variation of R_1, R_1

Results from varying R_1, R_1 are shown in Table 4. Almost any small non-polar substituent provides good inhibition of NRII and antibacterial potency. There is a small diminution of antibacterial activity as the R_1 substituent grows too large. Polar substituents (last three entries) cause a significant loss of activity.

The Effect of the Phenolic Groups

Table 5 displays the results from three series featuring modification of the OH groups thought to be essential from previous reports (Garchar et al., 1993). In the first series, the OH is replaced with NH_2, causing a loss of activity vs NRII and bacterial growth. In the second series the effects of successive alkylations are shown. Dialkylation is as deleterious as complete removal of the phenolic groups in that both modifications engender a complete loss of all activity. The final entry suggests that the para phenols are most effective for inhibition of NRII although the MICs for the meta isomer are quite respectable.

The Effect of Polar Solubilizing Substituents

Given our desire to reduce the overall lipophilicity of these agents and the suggestion (from Table 4) that such changes at R_1 reduce potency, we attempted to place polar substituents more remote to the phenolic groups (Tables 6 and 7). All such efforts failed to retain any significant anti-NRII or antibacterial activity. Particularly disconcerting was the decreased activity when we attempted to bury the polar substituent within lipophilic groups, as was the case for entry 4 (Table 6) and entries 1, 4 and 5 in Table 7.

In summary, R_2 and R_3 optimized to large lipophilic groups while R_1 and R_1 optimized to smaller lipophilic substituents. The para phenols were essential for inhibition of NRII, and all attempts to reduce the lipophilicity with polar groups while maintaining activity failed.

ANTIBACTERIAL PROFILE OF THE DIPHENOLIC METHANES

The two most active compounds, PD163892 (Table 2) and PD164592 (Table 3), were chosen for additional antibacterial characterization. Given the importance of the phenolic groups we monitored the MICs in the presence of metals (100 mM Ca^{++} or Mg^{++}) and as a function of pH 6–9. No effects were observed.

Since the HKs are not essential proteins, we theorized earlier that the inhibitors of HKs might not be cidal. Both PD compounds were bactericidal in *Enterococcus faecium, S. aureus* and *S. pyogenes* at concentrations 1–4 dilutions above their MICs. (True for all actives tested). PD164592 retains the antibacterial activity vs ciprofloxacin/methicillin resistant *Staphylococcus aureus* and vancomycin resistant *Enterococcus faecium* as shown in Table 8.

Table 6. Structure activity of the diphenolic methanes: Attempts to place polar substituents remote to the phenolic groups

Structure	Enzyme (μM or %) NRII IC$_{50}$ (% Inh)	Antibacterial data MICs (μg/mL)				
		E. coli	*E. coli LKY*	*B. subtilis*	*S. aureus*	*S. pyogenes*
	77 (55)	256	32	128	64	256
	(20)	>64	64	16	16	>64
	(4)	>256	>256	>256	>256	>256
	(10)	64	64	16	16	4

We next tested the PD compounds for *in vivo* efficacy in the acute mouse infection model (Sesnie et al., 1989) vs *S. pyogenes* where the MIC was 1.0 μg/ml. Neither single nor multiple dosing, orally or subcutaneously produced any protective effects. We were not surprised by the results, since we anticipated that protein binding for these lipophilic agents might be very high. Indeed, the MICs of both PD compounds were increased to >64 μg/ml by the addition of human serum albumin or BSA. Before we devised a strategy to reduce protein binding, we sought to confirm the desired mechanism of action.

Table 7. Structure activity of the diphenolic methanes: Attempts to place polar substituents within the cyclohexane ring

Structure (X)	Enzyme (μM or %) NRII IC$_{50}$ (% Inh)	Antibacterial data MICs (μg/mL)				
		E. coli	*E. coli LKY*	*B. subtilis*	*S. aureus*	*S. pyogenes*
S	>200 (1)	>64	32	32	32	16
SO$_2$	(0)	>64	>64	>64	>64	>64
N	>200 (0)	>64	>64	>64	>64	>64
NCH$_2$Ph	>200 (23)	>64	>64	>64	>64	>64
N-*t*-Bu	(3)	>64	>64	>64	>64	>64
N-CO$_2$Et	(0)	>64	>64	>64	>64	>64

Table 8. The antibacterial activities [MICs (μg/mL)] of PD164592 vs resistant organisms

Strain	Compounds		
	Ciprofloxacin	Methicillin	164592
S. aureus			
WT			
MR	0.1	0.05	1
QRMR	0.5	16	4
	>64	32	4
	Vancomycin	Teicoplanin	164592
E. faecium			
Van S$^+$	>4096	>512	2

MECHANISM OF ACTION

The two biggest questions still remained: do these compounds, which clearly inhibit NRII, have any effect on the actual two-component pathways in bacteria; and is the MIC (or the MBC) a result of inhibiting such pathways? The most direct approach to address these issues was to raise mutants and hopefully map the resistance to alterations in some HK genes. Unfortunately, this approach was obviated when no passage mutants could be harvested. The second and more challenging approach was to examine the active and inactive agents in various assays designed to monitor the output of the two-component pathways. This task was complicated since the active compounds killed the bacteria that were used in such assays.

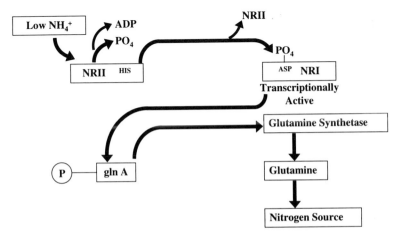

Figure 2. A depiction of the nitrogen regulation two-component pathway where NRII is the kinase and NRI is the response regulator.

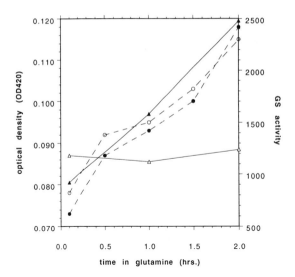

Figure 3. Measurement of glutamine synthetase (GS) activity as a function of cell growth in *E. coli*. Time is measured in hours from first glutamine synthetase sampling. The *E. coli* was grown in a nitrogen poor media to stimulate GS production with and without drug. (- - -) control growth curve of *E. coli*; (——) control levels of glutamine synthetase activity of cells; (- - -) growth cells treated with 16 μg/ml of PD009094; (Δ——) glutamine synthetase levels of cells treated with 16 μg/ml of PD009094.

Table 9. The effects of certain NRII inhibitors in functional two-component pathway assays

Compound	GS inhib[1] NRII	Gro inhib[2] PhoR	Swarm inhib[3] CheA	%NRII inhib
				98
	Yes	Yes	Yes	
				100
	Yes	Yes	Yes	
				0
	No	No	No	
				0
	No	No	No	

1. Inhibition of Glutamine Synthetase production.
2. Inhibition of growth under PhoR control of phosphate assimilation.
3. Inhibition of bacterial swimming (swarm) toward the outer edges (nutrient rich) of a gradient nutrient

The Effect of the Diphenolic Methanes on Two-Component Pathways

NRII is part of the nitrogen regulation pathway depicted in Figure 2 and described in several reviews (Stock et al., 1989; Bourret et al., 1991). A functional NRII senses nitrogen starvation and begins the cascade to activate the promotor (P) of glnA, resulting in increased levels of glutamine synthetase and ultimately glutamine which serves as the cell's nitrogen source. Inhibition of NRII, in a nitrogen poor media, should cause a direct decrease in glutamine synthetase levels, as measured by standard glutamine synthetase assays. This concept (illustrated in Figure 2) is complicated by cross talk and small molecule phosphorylation of NRI. A mutant *E. coli* was designed to minimize the effects of crosstalk by removing the genes controlling the acetyl phosphate small molecule phosphorylation pathway (unpublished results). The results from treatment of this *E. coli* with PD009094 (Table 2) is shown in Figure 3. The conditions were standardized in nitrogen poor media, in which the cells grow with a proportionate increase in glutamine synthetase levels. At 16 μg/ml of PD009094 (1/2 MIC) the cells continued to grow, but glutamine synthetase production was halted. At one dilution higher the bacterial growth was inhibited.

Encouraged with this result, we then proceeded to design similar functional assays to assess the effects of the compounds in the phosphate assimilation (Stock et al., 1989) and the chemotaxis (Stock et al., 1992) pathways. In the former case cells were monitored for growth inhibition in a PhoR dependent growth assay. In the latter case the inhibition of *E. coli* swimming (swarm) response in a nutrient gradient media, where the nutrients were more dense toward the outer edges, was measured relative to a no drug control. Table 9 shows the results for all three assays together. In every instance the compounds that strongly inhibited NRII also displayed inhibition of the other two-component pathways, and the inactive compounds vs NRII were inactive vs the other pathways.

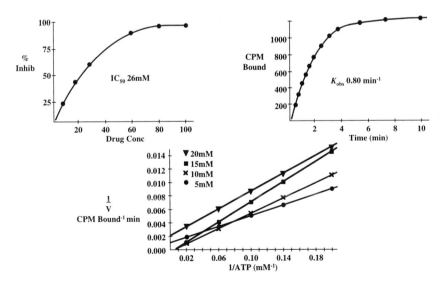

Figure 4. Enzyme kinetics of NRII and the effects of PD009094. In panel 1 the % inhibition of NRII is plotted vs increasing concentrations of PD009094. In panel 2 the autophosphorylation of NRII in the absence of drug is shown K_{obs} 0.80 min^{-1}. In panel 3, a double reciprocal plot showing the lack of competitive inhibition is shown. The lines for a competitive inhibitor would intersect at a single point.

Enzyme Kinetics: The Diphenolic Methanes and NRII

Following the general procedures of Stewart (1997) and Fisher (1996), the effects of these inhibitors on the autophosphorylation of NRII were measured (Figure 4). The autophosphorylation reaction occurs very rapidly and is first order with respect to ATP. With longer times the phosphorylated enzyme loses phosphate by multiple mechanisms. The compounds are not competitive with ATP.

Macromolecular Synthesis Inhibition and Killing Kinetics

In *E. coli* and *B. subtilis*, the active diphenolic methanes completely inhibited protein, DNA, and RNA synthesis at concentration 2–4 times their MICs. Even approaching the MIC, the inhibitory curves all moved in parallel. We examined our library of standard drugs in this assay and only polymyxin fit the same profile, suggesting a membrane perturbation component to the mechanism of action.

We then examined the killing kinetics of the active compounds at 1/4, 1 and 4 times the MIC. All of the active compounds tested showed a rapid (one hour) 4–5 log reduction of viable bacteria at the MIC with no rebound over time. The control and 1/4 MIC curves were superimposable. This is consistent with the glutamine synthetase experiments in which the cells grew well at 1/2 MIC.

Uptake of Propidium Iodide

Given the suggestion of membrane perturbation and the lipophilicity of the compounds, we examined the three most active agents and a few inactives for propidium iodide uptake. Compounds which disrupt bacterial membranes permit the rapid uptake of this fluorescent dye into the cell. The cells were treated with drug and dye and were counted to 50,000 cells. After one hour at the MIC concentration, all of the active compounds showed a 13–16 fold increase in mean fluorescence over control (no drug) cells. Over 90% of the treated cells showed the effect. Even after 5 minutes, 27% of the cells were already taking up the dye with a mean fluorescence of 2X over control. Inactive compounds gave fluorescence much nearer control. These results are highly consistent with membrane disruption as at least one component of the antibacterial action of the diphenolic methanes.

CONCLUSION

This work reveals a new class of compounds selected for their inhibition of bacterial two-component signalling, targeting NRII as a prototype bacterial histidine kinase. The inhibitory effects for NRII were selective relative to the lack of effect vs several mammalian tyrosine kinases. More significantly this research clearly demonstrated that a two-component signalling inhibitor at the enzyme level could indeed have effects on two-component pathways in bacteria. Unfortunately the compounds themselves displayed a second, less desirable mechanistic component, namely membrane perturbation, which along with high protein binding limited their potential utility. Nonetheless, this work does support two-component signalling as a *bona fide* target in antibacterial drug design.

REFERENCES

Atkinson, M.R. and Ninfa, A.J., 1993, Mutational analysis of the bacterial signal transducing protein kinase/phosphatase nitrogen regulator 11 (NR11), *J. Bacteriol.* 175:7016.

Berkowitz, F.E., 1995, Antibiotic resistance in bacteria, *Southern Med. J.* 88:797.

Bourret, R.B., Borkovich, K.A., and Simon, M.I., 1991, Signal transduction pathways involving protein phosphorylation in prokaryotes, *Ann. Rev. Biochem.* 60:401.

Chu, D.T.W., Plattner, J.J., and Katz, L., New approaches in antibacterial research, *J. Med. Chem.* 39:3853.

Cohen, M.A., Griffin, T.J., Bien, P.A., Heifetz, C.L, and Domagala, J.M., 1985, *In vitro* activity of CI-934, a quinolone carboxylic acid active against gram positive and gram negative bacteria, *Antimicrob. Agents Chemother.* 28:766.

Cormican, M.C. and Jones, R.N., 1996, Emerging resistance to antimicrobial agents in gram positive bacteria, *Drugs* 51:Suppl. 1:6.

Demers, J.P., Bernstein, J.I., Fernandez, J.A., Foleno, B.D., Frago-Spano, S.A., Hlasta, D.J., Johnson, S.G., Kanojia, R.M., Klaubert, D.H., Loeloff, M.J., Sheppard, C.M., Webb, G.C., Weidner-Wells, M.A., and Barrett, J.F., 1997, The identification of RWJ-49815, a novel inhibitor of bacterial two-component regulatory systems and a potent gram positive antibacterial, 37th Interscience Conference for Antimicrobial Agents and Chemotherapy, Toronto, Canada, Sept 28-Oct 1, Abst F-227.

Desnottes, J.F., 1996, New targets and strategies for the development of antibacterial agents, *Trends in Biotechnology* 14:134.

Domagala, J.M. and Sanchez, J.P., 1997, New approaches and agents to overcome bacterial resistance, in: *Annual Reports in Medicinal Chemistry*, J.A. Bristol, ed. Academic Press, New York 32:111.

Edmund, M.B., Wenzel, R.P., and Pasculle, A.W., 1996, Vancomycin resistant Staphylococcus aureus: perspective on measures needed for control, *Ann. Intern. Med.* 124:329.

Fisher, S.L., Kim, S.K., Wanner, B.L., and Walsh, C.T., 1996, Kinetic comparison of the specificity of vancomycin resistant kinase VanS for two response regulators VanR and PhoB. *Biochem.* 35:4733.

Garchar, H.H., Kalola, S.H., and Parsania, P.H., 1993, Synthesis and evaluation of bisphenol C and its derivatives as potential antibacterial and antifungal agents, *Asian J. Chem.* 5:340.

Gaynes, R. and Lynch, J.P., 1991, Nosocomical pneumonia: treating the hospital killer, *Intern. Med.* 12:October, 23.

Hagman, H.M. and Strausbaugh, L.J., 1996, Vancomycin resistant enterococci, Postgraduate Med. 99:60.

Haldimann, A., Prahalad, M.K., Fisher, S.L., Kim, S.K., Walsh, C.T,, and Wanner, B.L. 1996, Altered recognition mutants of the response regulator PhoB: a new genetic strategy for studying protein-protein interactions, *Proc. Natl. Acad. Sci.* 93:14361.

Howe, R.A., Brown, N.M., and Spenser, R.C., 1996, The new threats of gram positive pathogens: re-emergence of things past, *J. Clin. Pathol.* 49:444.

Jones, R.N., 1996, Impact of changing pathogens and antimicrobial susceptibility patterns in the treatment of serious infections in hospitalized patients, Am. J. Med. 100: Suppl 6A:6A-3S.

Koshland, D.E., 1992, The microbial wars, *Science* 257:1021–1078.

Koshland, D.E., 1993, The two-component pathways come to eukaryotes, *Science*, 262:532.

Kumin, C.M., 1993, Resistance to antimicrobial drugs - a worldwide calamity, *Ann. Intern. Med.* 118:557.

Licata, L., Melton, J.L., Fernandez, J.A., Frechette, R.F., Beach, M., Webb, G., Lawrence, L.E., Barrett, J.F., and Frosco, M.B., 1997, The *in vitro* characterization of a novel class of antibacterial agents that inhibit bacterial two-component systems, 37th Interscience Conference for Antimicrobial Agents and Chemotherapy, Toronto, Canada, Sept 28-Oct 1, Abst F-226.

Lukat, G.S., McCleary, W.R., Stock, A.M., and Stock, J.B., 1992, Phosphorylation of bacterial response regulator proteins by low molecular weight phospho-donors, *Proc. Natl. Acad. Sci.* 89:718.

Macielag, M.J., Bernstein, J.I., Demers, J.P., Dow, T., Foleno, B., Goldschmidt, R., Guan, J., Hilliard, J.J., Hlasta, D.J., Johnson, C.E., Johnson, S.G., Kanojia, R.M., Loeloff, M., Ohemeng, K.A., Russel, R.K., Sheppard, C.M., Frago-Spano, S.A., Sui, Z., Weidner-Wells, M.A., Werblood, H. and Barret, J.F., 1997 Antibacterial salicylamides that inhibit bacterial two-component regulatory systems, 37th Interscience Conference for Antimicrobial Agents and Chemotherapy, Toronto, Canada, Sept 28 - Oct 1, Abst F-228.

McCleary, W.R. and Stock, J.B., 1994, Acetyl phosphate and the activation of two-component response regulators, *J. Biol. Chem.* 269:31567.

Parkinson, J.S. and Kofoid, E.C., 1992, Communication modules in bacterial signalling proteins, *Ann. Rev. Genet.* 26:71.

Pinner, R.W., Teutsch, S.M., Simonsen, L., Klug, L.A., Graber, J.M., Clark, M.J., and Berkelman, R.L., 1996, Trends in infectious diseases mortality in the United States, *JAMA* 257:189.

Report 1995, Report of the ASM task force on antibiotic resistance, public and scientific affairs, 1325 Massachusetts Ave. N.W., Washington, D.C. 20005–4171.

Roychoudhury, S., Zielinkski, N.A., Ninfa, A.J., Allen, N.E., Jungheim, L.N., Nicas, T.I., and Chakrubarty, A.M., 1993, Inhibitors of two-component signal transduction systems: inhibition of alginate gene activation in Pseudomonas aeruginosa, *Proc. Natl. Acad. Sci.* 90:965.

Schwartz, M.N. 1994, Hospital acquired infections: diseases with increasingly limited therapies, *Proc. Natl. Acad. Sci. USA*, 91:2420.

Sesnie, J.A., Fritsch, P.W., Griffin, T.J., Heifetz, C.L., Leopold, T.E., Shapiro, M.A., and Vincent, P.W., 1989, Comparative chemotherapeutic activity of new fluorinated quinolones and standard agents against a variety of bacteria in a mouse infection model. *J. Antimicrob. Chemother.* 23:729.

Setti, E.L., Quattrocchio, L., and Micetich, R.G., 1997, Current approaches to overcome bacterial resistance, *Drugs Future* 22:271.

Shimi, I.R., Shoukry, S., and Zaki, Z., 1976, 4,4′-Isopropylidine-bis[2-isopropyl]phenol, a new inhibitor for cell wall formation of B. subtilis, *Antimicrob. Agents Chemother.* 9:580.

Spivack, J., Leib, T.K., and Lobos, J.H., 1994, Novel pathways for bacterial metabolism of bisphenol A., *J. Biol. Chem.* 269:7323.

Stewart, R.C., 1997, Kinetic characterization of phosphotransfer between CheA and CheY in the bacterial chemotaxis signal transduction pathway. *Biochem.* 36:2030.

Stinson, C.C. 1996, Drug firms restock antibacterial arsenal, *Chem. Eng. News.* Sept 23:75.

Stock, J.B. Ninfa, A.J., and Stock, A.M., 1989, Protein phosphorylation and regulation of the adaptive response in bacteria, *Microbiol. Rev.* 53:450.

Stock, J.B., Surette, M.G., McCleary, W.R., and Stock, A.M., 1992, Signal transduction in bacterial chemotaxis, *J. Biol. Chem.* 267:19753.

Strauch, M.A., de Mendoza, D., and Hoch, J.A., 1992, cis-Unsaturated fatty acids specifically inhibit signal transducting protein kinase required for initiation of sporulation in B. subtilis, *Mol. Microbiol.* 6:2909.

Subramaniam, G., Savithri, R., and Thambipillai, S., 1989, Synthesis and antifungal activity of bisphenolic derivatives, *J. Ind. Chem. Soc.* 66:797.

Swanson, R.V., Alex, L.A., and Simon, M.I., 1994, Histidine and aspartate phosphorylation: two-component systems and the limits of homology, *TIBS.* 19:485.

Travis, J., 1994, Reviving the antibiotic miracle? *Science* 264:360–393.

Wanner, B.L. 1992, Is cross regulation by phosphorylation of two-component response regulator proteins important in bacteria? *J. Bacteriol.* 174:2053.

INDEX

AAC, 34
AAC(1), 39
AAC(2'), 39, 40
AAC(3), 34, 39, 41
AAC(6'), 40, 55, 58
AAC(6')-APH(2''), 34, 39, 54, 56
AAC(6')-I, 34
AarA, 40
AarB, 40
AarC, 40
AarD, 40
AarP, 40
ABC transporters, 106, 145, 148, 149, 153, 167, 186
Acetyl phosphate small molecule phosphorylation
    pathway, 283
Acetyltransferases, 34
ACR1, 165
ACR2, 165, 166
ACR3, 165, 176, 177
Acyl-D-Ala-D-Ala, 73
Adherence, 270
Aeromonas spp, 90
Aeruginosa, 31
AhpC, 122
AIDS, 225
AlrA, 132
Alanine racemase, 210
Alginate two-component pathway (AlgR2/AlgR1),
    272
6α-hydroxymethylpencillanate, 88
Amethopterin, 103
Amidines, 272
Amikacin, 13, 29, 39, 40, 43, 44, 49, 125
7-aminocephalosporanic acid, 83, 243
Aminoglycoside-aminocyclitol antibiotics, 27
Aminoglycosides, 3–4, 27, 125
6-aminohexose ring, 29, 38
6-aminopenicillanic acid, 76, 83
Aminothiazolyl cephalosporins, 83
Amoxicillin, 9, 76, 80, 83
Ampicillin, 10, 80, 81

Ampicillin-resistant gram-negative pathogens, 79
Anaerobic bacteria, 225
AnsA, 128
ANT, 34,
ANT(2''), 34, 35, 57
ANT(3''), 35
ANT(4'), 35, 36, 45, 49
ANT(6) 34, 35
ANT(9) , 35
ANT(9)-Ia, 35
ANT(9)-Ib, 35
Antibiotic transport, 32
Antifolate, 99, 107, 108
Antimonite, 106, 164, 166
Antimony, 159
Antimycobacterial activity, 224
Anti-pseudomonal activity, 83
Antiturbecular agents, 226
Antituberculosis Drug Resistance Surveillance, 12
Antituberculosis drugs, 13, 225
APH, 34
APH(2''), 43, 53
APH(3'), 42, 43, 55
APH(3')-IIIa, 34
APH(3''), 54
APH(4), 43, 54
APH(6), 43, 54
APH(7''), 43, 54
APH(9), 43, 54
Apramycin, 29, 39, 42
Aqiofex aeolicus, 184
Arbekacin, 39, 53
Arabinogalactan, 126
Arabinosyltransferases, 126
Archaca, 184
Archaeoglobus fulgidus, 184
ars operon, 166
arsA, 167
ArsA, 167–175
ArsB, 167, 169, 172–177
ArsC arsenate reductase, 165, 166

arsD, 167
Arsenate, 159, 165, 166
Arsenicals, 159, 160, 161
Arsenite, 106, 159–166
arsR, 167
Azetidines, 228
Azetidinylphenyloxazolidinones, 233
1-azetdinylphenyloxazolidinones, 228
[3-H]-azidobenzyl derivative, 31
Azithromycin, 225
Azlocillin, 83
Aztreonam, 11, 82, 84–85

β-lactam(s), 136, 205
    antibiotics, vi, 71, 73, 75, 76, 200
    resistant streptococci, 269
β-lactamase(s), 71, 72, 73, 79, 87, 136, 199, 240
    Class A , 11–12, 72, 81, 83, 85–86
    Class C, 11, 80, 83
    inhibitor combinations, 82, 85
    inhibitors, 86, 91, 270
    mediated resistance, 10, 84
β-γ-methyleneadenosine, 36
Bacilli, 116
Bacillus subtilus, 184, 210, 276
Bacterial
    adaptation/survival, 186
    histidine kinase, 284
    membranes, 284
    protein synthesis inhibitors, 227
Bactericidal, 279
Bacteroides fragilis, 73, 90, 225, 261
Benzylpenicillin, 71, 76, 84
Bleomycin, 3
Borellia burgdoreri, 184
Butirosin, 29, 39, 41, 43, 44, 51, 52
    A, 49

Capreomycin, 133–134
Carbamate-linked quinolonly
    lactams, 242
    penems, 248, 250
Carbapenem, 11, 79, 86, 88, 90–91
Carbapenem-hydrolzying β-lactamses, 90
Carbonyl cyanide-*m*-chlorophenyl-EDP-1, 31
Carbonyl cyanide-*m*-chlorophenyl-hydrazone (CCCP),
    31
Casein kinases, 47
Catalase-perioxidase enzyme, 119
Cefepime, 85–86, 91
Cefoperazone, 81, 83
Cefotaximases, 85
Cefotaxime, 85, 259
Cefpirome, 91
Ceftazidimases, 85
Ceftazidime, 83–85
Ceftriaxone, 83
Cell wall, 202

Cell wall permeable (imp minus), 276
Cephaloridine, 76, 84
Cephalosporin(s), 3, 82, 200
    C, 76
Cephalosporinase(s), 79, 80
Cephalothin, 76, 82
Chemoprophylaxis, 13
Chemotaxis, 283
Chloramphenicol, 3, 227
Cidal agent, 199, 200
Cilastatin, 87
Ciprofloxacin, 117, 130, 221, 242, 250, 253
Cis fatty acids, 272
Citrobacter freundii, 11
Clavam, 80
Clavulanate, 79, 80, 81
Clavulanic acid, 79–83, 85, 199
Cma1, 136
Cma2, 136
Combinatorial chemistry, 189
Conjugation, 18
Cryptosporidium parvum, 105
Cyclic-AMP-dependent protein kinase (cAPK), 45,
    46, 47
Cyclic peptide, 133
Cycloserine, 117, 132
Cytochrome P4450, 192
Cytotoxic agents, 201

dhfr, 104, 108
D-Ala, 73, 74
D-Ala-D-Ala ligase, 200
D-alanine, 132
D-alanyl-D-alanine, 212
    synthase, 132
D-amino acid(s), 210
    ligase, 209
D-cycloserine, 132, 135
D-Glu, 73
D-glumate, 132, 209
D,L-diaminopimelate, 132
DNA polymerase β, 38
Deanimated aminoglycosides, 52
2-deoxystreptamine ring, 27, 38
Diaminopimelate, 73
Dibekacin, 29, 39, 55
3,4-difluoronitrobenzene, 228
Dihydropteroate synthase, 100, 101
Dihydrofolate
    reductase, 99, 101
    synthase, 100, 101
Dipeptidase, 87
Diphenolic methanes, 274
DNA gyrase, 253
DNA or RNA binding motif, 270
Dodecymaltoside, 21
Domagk, Gerhard, 115
DrrAB, 149, 150
Drug efflux, 19

EDP-II, 31
Efflux mechanisms, 92
Ehrlich, P., 83, 109, 159
EmbA, 126
EmbB, 126
EmbCAB, 126
EmbR, 126
Empirical method, 213
EmrE, 148
Endocarditis, 10
Energy-dependent phase (EDP-1), 30
Enoyl reductase, 119
Enolpyruvyl shikimate phosphate (EPSP) synthase, 205
Enterobacter cloacae, 205, 246–247, 251, 252–254, 256
  P99, 79
Enterobacteriaceae, 76, 83–85, 90
Enterococci, 2
Enterococcus-faecalis, 219, 225, 246–247, 251–252, 254, 256, 261
Enterococcus-faecium, 10, 219, 225, 261, 279
Envelope function, 270
Eperezolid, 222, 223–224, 227–228, 233, 235
EPSP synthase, 205, 206
Erbstatin, 55
Erythomycin, 197
ESBLs, 73
Escherichia coil (E. coli) i, 11, 79, 87, 187, 246–247, 251–252, 254, 256, 261, 263
  E. coli LKY, 276
  genomic library, 188
  K-12, 184, 186
Ethambutol, 12–13, 115, 117, 125–127
Ethionamide, 115, 117, 133–134
Eubacteria, 184
Eucaryotic orthologs, 200
Eukaryotes, 184
Everted membrane vesicles, 19, 162
Evolution, 75
Evolution of β-lactamases, 79
Expanded-spectrum cephalosporins, 11, 83, 85–86, 91
Expanded-spectum penicillins, 83–84
Extended-spectrum β-lactamases (ESBLs), vi, 12, 73, 79, 85

Fem proteins, 270
First-generation cephalosporins, 76, 85
Flavoprotein reductase, 207
Fleming, A. 1
Fleroxacin, 259
Fluorescent dye, 284
Fluoroquinolones, 13, 117, 130–131, 136
Fluorosulfonylbenzoyladenosine (FSBA), 44
Folate, 101, 106, 107, 108
Folate cofactors, 132
Folic acid, 3, 100
Formimidoyl-thienamycin, 86
Fortimicin, 29, 39
Functional classification, 72

glpF, 166
GlpF, 174
γ-Glutamylcysteine synthetase, 162, 164
Genestein, 56
Genomic libraries, 184
Genomics, vi
Gentamicin, 29, 30, 31, 35, 39, 40, 41, 43, 58, 59, 125
  B, 42
  C1, 42, 53
Glutamae reacemase (MurI), 210
Glutamine, 281
Glutamine synthetase, 281, 284
Glutathione, 107, 165
Glutathione-S-transferase
Glycopeptide antibiotics, 2
Glycosyltransferase, 127
Golden age of antibiotic, 183
Gonococcal infections, 79
Gram-negative organisms, 225
Gram-positive bacteria, 76, 202
gshI, 163, 164
GyrA, 130
GyrB, 131
Gyrase, 130

H locus, 106
Haemophilus influenzae, 187, 225
  Rd, 184
Helicobacter pylori, 184
Histidine kinase (HK), 270
  NR II, 273
  EnvZ and VanS, 274
Histidine protein kinases, 200
HIV-infected patients, 12
HK/RR pairs, 271
HlyB, 149
Homlogy, 75, 186
5-(hydroxymethyl)oxazolidinone(s), 223, 228, 230
7-Hydroxytropolone, 57
Hygromycin, 29
  B, 54

IMI-1 β-lactamase, 91
Imipenem, 11, 82, 86–90
InhA, 119, 122
InhA-encoded enoyl reductase, 133
Inhibitor-resistant TEM, 82
  derived enzymes (IRTs), 82, 86
Integrons, 4
Interones, 102
Intrinsic resistance, 117
IRORI SMART, 190
Isoquinolinesulfonamides, 56
Isepamicin, 29, 39, 41, 43
Isoniazid, 12–13, 115–117, 122, 128, 133, 135, 224
Isothiazalone I, 272
In Vivo Expression Technologies (IVET), 187
Izumenolide, 79

K. pneumoniae, 247
Kanamycin, 13, 29, 30, 37, 42, 43, 54, 55, 56, 125
  A, 51, 52
  B, 42, 53
KatG, 119, 122
Kinetic isotope effects, 212
Klebsiella aerogenes, 79
Klebsiella oxytoca, 79, 84–85
Klebsiella pneumoniae, 11, 79, 247, 263
  CR, 246–247, 251–252, 254, 256
  CS, 246–247, 251–252, 254, 256
Koch, Robert, 115

L-asparaginase, 128
LfrA, 131
LacZ, 187
Lederberg, J., 5
Legionella gormanii, 90
Leishmania major, 105
Leishmania, 105–8, 160, 163, 164
Leishmaniasis, 105, 160
Leprosy, 123
Levo-floxacin, 130
Lincomycin, 227
Lincosamide, 33
Lincosamines, 3
Linezolid, vi, 225, 226, 227, 228, 233, 235
Lipinski rule of 5, 192
Lipoic acid, 160
Lipoarabinomannanm, 126
Lipopolysaccharide, 202
Listeria monoctyogenes, 187
Lividomycin, 29, 39, 43, 51, 53, 55
  A, 44
LmrA, 149, 150, 153
LmrP, 146, 147, 153

M. avium, 126
M. avium complex, 225
M. bovis, 128
M. smegmatis, 126–127, 131
M. tubeculosis, 13, 122, 124, 225, 226
  enoyl reductase, 121
Macrolide(s), 3, 33, 199, 200
Macrophage phagolysosomes, 128
Magic bullet, 83
Maltose binding, 211
MAP kinase, 47
MarA, 40
MDR1, 148
MecA, 270
Mechanism-based inactivators, 73
Melarsoprol, 160, 162
Membrane perturbation, 284
Meropenem, 89, 255
Metallo-β-lacamases, 73, 88–91
Metalloid, 159
Methanobacterium thermoautotrophicum, 184

Methanococcus fannaschii, 184
Methicillin, 8, 78
  resistance, 270
Methicillin-resistant
  staphylococci, vi, 9–10
  Staphyloccocus aureus (MRSA), 8, 91, 197
  Staphylococcus epidermidis, 219
  susceptible staphylococci, 10
Methotrexate, 100
Methyl transferases, 136
MexB, 146, 147
Mezlocillin, 83
Microsome/hepatocyte, 192
M. leprae, 123
Mobile genetic elements, 2
Molecular modeling, 88
Molecular targerts, 185
Monobactam aztreonam, 83
Monobactams, 73
Monoclonal antibody, 241
Monurol™ (fosfomycin tromethamine), 205
Moraxella catarrhalis, 225
MRCS *S. aureus*, 247
MRP, 149, 150
MRSA, 9, 11, 92, 225
MSCR *S. aureus*, 250
Multidrug
  antibiotic therapy, 115
  efflux pump, 103
  resistance associated protein (MRP), 165
  resistance, 17
  therapy, 12
  transporters, 145, 151, 153
  treatment regimens, 123
Mutlidrug-resistant
  M. tuberculosis, 219
  plasmids, 79
  tuberculosis, 12–13
Mur enzymes, 212
Mur-A, 202
Mur-B, 207, 212
Mur-C, 209, 212
Mur-D, 209, 212, 213
Mur-E, 207, 210, 212
Mur-F, 209, 210, 212
Mur-Z, 204
Murein intermediates, 212
Murein sacculus, 202
Mycobacterial porins, 117
Mycolic acids, 119, 135
Mycoplasma genitalium, 184
Mycoplasma penumoniae, 184
Mycobacterium tuberculosis, 12, 115–116, 187, 206, 219

N-acetyltransfer, 33
N-gonorrhea, 79
NMP-transferase, 38
Nalidixic acid, 129

Neamine, 51, 52
Neomycin, 27, 29, 30, 39, 43, 44, 58
Nephrotoxicity, 58
Netilmicin, 29, 39, 43
NfxD, 130
Nicotinamidase, 128
Nicotinamide, 127
Nitrogen regulation pathway, 281
NMC-A enzyme, 90
Non-tuberculous mycobacteria, 125
Nocardia, 119
NorA, 131
Nucelotidyl-transferases, 34

O-acetylated-peptidoglycan, 40
O-nucleotideyltransfer, 33
Ω-loop, 85
O-phosphoryltransfer, 33
Ofloxacin, 117, 130–131
Olivanic acids, 79
Olivanic family, 86
Ototoxic, 58, 59
Outer membrane, 202
Oxacillin, 8, 76
Oxazolidinone(s), vi, 220, 221, 222, 225, 227–228, 230–231, 234

P-glycoprotein , 148, 151, 153, 160, 167
ParC, 130–131
ParE, 130
Parallel tagging, 189
Paromomycin, 29, 30, 39, 53, 55, 125
PBPs, 73, 74, 75, 76, 78, 81, 87
PBP-1, 253
PBP 1a, 87
PBP 1b, 87
PBP-2, 87, 253
PBP-3, 253
Para-aminosalicyclic acid (PAS), 117, 132
Partition ratio, 80
Penicillin(s), 3, 9, 73, 76, 80, 82, 197, 200, 219
  binding-protein(s) (PBP), 73, 92, 199, 202, 240
  and cephalosoporin-resistant *Streptococcus penumo-*
    niae, 219, 225, 226
  G, 8, 71, 74
  resistant streptococci, vi, 76
Pentostam, 160, 162
Peptidoglycan, 73, 74, 126, 202
Pgp, 149–153, 162
Phenolphthiocerol, 136
Phenyloxazolidinones, 235
Phosphate assimilation, 283
Phosphatidylinositol-4,5-bisphophshate, 59
Phosphinate inhibitors, 200
Phosphonates, 3
Phosphoenolpyruvate (PEP), 202
Phosphoryllase kinase, 47
Phosphotranserases, 3

Phototoxicity, 259
Phthiocerol, 136
Piperacillin, 80, 81, 82, 83
Piperazine ring, 221
Piperazinyloxasolidinones, 222
Piperazinylphenyloxazolidinone, 223
Piperidin-1-ylphenyloxaolidinone, 234
Plasma-mediated β-lacatamases, 79, 80
Plasmid, 18
Plasmid-borne resistance, 11
Plasmodium falciparum, 105
PncA, 128
Polyglutamylation, 104
Prokaryotic translation, 227
Proline racemase, 210
Promoter gene AlgD, 272
Propidium iodide, 284
Protein secretion, 270
Protein synthesis inhibitors, 199
Proteoliposomes, 21
Proteus mirabilis, 246, 247, 251, 252, 254, 256
Protozoa, 104, 105
PSE-2, 72
Pseudomonas, 205
Pseudomonas aeruginosa, 11, 83, 90, 92, 261, 263,
    272
  CR, 246, 247, 251, 252, 254, 256
  CS, 246, 247, 251, 252, 254, 256
PurA gene, 187
Pyrazinamidase, 128
Pyrazinamide, 13, 127–128, 135
Pyrazinoic acid, 128
Pyridoxal cofactor, 210
Pyrrolidine, 233
Pyrrolidinylphenyloxazoidinones, 229

QacA, 148
QacB, 148
QacC, 146–148
Quaternary imidazole **2**, 272
Quercertin, 56
Quinoline(s),v, 131, 200, 221
  antibacterials, 129, 221

R-glycidyl butyrate, 223
Random BiBii, 41, 42
Renal dehydropeptidase, 87, 89
Resistant mutants, 117
Response
  domain, 270
  regulator, 270
Ribosomal modifying enzymes, 270
Ribosomal S12 protein, 124
50S ribosomal subunit, 227
Ribostamycin, 29, 39, 43
Rifabutin, 123
Rifampicin, 115–117, 122, 124, 135
Rifampin, 12–13, 200

Rifamycin, 122
Rifapentin, 123
RNA polymerase, 123
RpoB, 123–124
RpsL gene, 124–125
16S rRNA, 124
Rrs, 124–125
RTEM, 79
Runge-Kutta alogrithim, 213

S. clavuligerus, 80
S. maltophilia, 90–91
Saccharomyces cerevisiae, 165, 184
Salicylamide **4**, 272
Salmonella paratyphi B, 79
Salmonella typhimurium, 79
  purA mutants, 187
SAR by NMR, 191
Scavenger pathways, 212
Secondary-amine-linked quinolonyl lactams, 244
Secondary multidrug transporters, 14
Semidormant, 116
Semi-synthetic penicillins and cephalosoporins,
  76
Sensor
  domain, 270
  protein, 270
Sequence alignment, 75
Serial passage resistance experiments, 256
Serine β-lactamases, 88, 90
Serine-dependent β-lactamases, 88
Serratia marcescens, 11, 90
SHV β-lactamase, 12, 72, 73, 83–86
SHV-derived inhibitor-resistant β-lactamase, 82
Signature tagged mutagenesis (STM), 187
Sisomicin, 29, 39, 42, 43
Sme-1 β-lactamase, 90–91
Solid phase synthesis, 190
SoxS, 40
Sparfloxacin, 117, 130
Spectinomycin, 29, 30, 32, 34, 35, 43, 54, 55
Spheroplast, 205
Split and mix procedure, 189
Staphylococci, 76, 205
Staphylococcus auerus, 88, 92, 185, 219, 225, 233,
    234, 247, 261, 269, 276, 279
  MRCR, 246, 247, 251, 252, 254, 256, 263
  MRCS, 246, 247, 251, 252, 254, 256
  MRSA, 261
  MSCR, 246, 247, 251, 252, 254, 256
  MSCS, 246, 247, 251, 252, 254, 256, 263
  resistant, 261
Staphylococcus epidermis, 9, 205
Staphylococcus haemolyticus, 9, 11
Staphylococcus saprophyticus, 246, 247, 251, 252,
    254, 256
Strains resistant, 225
Streptococcal infections, 76

Streptococcus pneumoniae, 92, 246, 247,249, 252,
    254, 256, 261, 263
  PR, 261
Streptococcus pyogenes, 246, 247, 251, 252, 254, 256,
    276, 279
Streptogramins, 3, 33
Streptomyces clavuligerus, 79
Streptomyces mediterranei, 122
Streptomycetes, 3
Streptomycin, 13, 27, 29, 32, 34, 35, 43, 117,
    124–125, 134, 197
Streptomycin-resistant strains, 13
Structure-activity relationship, 190
sul, 102
Sulbactam, 80, 81, 82, 83
Sulfonamides, 100, 101, 102
Sulphonamides, 3, 132
Swarm response, 283
Synechoystis sp., 184
Synergistic activity, 80
Syphillis, 197

Tazobactam, 80, 81, 82, 83
Teichoplanin, 2
TEM β-lactamases, 12, 73, 79, 81–86, 88–89,
    91
Tet protein, 20–23
Tetracycline(s), 3,17, 19, 147–148, 199, 200
Tetracycline resistance, 79
Theorell-Chance, 44
  kinetic mechanism, 36
Thienamycin, 86–87
Thiomorholinylphenyloxazolidinones, 223
Thiostrepton, 33
Third-generation cephalosporin, 9
Thrombine, 211
Thromboxane, 58
Thymidylate synthase, 99,101
Ticarcillin, 80
Toxoplasma gondii, 105
Tobramycin, 29, 31, 42, 55, 57
Topoisomerase I, 130, 188
Trans-activating factors, 40
Transduction, 18
Transformation, 18
Transmembrane electrical potential ($\Delta\psi$), 31
Transpeptidase reaction, 73
Transpeptidation, 73, 74
Transposable elements, 2
Transposition, 18
Trimethoprim, 3, 99, 101, 102
Trimetrexate, 104
Tuberactinomycins, 133
Two-component
  signalling, 270
  transduction, vi
Trypanosoma cruzi, 107
Trypanothione reductase, 160
Trypanothione, 107, 160, 162, 163, 164

Tyrosine kinases, 284
Tyrphostin, 55
Tuberactinomycines, 134
Tuberculosis (TB), 12, 115–116, 197, 219

UDP-GlcNAc, 212
UDP-MurNAc-L-alanine, 209
UDP-MurNAc-pentapeptide, 212, 213
UDP-MurNAc-peptide, 213
UDP-N-acetylglucosamine (UDP-GlcNAc), 202
Ureidopenicillins, 83

Vacuum cleaner hypothesis, 153
vanA, 2
vanB, 2
Van proteins, 271
VanS/VanR, 271, 272

Vancomycin , 2, 3, 9–11, 184, 197, 200, 212, 219,
    225, 226, 233, 234
    intermediate-resistant *S. aureus* (GISA), 10, 220
    resistance, 10–11, 270
Vancomycin-like activity, 222
Vanomycin-resistant
    enterococci (VRE), vi, 198, 259
    Enterococcus faecalis, 219
    Enetrococcus faecium, 226, 259
    Staphylococcus aureus, 184
    strains, 10
VicA, 134
Viomycin, 134
Viridans streptococcus, 246, 247, 251, 252, 254,
    254
VISA strains, 225
VREF strains, 225